CULTURAL CONCEPTIONS OF MENTAL HEALTH AND THERAPY

D1488375

CULTURE, ILLNESS, AND HEALING

Studies in Comparative Cross-Cultural Research

VOLUME 4

CULTURAL
CONCEPTIONS
OF MENTAL
HEALTH AND
THERAPY

Edited by

ANTHONY J. MARSELLA

University of Hawaii, Honolulu

and

GEOFFREY M. WHITE

East-West Center, Honolulu

D. REIDEL PUBLISHING COMPANY

A MEMBER OF THE KLUWER ACADEMIC PUBLISHERS GROUP

DORDRECHT / BOSTON / LANCASTER

Library of Congress Cataloging in Publication Data
Main entry under title:

Cultural conceptions of mental health and therapy.

   (Culture, illness, and healing ; v. 4)
   Includes bibliographies and indexes.
    1. Psychiatry, Transcultural. I. Marsella, Anthony J.
II. White, Geoffrey M. III. Series.
RC455.4.E8C8   362.2'042   82-3674
ISBN 90-277-1362-6   AACR2
ISBN 90-277-1757-5 (pbk)

Published by D. Reidel Publishing Company,
P.O. Box 17, 3300 AA Dordrecht, Holland.

Sold and distributed in the U.S.A. and Canada
by Kluwer Boston Inc.,
190 Old Derby Street, Hingham, MA 02043, U.S.A.

In all other countries, sold and distributed
by Kluwer Academic Publishers Group,
P.O. Box 322, 3300 AH Dordrecht, Holland.

D. Reidel Publishing Company is a member of the Kluwer Group.

Reprinted in 1984, 1989 with corrections

3—19—91

TABLE OF CONTENTS

SECTION IV: ISSUES AND DIRECTIONS

To Joy and Nancy —
Our Wives, Partners, and Friends

PREFACE

Within the past two decades, there has been an increased interest in the study of culture and mental health relationships. This interest has extended across many academic and professional disciplines, including anthropology, psychology, sociology, psychiatry, public health and social work, and has resulted in many books and scientific papers emphasizing the role of sociocultural factors in the etiology, epidemiology, manifestation and treatment of mental disorders. It is now evident that sociocultural variables are inextricably linked to all aspects of both normal and abnormal human behavior.

But, in spite of the massive accumulation of data regarding culture and mental health relationships, sociocultural factors have still not been incorporated into existing biological and psychological perspectives on mental disorder and therapy. Psychiatry, the Western medical specialty concerned with mental disorders, has for the most part continued to ignore socio-cultural factors in its theoretical and applied approaches to the problem. The major reason for this is psychiatry's continued commitment to a *disease* conception of mental disorder which assumes that mental disorders are largely biologically-caused illnesses which are universally represented in etiology and manifestation. Within this perspective, mental disorders are regarded as caused by universal processes which lead to discrete and recognizable symptoms regardless of the culture in which they occur.

However, this perspective is now the subject of growing criticism and debate. Cross-cultural studies have provided extensive data challenging the adequacy of the disease model. Based on data from virtually every continent in the world, researchers are now suggesting that culture is not simply incidental to mental disorder and therapy. Rather, it is a basic variable which interacts with biological, psychological and environmental variables in determining the causes, manifestations, and treatment of the entire spectrum of mental disorders. In this respect, all behavior is culturally related and all mental disorders and therapies are culture specific.

The purpose of the present book is to provide scholars and practitioners with a resource which articulates the importance of sociocultural variables in mental health through a survey of cultural conceptions of the person, mental disorders, and indigenous therapies in selected Asian and Pacific societies. This comparative perspective demonstrates that mental disorders have personal meaning and social significance only within cultural context, and that the very notion of "mental disorder" derives from a particular (Western) cultural and historical tradition. The reader should be alerted to the ethnocentric connotations of the phrases "mental health" and "mental disorder" which are used in this book as a convenient device to avoid awkward qualifications.

As the editors of this volume, we have attempted to capture both the controversy and the promise that represents the field of culture and mental health today by compiling a series of 16 original papers by major scholars and practitioners in the area. The papers have been prepared by anthropologists, psychiatrists, psychologists, and regional study specialists. This broad representation of writers and viewpoints offers readers a multidisciplinary perspective which best typifies the current state of the field. The anthropological perspective is emphasized in order to highlight the problems and prospects for the ethnographic study of culture and mental health as a human and scientific enterprise.

Since this book was first published in 1982 there has been a growing revival of interest in cultural and psychological studies of the self, marked by a number of recent volumes dealing with culture and self. These developments show clearly the theoretical significance of the present volume's concern with mental health as an acute focus for illuminating cultural conceptions of the person, seen through episodes of illness or disorder. The studies included here approach mental disorder as a culturally constructed phenomenon, rather than as a pre-defined clinical entity divorced from the natural contexts of social life. By focusing on the ways mental health and disorder are articulted in language, symbol and interaction, the papers which follow make significant contributions not only to the study of personal dysfunction but to an emerging new perspective on culture, psychology and social life.

This book is divided into four main sections: (1) Cultural Conceptions of the Person and Health, (2) Cultural Conceptions of Mental Disorder, (3) Cultural Conceptions of Therapy, and (4) An Overview of Issues and Directions. The first and the last sections of the book offer overview papers on the literature and basic issues in this field; while the second and third sections offer specific examples from Asian and Pacific cultural traditions. The separation of papers into these two sections (one focusing on "conceptions of mental disorder" and the other on "conceptions of therapy") reflects a difference of emphasis in these papers, rather than a division in subject matter, as the papers themselves demonstrate. The result of blending recent theoretical statements with well-documented ethnographic research will, we believe, give the reader a firm foundation for understanding the richness and variety of cultural conceptions of mental disorder, and for integrating the role of culture in various aspects of mental health. If we have been successful in our effort, the reader will emerge with a substantive basis for adopting a new and broader framework for under-standing and treating the age-old problem of mental disorder.

Section I of the book consists of four papers which summarize and evaluate current research on cultural conceptions of the person and health. In Paper 1, White and Marsella provide a rationale and perspective for the book by discussing the issues for mental health research which emerge when conceptions of dis-order are shown to be closely integrated with cultural conceptions of the person and other types of ethnopsychological understanding. Fabrega, in Paper 2, offers a detailed analysis of the assumptions underlying the contrasting bio-

medical and ethnomedical perspectives of the person and health. This is followed
in Paper 3 by White's examination of methodological and theoretical developments which have emerged from ethnographic investigations of cultural
knowledge of illness. In Paper 4, Shweder and Bourne present a comparative
analysis of the concept of person in two cultures; and describe the relative
merits and deficiences of universalist, evolutionist and relativist theories in
cross-cultural research.

Section II focuses on cultural conceptions of mental disorder. It includes five
papers. In Paper 5, Good and Good argue for a meaning-centered concept of
illness rather than a disease and symptomatology model. They offer an analysis
of the Iranian concept of "fright illness" using a semantic-network model to
support their position. Paper 6, by Gaines, contends that even Western psychiatry is guided by implicit models of the self and madness which derive from
specific cultural traditions rather than universal features of disease. Clement,
in Paper 7, gives a reformulation of approaches to "ethnoscience", and provides
an analysis of Samoan concepts of mental health and disorder based on her
fieldwork in this Polynesian culture. In Paper 8, Lock analyzes Japanese conceptions of mental health based on both popular and traditional understandings
about illness, some of which she represents in a network model of certain key
ethnopsychological concepts. This is followed in Paper 9 by Obeyesekere's
discussion of Ayurvedic notions of mental health and disorder, many of which
go back more than 5,000 years in history, with particular attention to the use
of Ayurvedic theory for the purposes of observation and experimentation.

Section III concerns cultural conceptions of therapy. It includes five papers.
In part 10, Connor focuses on Balinese traditional healers and approaches to
therapy. She discusses a number of case studies to illustrate linkages between
Balinese conceptions of the person and therapeutic processes. In Paper 11, Takie
Lebra carefully analyzes the intricate relationships between Japanese cultural
conceptions of selfhood and therapy processes in a religious cult. Wu offers a
discussion of the role of emotion in traditional Chinese therapies in Paper 12,
based on ethnographic observations and case material drawn from classical
texts. This is followed in Paper 13 by William Lebra's detailed examination of
Okinawan shamanistic therapies based on an analysis of conversational exchange
between healers and clients, recorded during his extensive studies of shamans
and other indigenous healers. Murase, in Paper 14, analyzes the Japanese concept
of *sunao* as representing important social ideals which underly indigenous
Japanese therapies, particularly *Naikan* and Morita therapy.

Section IV is the final section. It consists of two overview papers. Pedersen
discusses the intercultural context of cross-cultural counseling and psychotherapy in Paper 15. And in Paper 16, Marsella offers an overview of the field
of culture and mental health with special emphasis on its historical development, major issues, and current status.

All of the papers in the book were first presented at a conference on "Cultural
Conceptions of Mental Health and Therapy" which was held on June 2—6, 1980,

in Honolulu, Hawaii at the East-West Center. The conference was co-sponsored by two federally-funded research and training projects: "Culture and the Inter-active Process" (Culture Learning Institute, East-West Center) directed by David Wu, Geoffrey White and Jerry Boucher, and "Developing Interculturally Skilled Counselors" (NIMH # T24–15552–02) directed by Paul Pederson and Tony Marsella. All of the papers were revised and updated for final publication. A second volume of papers by other conference participants, *Mental Health Services Across Cultures*, is forthcoming under the editorship of Paul Pedersen, Tony Marsella and Norman Sartorius. The focus of the second volume is the application of cultural variables to human service delivery systems.

The editors wish to express their deep gratitude and appreciation to a number of individuals who helped make both the conference and the publication of this book possible including the administrative staff of the Culture Learning Institute; the secretaries who patiently typed and retyped the many manuscripts, especially Jenny Okano, Charlene Fujishige, June Gibson, and Gary Kawachi; Bonnie Ozaki, who compiled the index; our publication editors, Martin Scrivener, Arthur Evans and especially Arthur Kleinman, who offered patience, criticism, and encouragement at just the right times; and lastly, the chapter authors who responded to our suggestions on content and style with co-operation and grace. Without the assistance of all these people the publication of this book would not have been possible. Lastly, the order of editorship for this volume was decided by a coin flip; both editors contributed equally to the volume's completion.

Honolulu, 1984   ANTHONY J. MARSELLA
                                                       GEOFFREY M. WHITE

SECTION I

CULTURAL CONCEPTIONS OF THE
PERSON AND HEALTH

GEOFFREY M. WHITE AND ANTHONY J. MARSELLA

1. INTRODUCTION: CULTURAL CONCEPTIONS IN MENTAL HEALTH RESEARCH AND PRACTICE

The notion of "cultural conceptions of mental health" refers to common sense knowledge which is used to interpret social and medical experience, and which plays an important role in shaping both professional and everyday views of mental disorder. A growing amount of cultural and psychiatric research is showing that illness experience is an *interpretive* enterprise which is constructed in social situations according to the premises of cultural theories about illness and social behavior generally. Despite the large number of anthropological and psychiatric studies which have offered accounts of cultural beliefs about mental disorder, these accounts have generally been secondary to more broad ethnographic and clinical objectives of research. We still know very little about the symbolic and cognitive organization of common sense understandings about mental disorder which give illness experience cultural meaning and social significance. Research on these topics is essential for progress on answering fundamental questions about the universality and culture-specificity of aspects of mental disorder, its comprehension in human knowledge systems, and its significance for individuals and social communities. This book presents a series of papers whose primary objective is to examine conceptions of mental health as culturally ordered symbolic systems, and in so doing to draw attention to their relevance for understanding and treating mental disorder across cultures.

There is a substantial tradition of cross-cultural research which has described beliefs and practices connected with mental disorder in different societies (Opler 1959; Kiev 1964; Plog and Edgerton 1969; Caudill and Lin 1969; Westermeyer 1976). In describing contrastive conceptions of mental disorder, ethnographic research highlights the role of cultural knowledge in shaping illness and deviant behavior. The juxtaposition of different conceptions *between* cultures illuminates the interpretive aspects of disorder *within* any single culture. It is now well known that apparently similar illness events may be interpreted in highly variable ways depending upon the cultural theories available for reasoning about them. In the case of psychiatric illnesses which are recognized on the basis of verbal reports about thoughts, affect or personal outlook, etc., common-sense interpretations of behavioral and somatic events are central to both psychiatric diagnosis and ethnographic description.

The richness and complexity of cultural meanings in ordinary interpretations of disorder have been underscored by cross-cultural research which faces difficulties in both linguistic and conceptual translation in order to represent illness episodes as meaningful social events. Expressions of psychiatric illness in thought and behavior are of necessity mediated by the symbolic forms of language and culture. In general, however, interest in *how* personal or social meanings of

3

A. J. Marsella and G. M. White (eds.), Cultural Conceptions of Mental Health and Therapy, 1–38.

illness are constituted through cognitive and social processes has been secondary
to more direct research on the behavioral manifestations of particular types of
disorder and on "ethnopsychoses". Researchers have tended to treat cultural
constructs as an independent variable which can be used to explain observed
differences in behavioral or psychiatric phenomena (a similar point is made by
Young, 1976:5). Much of the cross-cultural, psychiatric research to date has
proceeded with quite simple assumptions about the role of ordinary language or
vernacular terms in "labeling" forms of abnormal behavior or psychological
disturbance, with little recognition of the creative power of language used in
social context and of the extent to which illness terms and concepts are embedded in wider cultural systems of knowledge about social behavior.

Because few ethnographic studies have focused explicitly on the conceptual
organization of cultural knowledge about mental disorder, or on culturally
appropriate ways of talking about disorder in social contexts, there has been
little convergence of methodological approaches which would help resolve the
formidable problems of analysis and representation involved in rendering
accounts of cultural conceptions of mental disorder. The result has been that
there is a great deal of uncertainty and debate about the recognition and universality of major psychoses such as depression and schizophrenia (see Singer 1975;
Kleinman 1977; Murphy 1976 and Marsella 1978, 1980), as well as about the
psychiatric significance of well-known "culture-bound" syndromes (see, for
example, Simons' (1980) discussion of *latah*, and the Goods' discussion of *susto*
in this volume). Debate on these issues is less fruitful than it would be with more
adequate information about the social and symbolic organization of cultural
knowledge of mental disorder.

The perspective taken here sees the symbolic ordering of illness in terms of
indigenous meanings and folk models as a primary factor in mental health
research and practice. This perspective is consistent with the largely interpretive
and cognitive thrust of the most influential theories of culture developed in
American anthropology during recent decades (e.g., Goodenough 1971; Geertz
1973; Keesing 1976). Methodological parallels to these developments began with
approaches variously termed "the new ethnography" or "ethnoscience" which
adapted linguistic models for the study of cultural systems (Pike 1954) and
focused largely on the semantic organization of terminological domains. These
approaches were concerned particularly with bringing a new measure of descriptive adequacy to the task of discovering and representing cultural knowledge as
a cognitive system (Frake 1969). The focus upon conceptual organization and
meaning in language, together with the attempt to inject a greater degree of rigor
into ethnographic description, seems well suited for the task Kleinman (1977)
calls the "new transcultural psychiatry", which devotes greater attention to the
symbolic structuring of cultural conceptions of mental disorder as an essential
component of mental health research and practice. Several of the chapters in the
present volume (White; Good and Good; Clement) discuss directly the usefulness
and limitations of the ethnoscience perspective in providing an ethnographic

base for such a "new transcultural psychiatry", and point to recent developments in cognitive anthropology (e.g., Frake 1980; D'Andrade 1981) and hermeneutics (e.g., Rabinow and Sullivan 1979) which address these limitations.

The papers in Parts II and III of this book describe symbolic and social contexts in which mental disorder is perceived, talked about and treated in a variety of Asian and Pacific cultures, as well as in Western psychiatry. In doing so, these studies demonstrate that cultural knowledge about mental disorder is embedded in a conceptual universe which is composed of a wide range of premises about the nature of persons and social behavior which do not pertain solely to illness or even abnormality. Ethnographic accounts of the personal and social meanings associated with mental disorder, necessarily go beyond descriptions of the meanings of terms or categories of illness to folk models which structure the interpretation of social and bodily events.

The comparisons, both implicit and explicit, given in these studies of different modes of interpreting mental disorder provide insight into the influence of culturally constituted understandings on psychiatric concepts in Western societies, where the significance of cultural constructs often goes unrecognized. Implicit theories of illness are usually regarded as relevant topics for research in non-Western societies where they are termed "cultural" (rather than simply "implicit", "common sense" or "lay" conceptions) and where modes of explanation and treatment often differ from the biomedical and psychological modes prevalent in the Western world. However, the very notion of "mental illness" as a domain of behavioral and medical experience is a product of specific cultural and historical traditions which regard certain forms of behavioral dysfunction as essentially psychological and medical in nature (see Simon 1978 and Neugebauer 1979). The component words of the phrase "mental illness"[1] reflect underlying assumptions which generally locate the causes of disorder in individual minds, personalities and neuroanatomies, and which view appropriate treatments as analogous to the treatment of medical disorders generally. As incorrigible as these basic suppositions seem in the context of modern medicine and psychiatry, they are predicated on assumptions about the nature of persons and social behavior which are symbolic constructions and which contrast with the symbolic constructions of other cultures. Even in Western societies, many forms of psychosocial distress can only be termed "mental" or "illness" in a metaphorical sense at best (Sarbin 1969). Some of the cultural influences on prevalent models of mental disorder in Western psychiatry are discussed in the papers by Fabrega, Gaines, Marsella and White. Additional areas of clinical relevance for cultural assumptions are reviewed below.

CLINICAL RELEVANCE OF CULTURAL CONCEPTIONS

The fact that many of the theoretical and diagnostic constructs used in mental health research and practice are linked with culturally-constituted understandings about persons and illness indicates that ethnographic research is not only relevant to the analysis of "exotic" belief systems, but to the use and improvement of scientific theories as well (see Kleinman 1977; Fabrega, this volume). Thus, far from pursuing the exotic and unfamiliar, ethnographic research is concerned with bringing into awareness familiar, taken-for-granted and often unrecognized assumptions about mental disorder. As Lazare (1973:346) has written,

By making explicit the implicit, the decision-making process in clinical psychiatry can become more rational, a broader range of treatment modalities should be made available, and the communication between physicians should be enhanced.

Even when implicit cultural conceptions have little *intrinsic* clinical significance, they exert systematic influences on a variety of activities which are clinically relevant, including psychiatric assessment, epidemiological research and inter-action/communication between practitioner and client. This section outlines briefly some cultural influences on the former activities, while interactional and communicational issues are taken up in a later section of this paper.

Clinical Judgment

Other than the rise of the use of psychopharmaceutical medicines, it is the development of formal systems of classification which most symbolize the claims of psychiatric medicine to objective and scientific status. The most recent and comprehensive classification scheme, the third *Diagnostic and Statistical Manual* (DSM—III) of the American Psychiatric Association, represents an attempt to codify psychiatric nosology in terms of a standardized, public and reliable category system. A large number of diagnostic instruments, such as the Minnesota Multiphasic Personality Inventory (MMPI), the Brief Psychiatric Rating Scale (BPRS) and the Present State Examination (PSE) (Wing et al. 1974), have been developed to render quantitative and actuarial assessments of personality and psychiatric disorder. Such techniques provide an important means of standardizing observations and of checking the reliability of clinical judgments. However, these very data which are intended to systematize and validate diagnostic procedures also provide evidence of the influence of implicit cultural concepts on clinical judgment as a cognitive process.

Questionnaire surveys of attitudes about mental illness have found a strong convergence between popular views and those of mental health professionals (Nunnally 1961; Townsend 1978). This parallel suggests that clinical judgments may be rooted in common sense (cultural) understandings. A number of studies have explored this possibility by using the same diagnostic instruments to elicit clinical judgments from both professional and nonprofessional, lay respondents. Chapman and Chapman (1967) demonstrated that both clinicians and students draw the same clinical inferences about psychopathology from data recorded with the Mann Draw-A-Person test, even though the inferences are not warranted by a correlational analysis of the data. They conclude that common sense conceptions lead to the perception of "illusory correlations" in the data, perceptions which may not be substantially altered by professional training.

The possible cultural bases for "illusory correlations" in clinical judgments have been explored further in a series of studies by D'Andrade (1974), Shweder (1977) and Shweder and D'Andrade (1980). These studies have drawn upon categories from both the MMPI and the BPRS to compare clinical ratings with judgments obtained by simply asking naive subjects to rate the *meanings* of the categories used in making those ratings. The results of these comparisons show that the structure of clinical ratings and the structure of semantic judgments are highly correlated. Furthermore, studies of the semantic organization of vocabulary used to describe personality in a number of non-western languages (see White 1980) have shown that conceptual dimensions evident in personality lexicons across cultures closely parallel the structure of theoretical formulations used in "interpersonal diagnosis" (Leary 1957; McLemore and Benjamin 1979; Wiggins 1980). Shweder and D'Andrade (1980) conclude that this convergence reflects cultural conceptions of "what goes with what" which are encoded in memory structures and expressed in ordinary language used by professional and lay populations alike. Furthermore, they argue that these cultural conceptions exert systematic influences on clinical judgments, such that psychiatric ratings reflect *models* of behavior and affect more closely than *actual* patterns in behavior or psychopathology. A schematic representation of the results of studies supporting these hypotheses is shown in Figure 1 which depicts the strong interrelation between 'ratings' and 'semantic structure' (indicated by a '+'), and only weak correlations between behavior and both 'ratings' and 'semantic structure', (indicated by a '0').

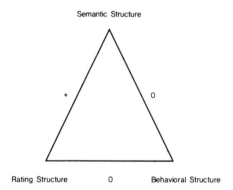

Fig. 1. Correlations among observed behavior, ratings of behavior and meanings of rating categories (adapted from Shweder and D'Andrade 1980:29).

Diagnostic testing is often viewed as an adjunct to medical decision-making which can improve the accuracy of clinical judgments, and the ways clinicians ordinarily "make sense" of psychiatric data. The most commonly recognized cognitive influence on clinical decisions is the limitation of information-processing *capacity*, as in the following passage:

In the role of interpreter of clinical data, the physician must contend with the limited size of working memory. . . . Algorithms, flow charts, decision trees, regression equations, and discriminant function analysis are techniques that increase the capacity for systematically processing large quantities of complex information and ensuring that all the data that should contribute to making a decision will be utilized (Elstein 1976:698).

This passage belies a view of medical cognition which presumes an "empiricist theory of language" as described in the papers by the Goods and Gaines in this volume, i.e., a view of category systems and rating scales as providing a direct and accurate reflection of clinical reality. However, studies of semantic and cultural influences on clinical judgment indicate that the predictive accuracy of psychiatric assessment is not only limited by the *amount* of information which can be processed, but also the *content* and *organization* of information which may be "systematically distorted" by implicit cultural models (Shweder and D'Andrade 1980).

There is a growing literature in cognitive psychology which demonstrates that people are not machine-like information processors who monitor the environment and systematically compute Bayesian probabilities or Pearson correlations in their heads (e.g., Nisbett and Ross 1979). Rather, people use cultural heuristics to reduce the size of a cognitive task by making selective use of available information (Tversky and Kahneman 1974), by ignoring the non-occurrence of events (Shweder 1977b) and by generally not looking beyond first-order main-effects in the interaction of relevant variables (Goldberg 1968). It is cultural knowledge which provides implicit rules specifying what to attend to (the "structures of relevance" described by Schutz (1970) and discussed by the Goods in their paper in this volume), how to take cognitive shortcuts, and how to make reasonable inferences in the face of complex, disparate and often contradictory information. Culture provides "structures of relevance" which determine what kinds of events or information are *salient* or noticeable, and hence serve to organize perception and interaction. Gaines' paper in this volume illustrates ways in which implicit cultural models among psychiatric residents influence what kinds of questions are asked and how much time is spent in the diagnostic process.

While studies cited above, using psychiatric rating data to compare professional and lay judgments, suggest that *some kind* of implicit cognitive or semantic processes influence clinical judgments, other studies which have made cross-cultural comparisons of both professional and lay perceptions indicate that it is, specifically, implicit *cultural* models which shape the perception of mental disorder among professional and lay populations alike. For example, Townsend (1978:9) surveyed popular and professional conceptions of mental disorder in Germany and America, and concluded that, except for an apparent effect of professional training in both countries in reducing negative stereotypes, "Mental health professionals in Germany and America resembled their lay compatriots in their conceptions of mental disorders more than they resembled each other."

Other studies which have compared clinical judgments of psychiatrists from different cultural and national backgrounds have turned up consistent contrasts in diagnostic styles which imply that shared models of disorder *within* cultures result in *between*-culture differences among mental health professionals. For example, a well-known study comparing hospital admissions in New York and London indicated consistent cross-national differences in the diagnosis of affective disorder (Cooper et al. 1972). More direct evidence for cultural differences in clinical judgment among psychiatrists comes from a series of studies by Leff (1974, 1977) who analyzed data from the International Pilot Study of Schizophrenia (WHO 1974) and found significant differences in psychiatrists' ratings of affect expressed by patients in the same videotaped interviews. Specifically, psychiatrists from "developed countries" tended to differentiate emotional states ("depression", "anxiety", "anger") expressed by patients from "developing countries" consistently more frequently than did "developing country" psychiatrists. After examining the degree of differentiation in *concepts* of emotion among psychiatrists, Leff concluded that "psychiatrists' preconceived notions about the differentiation of unpleasant affect . . . influenced their ratings of patients from developing countries" (1974:335).

The finding that implicit conceptions held by clinicians may bias diagnostic judgments with ethnically different patients underscores the point that psychiatric assessment does not consist of the recognition of disembodied diseases, but rather is constructed out of verbal reports and accounts offered by persons whose cultural conceptions, ways of speaking and social identities impact upon the diagnostic process. Just as cultural knowledge about illness provides expectations about "what goes with what" which have heuristic value in simplifying and making sense of symptom complaints, cultural knowledge about social identity consists of stereotypic conceptions which are likely to shape the perception of social behavior and illness. Parallels between social stereotypes and popular conceptions of mental illness imply that much of the research on social perception may also reveal processes which systematically shape clinical perception (cf. Townsend 1979). For example, several studies have shown that the meanings of personality attributions tend to shift according to the social identity of the person who is characterized (Kirk and Burton 1977; White 1978). There is a need for research which will examine the extent to which the perceived meanings of symptom complaints are affected by social factors such as age, sex, ethnicity or socio-economic status of the patient. Research on the conceptual integration of cultural knowledge of illness and of persons (social identities) would help to disentangle the role of various medical, conceptual, linguistic and interactional factors in producing observed differences in mental illness associated with sex (Broverman et al. 1970), ethnicity (Katz et al. 1969) and socio-economic status (Dohrenwend and Dobrenwend 1969; Derogatis et al. 1971). Since the study of socio-demographic variations in mental illness is the province of psychiatric epidemiology, the role of cultural conceptions in epidemiological research is discussed briefly below.

Epidemiology

Epidemiological research generally uses problem checklists, medical inventories and scheduled interviews, etc. to assess the prevalence and distribution of morbidity in specific populations. Thus, the influences of implicit cultural models on psychiatric observations are also likely to systematically affect epidemiological data in the direction of expectations of "what goes with what" according to cultural knowledge about illness and mental disorder. In addition to these cognitive influences on epidemiological data, cultural conceptions of mental disorder may also exert *social* influences on the expression and communication of symptom complaints. Thus, psychiatric data obtained through self-reports or interviewing about various symptom complaints are not simple *measurements* of observed conditions, but rather represent *interpretations* of events according to cultural rules for thinking and talking about illness in social situations.

Again, the role of implicit cultural models in psychiatric epidemiology is most evident and unavoidable in research in non-Western cultures. As Kennedy stated in his review (and Marsella emphasizes in his paper) of cultural psychiatry.

The methodological Achilles heel of many studies is in the diagnosis and appraisal of cases of mental disorder . . . due to . . . differential appraisal of similar behaviors . . . and problems of cross-cultural communication (1973:1184).

When a research instrument has to be translated into another language, the importance of meaning and "cultural connotations" of a set of verbal complaints or problem-statements becomes inescapable. Furthermore, linguistic translation does not necessarily entail cultural translation. For example, in a recent study with American and Hong Kong Chinese students,White (1982) shows that even though both groups perceive similar semantic relations among a set of symptom complaints, their explanations of those symptoms show distinct, culturally-patterned differences. These findings raise questions about the equivalence of translated versions of symptom checklists.

In recognition of the possibly unseen meanings and cultural connotations of problem statements used in epidemiological research, a number of recent studies have sought to use factor analysis as a statistical technique to uncover culture-specific patterns in epidemiological data (see Beiser et al. 1976 and Marsella, this volume). For example, factor analysis of the responses of Caucasian, Chinese and Japanese in Hawaii to a standardized depression checklist demonstrates that markedly different factor patterns characterize the responses of each ethnic group (Marsella et al. 1973). One such cultural contrast noted in this study was the appearance of more definite somatic factors in the Chinese responses, a finding which indicates that data derived from a seemingly straightforward symptom checklist may reveal more about culturally constituted modes of interpreting illness than about actual patterns of disorder.

Awareness of the central role of cultural factors in psychiatric assessment has led a number of investigators to suggest that cross-cultural studies of mental disorder, including the major psychoses such as schizophrenia or depression, must incorporate indigenous categories in research methodologies (Kleinman 1977; Marsella 1978). The problem of semantic and cultural influences on clinical judgment with any category system, as discussed above, adds a note of caution to attempts to use culturally-specific categories in epidemiological research. The difficulties in validating and generalizing from psychiatric rating data will not be lessened by the use of indigenous categories in survey techniques. These difficulties are also discussed by the Goods in their paper included in this volume.

In addition to the cognitive influences on perceiving and reporting symptom complaints, cultural conceptions also have a major impact on the social processes of communication and interaction involved in epidemiological research. Cultural differences in the personal and social meanings of certain complaints may lead to consistent differences in the way individuals express or report about illness in an interview situation. For example, Zola (1966) describes ethnic differences in presenting complaints associated with the same kinds of illness. Such differences, which may be related to both conceptual and sociolinguistic factors, will have an obvious skewing effect on epidemiological data. It is unclear, for example, whether reported sex differences in psycho-social distress are an accurate reflection of differential risk among males and females, or whether they reflect differences in male and female attitudes toward illness and sex roles (Nathanson 1975; Lee 1980). This confounding of the medical and cultural significance of epidemiological data makes clear the potential usefulness of more explicit models of how questions about illness are interpreted and responded to by members of particular social and cultural populations. Ethnographic accounts of cultural conceptions of mental illness among specific populations may help remove the interpretation of epidemiological findings from the realm of post-hoc speculation.

The foregoing discussion of the relevance of cultural conceptions of mental disorder for both clinical judgment and epidemiological research has suggested that implicit cultural models exert both cognitive and social influences on the process of psychiatric assessment. This discussion has pointed out several areas in which not only cultural knowledge of illness, but cultural knowledge about persons and social behavior may affect the perception and expression of symptom complaints. The mutual relevance of conceptions of mental disorder and cultural assumptions about personhood is emphasized throughout the papers in this volume. Some of the major themes relevant to the integration of common sense understandings about illness and social behavior are outlined below.

ISSUES IN MEANING AND REPRESENTATION

Disease and medicine have provided a convenient "domain" of specialized knowledge (termed ethnomedicine) about the world which has been analyzed and compared in a manner similar to other topical domains such as plants or animals. Since most cultures around the world exhibit well developed vocabularies for describing and talking about illness, ethnoscientific methods which focus on language and terminological domains have been used to represent cultural knowledge about disease in a wide range of societies (see Conklin 1972: 363–392). To a certain extent, cultural knowledge of mental disorder has also been studied by using lexical evidence to indicate where certain forms of disorder are "labeled" by vernacular terms. However, conceptions of disorder encompass cultural understandings about the nature of persons, minds, emotions, social interaction, etc., which cannot be construed as a bounded domain of specialized knowledge rooted in a limited phenomenological field such as the human body. The inclusion of these ethnopsychological constructs within the scope of ethnomedicine has important implications for the study of cultural knowledge of illness generally, whether psychiatric or otherwise.

As noted earlier, a number of papers in this volume, particularly those by White, Good and Good, and Clement, all discuss current approaches to the representation of cultural knowledge about illness by noting limitations in the traditional methods of ethnoscience. These chapters note a shift away from a reliance on models of illness concepts as lexical categories distinguished by "diagnostic features", toward a view of illness knowledge as embedded in coherent complexes of symbols which make up folk theories used to reason about and deal with illness in social situations. The Goods refer to the traditional concern with ostensive definitions (just as Clement discusses the ethnoscience focus on "referential meaning") of lexical categories as the "empiricist theory of language", which they decry as unable to explore the full range of conceptual associations which give cultural categories of illness their personal and social meaning. White makes a similar point in discussing "the case of the missing domain" and the developing interests of cognitive anthropologists in inferential processes used to construct accounts and make decisions about illness. He gives a number of examples of processual models which ethnographers have constructed to represent the types of interlinked inferences characteristic of folk theories.

The Goods' paper develops further their notion of "semantic network" proposed in earlier work (1977) to facilitate representation of the range of conceptual relations associated with important illness categories. They demonstrate the usefulness of semantic network models in representing the culturally-defined personal states and social experiences which coalesce in the Iranian concept of "fright illness". Margaret Lock also makes use of a semantic network model to represent the conceptual interrelation of important Japanese ethnopsychological constructs involved in popular conceptions of mental health. Her account shows the heuristic value of visual models in graphically portraying multiple conceptual relations which could not be as easily or effectively described in discursive form. These studies give an indication of greater contributions to our understanding of the cultural composition of concepts of mental health which may be expected as further research spells out procedures for gathering and representing ethnographic data in the form of semantic networks.

The use of semantic network models in rendering a "meaning-centered" account of popular illness categories is placed by the Goods in the philosophical context of hermeneutics and interpretive social science (see, for example, Geertz 1973; Ricoeur 1976 and Rabinow and Sullivan 1979). Despite the recent currency of the term "hermeneutic" (from the Greek *hermeneuein*, "to interpret"), appreciation of the role of interpretation in ethnographic research has a long history in cultural anthropology. However, the philosophical stance of the hermeneutic approach confronts squarely many of the issues which are most problematic for the scientific aspirations of social-science investigations of meaning in ordinary language or of folk knowledge. The hermeneutic perspective is valuable in focusing attention on, rather than minimizing, the interactive nature of interpretation and meaning as social constructions. While this approach offers a clearer sense of the problems in ethnographic interpretation, it has not so far been a source of solutions to the persistent difficulties of validating alternative models of folk knowledge (see Agar 1980) — difficulties which are likely to be particularly important if such models are to be incorporated in clinical research and assessment.

Although Geertz (1973) has opposed hermeneutic interpretations of cultural forms to symbolic representations based on cognitive rules (e.g., Goodenough, 1971), these approaches are not incompatible, as several of the papers in the present volume suggest (and see Frake 1980). For example, the hermeneutic perspective is consistent with Clement's conceptualization of "folk knowledge" in terms of representational forms associated with social institutions and transactions rather than with individuals; and the symbolic form of "network" models discussed by the Goods is quite similar to the type of "propositional" model derived by D'Andrade (1976) in representing American beliefs about illness, and discussed by White in his paper (although the procedures used to construct these two forms of representation are very different). At one level, the cognitive structuring of cultural knowledge of mental disorder provides the symbolic raw materials by which actors pose and counterpose interpretations (of illness) which, at another level, constitute meaningful social performances (see Harmon 1971).

While only the papers by the Goods and Gaines explicitly term their mode of analysis "hermeneutic", many of the papers included here show that an approach which focuses on the pragmatic aspects of meaning and interpretation is well suited to the study of conceptions of mental disorder which are most clearly expressed in interactive episodes of diagnosis, help-seeking and therapy. These papers also suggest that the episodic (or "script"-like, see Schank and Abelson 1977) structure of natural discourse about illness events provides an important framework for comparative research in cognition as well as in medicine and psychopathology. The widespread relevance of this episodic format is reflected in the fact that all of the ethnographic papers in Parts II and III of this book present cases of illness and treatment to represent the implicit "logic" of folk theories of mental disorder. Most of these chapters show that the description of a case, whether reported by the ethnographer or described in natural discourse, can be an effective way to discover the range of meanings associated with various symptoms and types of illness, without extensive reliance on a-priori definitions of what types of medical or social phenomena should be included in the observations. Because they are not constrained by such a-priori definitions, the portrayals which are given here underscore the relevance of ethnopsychological constructs in structuring cultural conceptions of mental disorder. Some of the major themes raised in the papers in this book, and promising topics for further research on the ethnopsychology of mental disorder, are outlined below.

ETHNOPSYCHOLOGY AND ETHNOMEDICINE

Conceptions of Person and Theories of Disorder

Cultural theories of mental disorder are, in a fundamental sense, about personal and social events. They draw upon cultural assumptions concerning the nature of ordinary personal experience and social interaction in order to interpret behavioral disturbances which are regarded as extraordinary, abnormal, or disruptive, etc. Thus, the comparative study of cultural knowledge of mental disorder stands to gain significant insights from examining the ways in which personal and social processes are conceptualized cross-culturally. While this broadening of scope may appear to diffuse the focus for comparative research on culture and mental health, it actually provides an incisive entry point into native symbol systems and promises considerable pay-offs for future research. Cultural theories of mental disorder lie at the intersection of conceptions of personhood and conceptions of illness, both of which are probably universal aspects of cultural knowledge. Just as Geertz (1976:225) has written that "The concept of person is, in fact, an excellent vehicle by means of which to examine this whole question of how to go about poking into another people's turn of mind ... ", so a people's conceptions of illness and behavioral dysfunction offer an excellent vehicle by which to examine their concept of person. It is in the context of illness events or episodes of disturbance that implicit premises about the nature of persons and ordinary social experience may become more "visible" or accessible to the researcher as they are expressed in natural discourse aimed at explaining, rationalizing or treating disorder (see Quinn (1980) for a more general statement about the functions of "folk theories" generally).

However, the notion of "person" (or self) is a highly abstract theoretical construct which does not lend itself in any simple or direct way to the purposes of comparative ethnographic research. To the contrary, abstract notions of "personhood" are susceptible to typification and reification in ways which may easily oversimplify or obscure the task of representing "another people's turn of mind". To be useful, the notion of implicit conceptions of person serves rather as a signpost for the interrelatedness or implicit coherence of more specific types of common sense understandings used to interpret behavioral events.

Most of the papers in the present volume describe ethnopsychological constructs which contribute to cultural theories of mental disorder without necessarily abstracting more fundamental principles which could be characterized as an implicit "theory" of personhood. The latter type of generalization is perhaps more easily portrayed on the basis of cross-cultural comparisons. The papers by Shweder and Bourne and by Gaines both discuss contrastive types of person concepts by comparing directly two different cultural traditions. What is important about both of these studies (for the purposes of the present volume) is that they postulate relations between broad cultural orientations toward social experience and more specific cognitive and behavioral phenomena relevant to folk theories of mental disorder. Shweder and Bourne make measured comparisons of cognitive aspects of person descriptions elicited from both Americans and Indians and find significant, patterned contrasts which they attribute to underlying differences in cultural premises about the individual in society. Specifically, they find that American subjects make greater use of individuated ("egocentric") constructs, such as personality attributions, in their accounts; while the Indian accounts show more evidence of context-specific and relational ("sociocentric") features of interaction. Their opposition of "egocentric" and "sociocentric" person concepts overlaps substantially with the "referential" and "indexical" concepts of selfhood described by Gaines (after Crapanzano, 1980) as characteristic of Protestant and Latin European traditions, respectively. (Although Gaines is distinguishing cultural conceptions within Western traditions, which may help to clarify the more usual practice of treating the West "as a single standard" of comparison as in the Shweder and Bourne paper.[2]) The presentation of the Latin self in social interaction tends to index a particular time, place and set of social relations, with the result that the self is less an object of reflection and abstraction than in the case of the "referential" Protestant self.

Gaines argues that the "referential" type person concept underlies forms of diagnosis and treatment in Western psychiatry, especially psychoanalysis. He describes cases showing that different assumptions about personhood and social reality among psychiatric residents may systematically affect their approach to treatment, as reflected in the time spent with patients in an emergency room setting. The point that implicit assumptions about the self and illness have systematic influences in Western psychiatry is developed further by Fabrega who suggests that features of the nosological system (such as the first-rank symptoms of schizophrenia), as well as the actual manifestations of psychiatric illness in Western societies, reflect cultural notions about "human psychology and causality". His statement that "contemporary Western psychology articulates a highly differentiated mentalistic self which is highly individuated and which looks out on an objective, impersonal and naturalistic world", echoes a number of the features of the "egocentric" and "referential" person concepts enumerated by both Shweder and Gaines. Most of the ethnographic papers in this book describe forms of non Western ethnopsychology which depart in a variety of ways from the above mentioned assumptions of psychiatric medicine.

Ethnographic descriptions of person concepts such as those by Shweder and Bourne and by Gaines are abstract characterizations of cultural modes of differentiating and organizaing the "behavioral environment" (see Hallowell 1955). The notion of "person concept" encompasses a culture's inventory of the psycho-social universe, together with the forms of reasoning used to interpret events in that universe. Most of the papers in Parts II and III of this volume describe recurrent themes in the ethnopsychological bases of cultural knowledge of mental disorder which suggest contrasts in the cultural form of person concepts. Among the topics which arise in a number of the papers and which provide conceptual anchor points for comparisons of conceptions of mental disorder, are: (1) relations among body, mind and environment, (2) emotions, (3) self-other relations, (4) causality, agency and responsibility, and (5) social images and social control.

Body, Mind and Environment

The human body provides potent metaphors and important constraints on the symbolic organization of understandings about the person, social action and health across cultures. The cultural systems described in this book all suggest that common sense understandings about body structure and functioning figure importantly into cultural views of selfhood and subjective experience. At issue particularly are the interfaces of body and environment on the one hand, and of body and subjective experience of self or mind on the other. The ethnographic papers in this book show indirectly that these interface points are conceptualized as far more distinct and impermeable in Western or biomedical views than in most of the Asian and Pacific cultures described here. The Ayurvedic, Balinese, Chinese and Japanese knowledge structures recounted here all reflect more holistic systems of belief which perceive symbolic correspondences between the body as microcosm and the universe (environment) as macrocosm. These systems evince a much higher degree of interaction and mutuality of cause and effect between body and environment than is the case for comparable Western notions. Both natural substances and energies, as well as supernatural forces may readily traverse the boundaries of body and person, such that bodily events are conceived as less separate from events in the environment, and psychological experience is less segmented from somatic conditions than in typical Western views. Because of this greater degree of segmentation, the typical Western view seems both more "naturalistic" in its conceptualization of body/environment relations, and more "psychological" in its conceptualization of body/mind relations.

The increased differentiation of psychological experience from somatic and social events in Western culture is a cornerstone for the development of the concept of "mental illness" itself. Fabrega writes here that the premise of Western biomedical theory that "the domain of the body contrasts with that of the mind" underlies basic distinctions between mental and physical illness and the development of medical subdisciplines such as neurology, psychiatry and internal medicine. To the extent that the psychiatric notion of "mental illness" is predicated on a segmentation of psychological processes from physical phenomena, the recognition by other cultures of an analogous class of mental disorders will hinge in part on similar ethnopsychological assumptions about body and mind, and their interrelation.

Many observers have noted the strongly dualistic or Cartesian assumptions about mind and body in Western cultural traditions, and have contrasted this orientation with Eastern traditions where such distinctions are said to be absent or minimal. The papers in this volume, particularly those which discuss Asian medical theories, are especially useful in delineating some of the cultural and cognitive bases for these frequently oversimplified contrasts. For example, most of these ethnographic accounts – of Ayurveda, Chinese and contemporary Japanese ethnomedicine – show that conceptual distinctions between bodily and psychological processes are important in Asian explanatory systems often characterized as non-dualistic. These accounts suggest that it is not the distinction of psychological processes, or of "mind" *per se*, but their place in explanatory reasoning about health and disorder which is culturally variant in important ways. In all of the Asian systems described here, psychological constructs are rarely perceived to operate independently of the body or the environment. Psychological variables such as feeling states or personality problems are not regarded as original causes of disorder, but as contributing, mediating or final causes among an array of interactive forces. Thus, in each Asian tradition, popular explanatory constructs are more appropriately characterized as "somato-psychic" in contrast to the familiar "psycho-somatic" mode of reasoning. Obeyesekere summarizes this succinctly in his observation that in the Ayurvedic tradition of medicine, "The major cause of mental illness is somato-psychic rather than psycho-somatic." However, he goes on to note that this does not derive from a lack of perception of psycho-somatic connections, which are frequently mentioned, but that " ... nowhere in Ayurveda is there a psychodynamic theory to explain these phenomena. By contrast, the somatic theory of the three *dosas* is always spelled out." These comments are echoed by Lock's assessment of East Asian medicine as showing

... a reductionistic somato-psychic emphasis of long historical standing such that for all problems, even where social and psychological components in disease causation are readily acknowledged, the physical manifestations of illness are the focus of treatment.

She notes that, by implication, traditional systems of medical classification did not differentiate a concept of mental health as distinct from physical health.

Cultural contrasts in comparisons of Western and non Western views of mind and body are closely tied with cultural modes of interpreting personal and social experience. A number of the papers characterize indigenous systems of belief as holistic in so far as they do not presume any sharp boundaries or discontinuities between the natural and the supernatural, the organic and the inorganic, or the physical and the mental. While these various orders of phenomena may actually be differentiated conceptually, they are perceived to be highly and continuously interactive. Natural elements, components of the body and states of mind are perceived to be interrelated as part to whole, or microcosm to macrocosm, and to be in continuous interaction such that energies are exchanged and the balance of cosmological forces (such as *yin* and *yang*) affected as change in one sphere affects change in another. Such interaction is commonly conceptualized in terms of supernatural forces (such as the Balinese 'sibling' spirits described by Connor), energies (such as the Japanese *ki* which Lock describes as exchanged continually between body and environment) or the balance and rhythm of cosmological principles (such as the East Asian *yin* and *yang* described by both Lock and Wu). One of the implications of such holistic systems of belief is that natural substances, especially food, and somatic factors gain greater primacy in explanatory system surrounding disorders of the person or mind. Here, then, are some of the cultural and symbolic bases of the somatic mode of presentation and explanation of illness complaints noted by psychiatric researchers in Chinese cultures (Marsella et al. 1973; Tseng 1975; Kleinman 1977).

Emotion

The largely symbolic and cognitive focus of the present volume may seem especially ironic in light of the fact that it is *emotion* which is generally regarded as a defining feature of many varieties of mental disorder. And in most theories of psychology and behavior, emotion is contrasted with and placed in opposition to cognition. Indeed, the opposition of emotion and cognition underlies some of the most basic ways of conceptualizing behavior and subjective experience in Western cultures. However, we are arguing that even our most basic conceptualizations are cultural constructions which are embedded in implicit theories of personhood and social reality. Research on cultural conceptions of mental disorder needn't be predicated on a dichotomous division of emotion and cognition, nor as focusing on cognition, but ignoring emotion.

Concepts of emotion do, however, occupy a somewhat priviledged status in cross-cultural research on conceptions of mental disorder. Certain aspects of affective experience are probably universal, as indicated by comparative research on facial expression of emotion (Ekman 1973) as well as on the lexical encoding of emotion cross-culturally (Boucher et al. n.d.). As many of the papers in this book make clear, *some form* of cultural understanding about emotion plays an important role in symbolizing significant forces which impinge upon the self in relation to its behavioral environment (Hallowell 1955). Emotion constructs are widely used to represent and reason about the relation of the person to somatic, psychological and social processes. Because emotion concepts are primary symbols of personal well-being, illness and disorder, they provide a critical focus for comparative research on cultural conceptions of mental disorder. However, in order to best exploit emotion as an access point for discovering the nature of cultural symbol systems, it is necessary to be aware of the taken-for-granted assumptions in Western theories of the person and mental disorder.

Emotional states are a major factor in psychiatric definitions of mental disorder, as in the distinction of "thought disorders" (e.g., schizophrenia) and "affective disorders" (e.g., depression). These distinctions, which are represented in the most recent psychiatric classifications of mental illness (as in the DSM-III), were first evident in Kraepelin's early typology of mental disorders. The Kraepelinian classification was influenced by Wundt's tripartite model of human psychology based on "cognition", "affect" and "will". However, far from being an accurate reflection of universal features of human experience, Wundt's influential theory is a relection of cultural assumptions about personhood and social behavior whose relation to universal structures of experience remains problematic. In the Western view articulated by Wundt, emotions are essentially physiological, not easily verbalized, and irrational. These features of emotion are in direct, complementary opposition to conceptions of thought as symbolic, expressable, and rational. To point to but one study of a non Western culture which illustrates the potential for a distinctly different ethnopsychology of emotion, Lutz's (1980) work on the Pacific atoll of Ifaluk shows that 'emotion' and 'thought' may be conceptualized as a true continuum. Comparative ethnographic research on cultural "theories" of the person and emotion is capable of providing a greater reflexive understanding of the "metaphors we live by" (Lakoff and Johnson 1980) as well as the "metaphors we do research by".

The papers in the present volume, which discuss cultural views of emotion, reveal intriguing parallels as well as important differences in the conceptualization of emotion cross-culturally. For example, a number of the papers describe conceptual oppositions of 'emotion' and indigenous notions of 'reason' or 'knowledge' which resemble popular Western notions quite closely. Lock's discussion of Japanese ethnopsychological understandings which juxtaposes Japanese terms for 'emotion', 'knowledge' and 'will' is surprisingly similar to the Wundtian schema mentioned above. Several of the accounts given in this book also describe metaphorical expressions of emotion as a force which may be directed inward toward the self or outward toward others; and which must be regulated, controlled or contained in order not to damage the self (as in Chinese beliefs about excess emotion, or the Iranian belief that the 'inner self' must be protected from emotional trauma) or disrupt social relations.

However, even in the cases where there are certain broad similarities in the conceptualization of emotion, there are distinct differences in the ways emotion constructs are used to reason about human experience. As might be expected from the above discussion of cultural differences in conceptions of "mind", "body" and "environment", the role of emotion constructs in cultural theories of the person or mental disorder may be highly variable across cultures. Once again, the degree of Western differentiation and segmentation of ethnopsychological constructs also applies to emotion concepts (see also Leff 1977). Given the dichotomous Western views of person and environment on the one hand, and of mental and physical processes on the other, emotions tend to be regarded as purely *psychological* processes which interact with other psychological processes such as thoughts and perceptions. In line with this view, emotional disturbances are frequently diagnosed and treated as a closed system. The Freudian hydraulic metaphor which views emotion as a deep, insurgent force within the individual expresses a conceptualization of emotion which is basically *intrapsychic* in nature.

In contrast with this strongly individuated theory of emotion, a number of the papers in this book describe systems of belief which regard emotions as integrated more closely with both interpersonal relations as well as somatic processes. The functional interdependence of affective and somatic processes is conceptualized especially clearly in many of the Asian cultures described here. For example, emotional experience is localized in particular regions or organs of the body, as in the Ayurvedic theory that emotional shock may block the channels of the heart and sense organs, or the Chinese and Japanese association of specific affects and particular internal organs, as discussed in Wu's review of the Chinese anatomy of emotion and in both T. Lebra's and Lock's discussion of the Japanese view of the stomach (*hara*) as the emotional center of the person. In addition, the ebbs and flows of emotion are conceptualized in terms of the *interdependence* of the person and affect as microcosmos and the macrocosmos, including social, supernatural and climactic conditions. This sort of interdependence is represented in terms of balance of energies and cosmological principles such as *yin* and *yang*.

Most of the papers, whether dealing with Asian or Pacific cultures, provide clear illustrations of theories of personhood which link emotions with psychological conflict. In other words, cultural explanations of emotional disorder in these societies is more relational or "sociocentric" (to borrow Shweder and Bourne's term) than in comparable Western explanations. The concern with maintaining interpersonal harmony and a balanced emotional state is expressed in both the Japanese tea ceremony mentioned by Lock and the Chinese ideal of *hsiu yang* described by Wu. Similarly, the papers by both Clement and White describe explanatory models in Pacific societies (Samoa and Santa Isabel, Solomon Islands) which are strongly situational in orientation. The mental disorders defined by Samoans as caused by "an excess of emotion" are generally attributed to a particular aggravating situation (e.g., loss of a loved one) and treated by removal of the offending circumstances. These analyses of situation-based reasoning about emotion is in basic agreement with Lutz's (1980) observations that Ifalukian emotions are defined in relation to social situations to a much greater extent than comparable American conceptions which are linked to internal and physiological bases.

Self and Other

Although the notions of 'person' and 'self' are often used interchangeably (and the papers in this volume draw no definitive distinctions between them), some clarification is possible (see, for example, Rorty 1976). Specifically, the notion of self entails a reflexivity and an opposition of 'self' and 'other' which 'person' does not. The ways in which a culture conceptualizes the opposition of self and other appears to have important consequences for its assumptions about illness and disorder. Notions of self and other provide a social analog to many of the dichotomous oppositions discussed above, such as "mind"/"body"/ "environment". As in the earlier discussion, the Western view of the self as a well-differentiated, distinct social entity contrasts sharply with the non-Western cultures described here. Once again, a greater degree of conceptual differentiation or segmentation (between self and other) characterizes Western notions in contrast with comparable Asian and Pacific ideas. This difference is alluded to in many of the ethnographic papers with phrases such as "unbounded" or "permeable boundaries" or "lack of clear demarcation", etc. used to describe indigenous views of self/other relations.

The comparative discussions of person concepts by Shweder and Bourne, and by Gaines, rely largely on characterizations of differences in self-other relations. Their use of boundary metaphors (such as the "discrete" or "inviolate" nature of the "egocentric" person concept) is important primarily as an indication of cultural differences in the implicit logic of reasoning about social interaction. Thus, the sharp boundaries of the Western person concept are associated with the perception of behavior as emanating from the individual as an autonomous social actor and as the principal locus of thought, feeling, motivation and action. Similarly, the "loose" or "permeable" boundaries of the "sociocentric" person are associated with the belief that behavior is a function of particular self-other relations among interdependent social actors.

Consistent with their description of the Western "egocentric" person concept, Shweder and Bourne show that Americans make greater use of individuated, psychological types of explanatory constructs (such as personality trait words) in describing social behavior. Their findings cast light on some of the cultural bases of the extensive "psychologization" of Western models of mental disorder and social behavior in general (White 1982). Fabrega and Gaines also point to specific influences of Western (or, in Gaines' terms, Protestant European) views of self-other relations on psychiatric models of illness and approaches to treatment. In so far as the self is more readily abstracted from social contexts and becomes an object of reflection, it is not surprising that the notion of psychology itself looms so large in both popular and professional views of social experience in Western society; that a great deal of concern focuses on personal identity or the ego as an integrated and continuous expression of the person; and that various forms of illness and mental disorder are characterized as disruptions in the unity or continuity of ego integration.

The importance of implicit assumptions about self-other relations for cultural views of personal adjustment and mental health is perhaps best illustrated in this volume through the juxtaposition of Western and Japanese views, as outlined in the papers by Lock, Lebra and Murase. While Lock's paper is dealing with popular beliefs in general, and the latter two are concerned with particular forms of therapy, they all describe aspects of cultural knowledge of mental disorder which is intensely interpersonal in its orientation. Lebra's description of the interpersonal dynamics of "self-accusation" and the attribution of responsibility for moral behavior is perhaps most revealing of the fluidity of the Japanese concept of the person in contrast with that in the West. She argues that these behaviors, as well as the ease of "identity exchange" in therapy rituals, make sense in light of the Japanese "belief that there is no clear cut demarcation line between self and other". The sharp contrast between Western concepts of self-other relations, as embodied in psychotherapy, and Japanese person concepts is further underscored in Murase's outline of social ideology associated with *Naikan* and Morita therapies which are fundamentally interpersonal in their goals and procedures. Murase lists a series of conceptual oppositions which contrast the Japanese ideal of the *sunao* person with the "ego" described in Western psychoanalytic theory. Many of the oppositions (such as "relationship-oriented" vs. "individual-centered" or "dependent" vs. "autonomous") closely resemble the contrastive person concepts described by Shweder and Bourne, and by Gaines. The extensive convergence of these comparative analyses attests to the relative similarity of very different concepts of person (Indian and Japanese) when compared with Western notions; and suggest that there may be a limited number of cultural solutions to the puzzle of self-other relations. This convergence also raises a cautionary note concerning the ease with which cultural contrasts may be enumerated based on semantic oppositions implicit in our language (many of the oppositions in Murase's comparisons reflect the bi-polar semantic differential scales "active vs. passive" and "strong vs. weak" (see Osgood et al. 1975 and White 1980)).

Causality, Agency and Responsibility

The above discussion of ethnopsychological constructs such as "mind", "body", "emotion", "self" and "other" indicates that much of the cultural variation surrounding these notions is connected with differing views of processes of interaction, i.e., with causal reasoning about what affects what, and about the sources of change and stability in behavioral experience. While certain general forms of causal inference are probably universal in symptom recognition and illness explanations (as in Obeyesekere's account of methods of observation and experimentation in more formal Ayurvedic medicine), the perception of specific causal agents appears both complex and highly variable across cultures. For example, Fabrega distinguishes between two interrelated types of etiological question – one about "causation" (why?), and one about "mechanism" (how?) – both of which may influence the construction of meaningful explanations and the attribution of responsibility (cf. Young 1976:17). As the previous sketch of person concepts suggests, Western explanatory models (both popular and professional) tend to locate the causes of mental disorder within individual psyches, and particularly with the self as a unitary social actor. In contrast, comparable Asian and Pacific models give proportionately greater weight to interdependent somatic processes, supernatural forces and social relations as causal agents. Even in some cases where these latter models perceive psychological causes of mental disorder, as in the emotional disturbances described by the Goods for Iran and Wu for Chinese, these illnesses are interpreted with analogical reasoning about imbalances which resemble the "logic" of somatic disorder.

Beliefs about the perceived power of unseen supernatural forces to traverse the boundaries of the person and effect both somatic and psychological/behavioral changes are widespread. In most of the cases reported here, supernatural forces assume an important role as causal agents in explanations of disturbed behavior. Such forces may take the form of personified spirits (as exemplified here by Samoan ancestral spirits, Japanese Gedatsu 'guardian spirits' and Balinese 'sibling spirits'), or of disembodied influences emanating from sorcerers or gods. In either case, the potential for multiple or alternative agents in the explanation of individual behavior contrasts sharply with the explanatory role of the unitary self in Western concepts of person. As Takie Lebra writes, "interchange with supernaturals expands a spectrum of role options" and adds considerable flexibility to the symbolic manipulation of social identity.

Beliefs about supernatural forces and beings have important implications for the attribution of responsibility in cultural explanations of mental disorder. Because most of the behavioral phenomena classed as extraordinary or abnormal are evaluated as socially and morally undesirable (with important exceptions, such as the Balinese 'blessed madness'), the perception of agency and the attribution of responsibility entail significant social consequences, particularly for the nature of others' response to the afflicted individual. For example, in Samoa, delirious behavior seen as the result of possession by an angry ancestral spirit is treated by spirit healers. However, if possession is doubted, the afflicted person is regarded as responsible and may even be beaten as a result. Similarly in Bali, irratic behavior by a child may be tolerated if it is perceived as the manifestation of personality traits of an ancestor reincarnated in the child. Such beliefs as these may function to alleviate culpability or stigma from the disordered individual, possibly shifting it to others.

The role of supernatural agents in cultural knowledge of mental disorder has the general effect of decentering the locus of causality from the individual as a unitary social actor (when compared with the role of psychological factors in Western explanatory models). This decentering has important analogs in interpersonal behavior in which the attribution of responsibility is much less bound by distinctions between self and other. Much of the above discussion of cultural contrasts in concepts of self and other can be stated more concretely in terms of the perception of agency and the attribution of responsibility which, as Young (1976:14) has argued, is one of the definitional hallmarks of illness events across cultures. When behavior is perceived to emanate from bounded individuals, agency and responsibility are attributed to *either* self *or* other. The extensive literature in attribution theory (see Jones et al. 1973) shows that much of common sense explanation of social behavior among Westerners presupposes a kind of inferential tradeoff between self and other, or between person and situation. However, numerous examples in this book suggest that many non-Western conceptions of personhood entail a greater blending of agency (and responsibility) between *both* self *and* other. This melding of responsibility for behavior is illustrated in Lebra's discussion of the Japanese self as a passive (rather than active) agent, whose actions are responsive to the moral demands and obligations of others, as represented linguistically in extensive use of "passive causative" constructions to express agency and the "allocentric" allocation of responsibility. Throughout this book there are numerous examples of explanatory models which may interpet illness or mental disorder as the result of socio-moral conflict or strained relations within a significant social group (e.g., family, village), rather than within an individual psyche. Even in cases where responsibility or blame is attributed to the afflicted individual, this type of interpersonal explanatory model may require that treatment or cure be focused on mending social relations, as in the apology rituals described by Clement and T. Lebra, the offerings to offended ancestral spirits mentioned by Connor and W. Lebra, and the 'disentangling' meetings discussed by White (see also Turner 1964). Gaines in his paper, and other studies of Western popular conceptions of mental disorder (Nunnally 1961; Townsend 1978), show that, in contrast with the above models, "individual responsibility" and "personal effort" are basic components of common sense Western notions of causation and cure. Their findings are echoed in Shweder and Bourne's citation of Selby's remark (1974: 62–66) that the "folk explanatory model that puts responsibility for morality and cure on the individual" is "deeply rooted in Western thought".

Social Images and Social Control

The above discussion of agency and responsibility indicates that cultural knowledge of mental disorder "packages" a great deal of information about the social and moral consequences of abnormal or disruptive behavior. As labeling theorists (Scheff 1966; Rosenhan 1973 and Waxler 1974) have shown, the ascription of mental disorder evokes culturally prescribed responses from others which structure the experience of the afflicted individual as he or she moves about in the social system. The study of conceptions of mental disorder becomes important as a means of determining what kinds of social reality are likely to be created by the interpretation of behavior as mentally disordered.

The ascription of mental disorder is in many ways cognitively and socially analogous to the perception of social identity generally. In both cases, categorization provides a conceptual basis for making inferences about additional behavioral characteristics and role expectations. Thus, an important question about the organization of cultural knowledge of mental disorder asks 'what are its culturally defined social identities?' and 'what are the similarities and differences in the cultural meanings associated with the identities of mental disorder (e.g., being "crazy", "bewitched" or "possessed", etc.) and other significant social identities?'

These questions are addressed directly by Clement in her description of the Samoan concept of 'madperson' in comparison with other types of social identity. These comparisons show that the 'madperson' " ... stands out as a prototype constituting a standard against which other roles may be compared, an embodiment or representation of important cultural themes ... " As a type of social identity, the Samoan notion of being "crazy" serves an important function in representing disvalued behaviors which are defined in opposition with culturally-defined forms of ideal social behavior. In contrast, the Samoan concept of a 'cultured person' condenses important positive social ideals. By thus examining cultural understandings about social behavior represented in these positive and negative prototypes, Clement is able to demonstrate that Samoan folk knowledge of mental disorder is structured by cultural definitions of desirable social behavior as, for example, 'cultured', 'wise' and, especially, 'respectful' (as shown through 'social sensitivity' and the appropriate use of 'proper speech').

Most of the papers in this volume describe evaluatively polarized behavioral images in which social ideals are contrasted with negative, socially-undesirable behavior associated with mental disorder. This type of evaluative polarization is built upon a conceptual dimension which is probably universal in interpersonal vocabulary (White 1980). In this book, Murase characterizes the Japanese concept of a 'sunao person' which represents an extensive amount of cultural knowledge about ideal forms of both intra- and inter-personal experience, and figures importantly in the goals of the Japanese therapies he describes. He notes that the attribution of "not being sunao" carries equally well understood negative implications. The Chinese ideal of hsiu-yang described by Wu represents the ability to maintain both emotional equanimity and interpersonal harmony; and the absence of these traits is associated with disruptive behavior and greater vulnerability to stress. As a last example, the Goods mention the Iranian belief that the "ideal person is one who keeps a pure and calm interior self ... negotiating outward relationships in such a way as to protect the inner self ... " Their paper shows that the cultural meanings of "fright illness" are constructed in part as a departure from this ideal behavioral image.

Other cross-cultural studies of folk knowledge of mental disorder have noted that social criteria, particularly behaviors regarded as disruptive or dangerous, are among the most salient in folk definitions of mental disorder (see, e.g., Westermeyer and Wintrob 1979). These findings are consistent with the arguments of labeling theorists who argue that the ascription of mental disorder functions largely to categorize disruptive behavior as deviant and thus invoke sanctions aimed at controlling or regulating that behavior. The papers included here suggest that this argument is a special case of the more general phenomenon in which cultural knowledge of mental disorder is structured in part by conceptual oppositions which represent both positive and negative behavioral ideals, and which may be embodied in contrastive prototypical identities.

Investigation of the culturally constructed social identities associated with mental disorder, as well as with positive social ideals, will contribute to our understanding of the social meanings and functions of images of "craziness". The attribution of mental disorder creates social realities which have a wide range of consequences for the person and the community. Important among these consequences are both the control of disruptive behavior regarded as deviant, as well as influences upon the actual course and outcome of illness episodes. Ethnographic data about the cultural meanings associated with common sense knowledge of mental disorder may provide a more informed basis with which to identify the social functions of illness attributions, and integrate them into a broader culture-based theory of illness and social action. It is only by examining the ways in which cultural knowledge of mental disorder is constituted within wider systems of meaning that it will be possible to discover cultural variables which influence the outcome of treatments (Waxler 1979), or which function to sanction undesirable social behavior. The papers in this volume suggest that a good place to begin to search for cultural variables which make a difference in this regard is with cultural conceptions of the person which include understandings about "mind", "body" and "environment", "emotions", "causality" and "responsibility", and "social images".

THEORY AND THERAPY

Much of the previous section has been devoted to articulating the point that illness experience is constituted by conceptual models of the person, including interrelated understandings about physiology, subjective experience, social relations and the macrocosmos. We have emphasized that cultural models are important as a means of interpreting illness which gives mental disorder personal and social significance. However, these same conceptual models also structure the *healing* process which is based on the interpretation of illness as a meaningful event which can be responded to in appropriate and effective ways, and which organizes interactions with others. Most of what has been written about interpretive models in the construction of illness applies directly to the construction of the healing process as well. In fact, cultural conceptions of illness and of healing are so closely integrated that they could hardly be studied independently. The formulation of meaningful explanations derives partly from knowledge about available treatments (Young, 1976; Blum, 1978); and the selection of treatments is implicated by causal reasoning used to interpret illness. Thus ethnographic research on conceptions of illness is illuminated by the investigation of healing forms; and understanding the therapeutic process requires research on the interpretation of illness (see White, this volume).

This interpretive view of healing implies that it is impossible to gain a full understanding of therapeutic processes through "biomedical or psychiatric reductionism" (Kleinman 1980:364; Marsella, this volume). There is a strong tradition of cultural research which has pointed to the role of symbolic and social factors which produce psychodynamic and especially cathartic effects in the client (e.g., Frank 1961; Prince 1976; Lebra 1976). Yet, we still understand little about how such symbolic and social factors are constituted within cultural systems of understanding about persons and behavior; and have made little progress in formulating a framework for comparative research capable of identifying universal and culture specific features of clinical activities. The papers in the present volume, particularly those in Section III, are aimed at penetrating the symbolic complexes which link treatment forms with cultural premises about personhood and social interaction. These studies demonstrate that such symbolic linkages systematically influence not only the nature of clinical encounters, but the whole process of illness as a personal and social experience, including (a) how appropriate treatments are conceptualized, (b) selection among treatments, (c) communication and interaction among patient and healer, and (d) the course and outcome of treatment. These topics are taken up briefly below.

Folk theories of mental disorder include postulates about appropriate paths for corrective action aimed at re-establishing positive or desirable patterns of experience and behavior. The symbolic links between interpretation of illness and plausible treatments constitute a range of meaningful responses to illness events which represent the temporal sequencing of cause and cure. This temporal sequencing gives folk theories of mental disorder their episodic structure which appears to be a universal format for the cognitive organization of folk theories of illness. The processual structure of folk theories provides a framework for their representation across cultures (Fabrega 1974; Kleinman 1974; Young 1976). Recent research in cognitive psychology suggests that a great deal of common sense knowledge is organized in episodic or "script"-like structures (Schank and Abelson 1977). As mentioned earlier, most of the ethnographic papers here (particulary those in Part III) use the case format for presenting illness episodes. Both Marsella and White discuss this processual structure in more general terms. Clement notes that Samoan "curing rituals and routines" constitute an important representational format for folk knowledge which is not included in her analysis. In this volume, the most explicit account of the episodic organization of a therapeutic interchange is W. Lebra's description of Okinawan shamanic therapy in terms of a routinized sequence of stages moving from diagnosis to prescribed remedy.

One of the major areas of clinical relevance of folk theories of mental disorder is their influence upon health-care decisions and the selection among alternative forms of treatment. (See Chrisman (1977) for a formulation of the place of explanatory models in the broader context of health-seeking behavior; and see Tversky and Kahneman (1981) for discussion of the influence of implicit "frames" on decision.) Ethnographic accounts of cultural modes of interpreting and explaining disorder can provide much-needed insight into socio-demographic variations in the utilization of health care services. Recent studies suggest that it is possible to develop cognitive models based on a limited number of cultural assumptions which "predict" health-care decisions quite well (Young 1979). However, the relation of explanatory constructs and actual health-seeking behavior may be quite loose and indeterminate. For example, Clement notes that when a new mental health program was introduced in Samoa, "folk knowledge was being used in the construction of expectations about the program, but it was not being used as sufficient information upon which to decide whether to use or continue using the program" (and see Kunstadter 1975).

As much of the discussion in this paper has indicated, the papers in this volume show that cultural reasoning about mental disorder creates a meaning-based rationale which exerts pervasive (if general) influences on the perception of appropriate remedies. For example, the contrastive explanatory modes characterized here as "psycho-somatic" and "somato-psychic" are rooted in different assumptions about the direction of causality linking physical and affective complaints, which in turn entail quite different approaches to treatment. Obeysekere notes that in Auyrvedic medicine, where "there is a systematic attempt to connect the cure to the theory of illness", the herbal prescriptions frequently used to treat emotional disturbance can be seen as entailments of the well-developed somatic and humoral theory of illness. And a number of the papers (especially Clement, Connor, Lebra, and Lebra) show that where there is an ideology of supernatural causes of illness, there are likely to be ritualized means for enlisting spiritual assistance in the process of diagnosis and treatment, usually involving specialized intermediary roles such as spirit mediums.

The accounts given in this book show that much of the cultural logic which interconnects indigenous notions of causality with appropriate forms of treatment is embedded in a framework of ethnopsychological understandings about the person and social behavior. This point is most clear in the contrast of Western conceptions of person and therapy described by Gaines and several of the non-Western cultures described here. As Gaines indicates, the use of "talk therapy" aimed at altering individual behavior though the individual's "insight" into his or her own personality is firmly rooted in a conception of the person as a distinct and independent individual, capable of self-transformation in relative isolation from particular social contexts. In contrast, Lock describes the Japanese notion of the "inner" self which is not easily verbalized and of personality which is largely unalterable. Consequently, the Japanese have little regard for "talk therapy" as a vehicle of therapeutic change. Where Japanese therapies do involve systematic individual self-reflection or introspection, as in *Naikan* Therapy described by Murase, it is with the goal of achieving a greater sense of empathy, identification and union with significant others, rather than a state of autonomy and independence as in the Western ego ideal.

The cultural logic of illness and therapy provides a symbolic basis for communication and interaction between patient and healer, and self and other generally, which probably has a substantial influence on the course and outcome of illness events (see Waxler 1979). Psychotherapy researchers have long suggested that the effectiveness of therapeutic intervention is strongly influenced by the relationship between therapist and client (Frank 1961; Prince 1976). Kleinman et al. (1978) describe a number of cases showing that, "a patient's explanatory model and view of clinical reality can be quite discordant with the professional model, producing misunderstanding and problems of clinical management" (254). For example, uncertainties about whether a clinician is acting as a "therapist" or a "diagnostician" may lead to conflict and miscommunication during the interaction which takes place during a mental status examination (Caughey 1978).

Research in social psychology has attempted to identify what facets of the practitioner-client relationship in psychotherapy contribute to improved outcome. Although some work in this area has investigated *what* constructs may be relevant to a client's view of therapy (e.g., Carr 1980; Higginbotham 1979), researchers have mostly used standardized rating data and focused on pre-defined experimental variables such as "cognitive complexity" which are susceptible to quantification but generally devoid of cultural content (Witkin et al. 1968). The papers in this volume indicate that cultural "content" in the form of knowledge of disorder based on fundamental conceptions of personhood provides the framework for much of what is understood and communicated in the course of therapeutic discourse. Connor gives a number of cases which illustrate her claim that, " . . . a crucial component of therapeutic processes is communication about the key symbols which operate in the conceptualization of the 'person'."

Therapeutic reality is constructed out of the interaction of patient and healer (and others) who "collaborate" to produce a plausible (meaningful) view of the causes of disorder and to determine appropriate courses of action. The success of the enterprise hinges largely on the ability of the interactants to synchronize and coordinate their conversational and nonverbal exchange. Such exchange requires a certain degree of sharing of linguistic and cultural knowledge by which interpretations are "negotiated" through questioning, answering and nonverbal interaction. For example, Wu mentions the importance of indirect and nonverbal expressions of emotion in Chinese social interaction where open or strong verbal displays of emotion are contrary to cultural ideals of harmony and equanimity. Furthermore, a Chinese patient's view of a clinical encounter may entail the belief that a competent doctor can make a diagnosis without extensive verbal interrogation.

Analysis of conversational exchanges in modern clinical settings shows that therapeutic interaction may take on stylized forms which go quite unrecognized (Labov and Fanshel 1977) William Lebra's description of Okinawan shamanistic therapy is perhaps the most detailed illustration in this book of the negotiation of interpretations of illness through ritualized conversational exchanges between shaman and client, whom Lebra regards as "jointly constructing a scenario". He shows that a successful shaman is a skilled performer who draws upon his own knowledge of local culture and social structure to make informed inferences about the causes of problems in order to construct diagnostic interpretations which will be accepted by his clients as likely causes of their distress. For example, he notes that because about 80% of the presenting complaints involve health problems, some clients who seek out a shaman for a "spiritual checkup" find themselves with previously unrecognized health disorders. A successful shamanic performance requires the collaboration of the client who must respond according to the conventions of the therapeutic context. To illustrate this, Lebra gives a number of examples of performative "misfires" in which the client does not cooperate in confirming the shaman's interpretation, and no diagnostic or therapeutic resolution is achieved.

Several of the papers discuss briefly the question of the effectiveness and validity of indigenous therapies. These topics pose important questions which can be addressed in future research aimed at evaluating the effects of differing modes of therapeutic intervention. There are, however, major unsolved methodological problems with any such research endeavor, and none of the papers in this volume attempts to evaluate the effectiveness of traditional healing. However, these papers do describe in some detail the symbolic bases by which illness is given meaning and placed in a culturally defined social context. In most cases, this process exerts persuasive influences aimed at transforming the person and illness to a more desired, positive state. William Lebra describes this process as the "emic validity" of Okinawan shamanic therapy which, as he states, is "cheap and accessible", provides a "congenial social setting", involves genuine emotional "catharsis" and renders prescriptions for actions with "hope for a positive outcome". Similar conclusions are drawn by Clement for traditional healing in Samoa (which is "sensitive to underlying and culturally unarticulated stressors in the client's environment"), and by Connor for Balinese healing (in which positive outcomes are linked with the abilities of patients and families to "understand the fundamentals of traditional therapies, and comprehend the significance of the major symbols invoked in the healing ritual"). Takie Lebra observes that for a therapy to be effective, its "repertoire of messages ... must be embedded in the culture of its client", and that by intensifying and amplifying familiar cultural themes it may be able to produce cathartic effects which give it "therapeutic leverage". She notes that both the religious Gedatsu therapy as well as the more secular Morita and *Naikan* therapies achieve their effect by tapping cultural themes in this way. Lock is somewhat less sanguine about the effectiveness of traditional healing involving the somato-psychic treatments which she describes as reductionistic such that, "if not administered in conjunction with appropriate social services" will not be likely to fulfill their potential. Although these descriptions of traditional healing and indigenous therapies do not come to a consensus about the effectiveness of traditional healing as a form of treatment for mental disorders, they do provide abundant evidence of the power of cultural symbols in establishing a basis for communication and interaction which can give the experience of mental disorder social meaning.

In pointing to the importance of shared, overlapping or complementary models of illness and therapy held by patient and healer, these papers raise questions about the effectiveness of Western psychotherapy among populations other than middle-class Caucasians (see Pedersen, this volume). There are a number of studies which have shown that it is, in fact, primarily White, middle-class and educated patients who are most often judged "suitable" for psycho-therapy ("talk therapy"), due largely to the greater perceived "psychological mindedness" of this population (Meltzer 1978). These findings are entirely consistent with the view of Western psychotherapy as an ethno-therapy which is a product of specific cultural traditions, and is best suited to communication and therapeutic interaction among individuals within those cultural backgrounds (Pande 1968). Connor, in her paper, questions the degree to which modern psychiatry can effectively treat disturbed individuals in Bali, given the gaps in cultural assumptions required for effective communication between therapist and client. In the absence of attempts to carry out research aimed at examining the differential effects of diverse therapies, answers to these questions may remain confined to folk intuitions about "what causes what" and "what leads to what" in the course of illness events. The studies which follow go a long way toward identifying the sorts of ethnographic models which will be required to discover and represent the cultural meanings and symbols which make a difference in the therapeutic process.

CONCLUSION

This paper has reviewed a number of issues which cross-cut the papers which follow. The intent has not been to derive conclusive statements about cultural conceptions of mental disorder, but rather to highlight recurring themes in these papers which point to areas of convergence in the ways mental disorders are interpreted cross-culturally. Perhaps the most prominent theme which emerges from these papers is the close integration of cultural conceptions of personhood with folk knowledge of mental disorder (or illness generally). These papers show that ethnomedical studies of illness events and ethnopsychological studies of person concepts have a strong mutual relevance — that a focus on folk theories of abnormal or disruptive behavior provides rich ethnographic data which may delineate the nature of cultural assumptions about persons and social action expressed in natural discourse; and that much of the "logic" of cultural reasoning about mental disorder can be represented in terms of premises about causality and social behavior.

In dealing primarily with cultural *knowledge* (or folk "theories") of mental disorder, this volume is examining one aspect of the broader concern with understanding the role of culture in the manifestation of illness and behavioral disturbance across cultures, as has been more common in previous compendia on culture and mental health. These papers are essentially cultural and symbolic in orientation. That is to say, they deal most thoroughly and extensively with the structure and manipulation of cultural constructs, and only by implication with the relation of these cultural variables to, say, the biological bases of mental disorder or the impact of social-institutional arrangements on illness events (although the papers by Fabrega and Marsella do locate the study of cultural conceptions of disorder within this wider sphere). This focus is not meant to imply that these latter variables are in any way secondary to the role of cultural knowledge in understanding, explaining or treating mental disorder. Rather, it serves to underscore the extensive role of cultural *interpretations* in mental disorder as a social and behavioral process; to point to their significance as an essential ingredient in healing; and to highlight the semantic quandries which can easily flaw cross-cultural psychiatric or ethnographic research attempting to represent indigenous meanings and folk theories. This paper has outlined some of the points at which these interpretive aspects of cultural knowledge impact upon mental health research and practice; has reviewed some of the methodological issues which challenge those who attempt to represent others' representations of mental disorder; and has pointed to a number of recurrent conceptual themes in folk knowledge across cultures which provide a perspective with which to better understand some of the cultural constraints on scientific and clinical practices aimed at understanding and treating disorder.

NOTES

1. Despite its ethnocentric connotations, the term "mental disorder" is used throughout this chapter as a convenient device for those forms of illness and behavior which are regarded cross-culturally as abnormal or disruptive and which usually require corrective action.
2. Although Gaines' distinction of varieties of 'Western' cultural traditions is much to the point and will hopefully give rise to a refinement of terminology now in use, the label "Western" is used in this chapter for reasons of brevity and convenience. However, where the label "Western" appears it would be more accurate to give it the reading "Protestant European". Further qualification and clarification of such global references is much needed.

REFERENCES

Agar, M.
1980 Hermeneutics in Anthropology: A Review Essay. Ethos 8:253–272.

Boucher, J., A. Ginorio, and M. Brandt
n.d. Emotion Lexicons of Eight Cultures. Unpublished manuscript. Culture Learning Institute. East-West Center. Honolulu, Hawaii.

Beiser, M., et al.
1976 Measuring Psychoneurotic Behavior in Cross-Cultural Surveys. The Journal of Nervous and Mental Disease 163:10–23.

Blum, J. D.
1978 On Changes in Psychiatric Diagnosis Over Time. American Psychologist 33:1017–1031.

Broverman, I. K. et al.
1970 Sex-role Stereotypes and Clinical Judgments of Mental Health. Journal of Clinical and Consulting Psychology 34:1–7.

Carr, J. E.
1980 Personal Construct Theory and Psychotherapy Research. In Personal Construct Psychology: Psychotherapy and Personality. A. W. Landfield and L. Leitner (eds.). New York: Wiley.

Caudill, W. and T. Lin, eds.
1969 Mental Health Research in Asia and the Pacific. Honolulu: University Press of Hawaii.

Caughey, J.
1978 Identity Struggles in the Mental Status Examination. Paper presented at the 77th Annual Meeting of the American Anthropological Association. Los Angeles, CA.

Chapman, L. and J. Chapman
1967 Genesis of Popular but Erroneous Psychodiagnostic Observations. Journal of Abnormal Psychology 72:193–204.

Chrisman, N. J.
1977 The Health Seeking Process: An Approach to the Natural History of Illness. Culture, Medicine and Psychiatry 1:351–377.

Conklin, H. C.
1972 Folk Classification. New Haven: Yale University Department of Anthropology.

Cooper, J. E., R. E. Kendall, and B. J. Gurland
1972 Psychiatric Diagnoses in New York and London: A Comparative Study of Mental Hospital Admissions. Maudsley Monograph No. 20. London: Oxford University Press.

Crapanzano, V.
1981 Text, Transference and Indexicality. Ethos 9:122–148.

D'Andrade, R. G.
1974 Memory and the Assessment of Behavior. In Measurement in the Social Sciences. T. Blalock (ed.). Chicago: Aldine-Atherton.
1976 A Propositional Analysis of U.S. American Beliefs About Disease. In Meaning in Anthropology. K. Basso and H. Selby (eds.). Albuquerque: University of New Mexico Press.
1981 The Cultural Part of Cognition. Cognitive Science 5:179–195.

Derogatis, L., et al.
1971 Neurotic Symptom Dimensions as Perceived by Psychiatrists and Patients of Various Social Classes. Archives of General Psychiatry 24:454–464.

Dohrenwend, B. P., and B. S. Dohrenwend
1969 Social Status and Psychological Disorder: A Causal Inquiry. New York: Wiley-Interscience.

Ekman, P.
    1973 Cross-Cultural Studies of Facial Expression. *In* Darwin and Facial Expression. P. Ekman (ed.). New York: Academic Press.
Elstein, A. S.
    1976 Clinical Judgment: Psychological Research and Medical Practice. Science 194: 696–700.
Fabrega, H.
    1974 Disease and Social Behavior. Cambridge: MIT Press.
Frake C. O.
    1969 The Ethnographic Study of Cognitive Systems. *In* Cognitive Anthropology. S. Tyler (ed.). New York: Holt, Rinehart and Winston, Inc. (originally published 1962)
    1980 Interpretations of Illness: An Ethnographic Perspective on Events and their Causes. *In* Language and Cultural Description. C. O. Frake, (ed.). Stanford: Stanford University Press.
Frank, J.
    1961 Persuasion and Healing. Baltimore: Johns Hopkins Press.
Geertz, C.
    1973 The Interpretation of Cultures. New York: Basic Books, Inc.
    1976 "From the Native's Point of View": On the Nature of Anthropological Understanding. *In* Meaning in Anthropology. K. Basso and H. Selby (eds.). Albuquerque: University of New Mexico.
Goldberg, L. R.
    1968 Simple Models or Simple Processes? Some Research on Clinical Judgments. American Psychologist 23:483–495.
Goodenough, W.
    1971 Culture, Language and Society. Addison-Wesley Modular Publication. Reading, MA: Addison Wesley.
Hallowell, A. I.
    1955 Culture and Experience. Philadelphia: University of Pennsylvania Press.
Harman, G. H.
    1971 Three Levels of Meaning. *In* Semantics: An Interdisciplinary Reader in Philosophy, Linguistics and Psychology. D. Steinberg and L. Jakobovits (eds.). pp. 66–75. Cambridge: Cambridge University Press.
Higginbotham, H. N.
    1979 Culture and Mental Health Services. *In* Perspectives on Cross-Cultural Psychology. A. Marsella *et al.* (eds.). New York: Academic Press.
Jones, E. E., et al.
    1972 Attribution: Perceiving the Causes of Behavior. Morristown, NJ: General Learning Press.
Katz, M., J. Cole, and H. Lowery
    1969 Studies of the Diagnostic Process: The Influence of Symptom Perception, Past Experience, and Ethnic Background on Diagnostic Decisions. American Journal of Psychiatry 125:109–119.
Keesing, R. M.
    1976 Cultural Anthropology: A Contemporary Perspective. New York: Holt, Rinehart and Winston.
Kennedy, J.
    1973 Cultural Psychiatry. *In* Handbook of Social and Cultural Anthropology. J. Honigmann (ed.), Chicago: Rand-McNally.
Kiev, A., ed.
    1964 Magic, Faith and Healing. New York: Free Press.

Kirk, L. and M. Burton
  1977 Meaning and Context: A Study of Contextual Shifts in Meaning of Maasai Personality Descriptors. American Ethnologist 4:734–761.
Kleinman, A.
  1974 The Use of "Explanatory Models" as a Conceptual Frame for Comparative Cross-Cultural Research on Illness Experiences and the basic Tasks of Clinical Care Amongst Chinese and Other Populations. In Medicine in Chinese Cultures. A. Kleinman et al. (eds.). Washington, D.C.: U.S. Government Printing Office.
  1977 Depression, Somatization and the "New Cross-Cultural Psychiatry". Social Science and Medicine 11:3–10.
  1980 Patients and Healers in the Context of Culture. Berkeley: University of California Press.
Kleinman, A., L. Eisenberg, and B. Good
  1978 Culture, Illness and Care: Clinical Lessons from Anthropologic and and Cross-Cultural Research. Annals of Internal Medicine 88:251–258.
Kunstadter, P.
  1975 Do Cultural Differences Make Any Difference? Choice Points in Medical Systems Available in Northwestern Thailand. In Medicine in Chinese Cultures. A. Kleinman et al. (eds.). Washington, D.C.: U.S. Government Printing Office.
Labov, W. and D. Fanshel
  1977 Therapeutic Discourse: Psychotherapy as Conversation. New York: Academic Press.
Lakoff, G. and M. Johnson
  1980 Metaphors We Live By. Chicago: University of Chicago Press.
Lazare, A.
  1973 Hidden Conceptual Models in Clinical Psychiatry. The New England Journal of Medicine 288:345–351.
Leary, T.
  1957 Interpersonal Diagnosis of Personality. New York: The Ronald Cress Co.
Lebra, W., ed.
  1976 Culture-Bound Syndromes, Ethnopsychiatry, and Alternate Therapies. Honolulu: University of Hawaii Press.
Lee, R. P.
  1980 Sex Roles, Social Status and Psychiatric Symptoms in Urban Hong Kong. In Normal and Abnormal in Chinese Culture. A. Kleinman and T. Lin (eds.). pp. 273–289. Dordrecht, Holland: D. Reidel Publishing Co.
Leff, J.
  1974 Transcultural Influences on Psychiatrists' Rating of Verbally Expressed Emotion. British Journal of Psychiatry 125:336–340.
  1977 The Cross-Cultural Study of Emotions. Culture, Medicine and Society 1:317–350.
Lutz, C.
  1980 Emotion Words and Emotional Development on Ifaluk Atoll. Unpublished Ph.D. Dissertation. Department of Anthropology, Harvard University.
Marsella, A. J.
  1978 Thoughts on Cross-Cultural Studies on the Epidemiology of Depression. Culture, Medicine and Psychiatry 2:343–357.
  1980 Depressive Experience and Disorder Across Cultures: A Review of the Liturature. In Handbook of Cross-Cultural Psychology. H. Triandis and J. Draguns (eds.). Boston: Allyn-Bacon.
Marsella, A. J., D. Kinzie, and P. Gordon
  1973 Ethnic Variations in the Expression of Depression. Journal of Cross-Cultural Psychology 4:435–458.

McLemore, C. W. and L. S. Benjamin
    1979 Whatever Happened to Interpersonal Diagnosis? A Psychosocial Alternative to DSM-III. American Psychologist 34:17–34.
Meltzer, J. D.
    1978 A Semiotic Approach to Suitability for Psychotherapy. Psychiatry 41:435–458.
Murphy, J.
    1976 Psychiatric Labeling in Cross-Cultural Perspective. Science 191:1091–1028.
Nathanson, C. C.
    1975 Illness and the Feminine Role: A Theoretical Review. Social Science and Medicine 9:57–62.
Neugebauer, R.
    1979 Medieval and Early Modern Theories of Mental Illness. Archives of General Psychiatry 36:477–483.
Nisbett, R. E. and L. D. Ross
    1979 Human Inference: Strategies and Shortcomings of Informal Judgement. Englewood Cliffs, NJ: Prentice-Hall.
Nunnally, J. C.
    1961 Popular Conceptions of Mental Health. New York: Holt, Rinehart and Winston, Inc.
Opler, M. K., ed.
    1959 Culture and Mental Health. New York: MacMillan.
Osgood, C. E., W. H. May and M. S. Miron
    1975 Cross-Cultural Universals in Affective Meaning. Urbana: University of Illinois Press.
Pande, S. K.
    1968 The Mystique of "Western" Psychotherapy: An Eastern Interpretation. Journal of Nervous and Mental Disease 146:425–432.
Pike, K. L.
    1954 Language in Relation to a Unified Theory of the Structure of Human Behavior, Part I. Glendale: Summer Institute of Linguistics.
Plog, S. C. and R. B. Edgerton, eds.
    1969 Changing Perspectives in Mental Illness. New York: Holt, Rinehart and Winston, Inc.
Prince, R.
    1976 Psychotherapy as the Manipulation of Endogenous Healing Mechanisms: A Transcultural Survey. Transcultural Psychiatric Research Review 13:155–133.
Quinn, N.
    1980 Notes for Workshop on Folk Theory. Unpublished Manuscript.
Rabinow, P. and W. Sullivan, eds.
    1979 Interpretive Social Science. Berkeley: University of California Press.
Ricoeur, P.
    1976 Interpretation Theory: Discourse and the Surplus of Meaning. Fort Worth: Texas Christian University Press.
Rorty, A.
    1976 A Literary Postscript: Characters, Persons, Selves and Individuals. In The Identities of Persons. A. Rorty, (ed.). Berkeley: University of California Press.
Rosenhan, D.
    1973 On Being Sane in Insane Places. Science 179:250–258.
Sarbin, T. R.
    1969 The Scientific Status of the Mental Illness Metaphor. In Changing Perspectives in Mental Illness. S. C. Plog and R. B. Edgerton (eds.). New York: Holt, Rinehart and Winston.

Schank, R. and R. Abelson
1977 Scripts, Plans, Goals and Understanding. Hillsdale, NJ: Lawrence Erlbaum Associates.

Scheff, T. J.
1966 Being Mentally Ill: A Sociological Theory. Chicago: Aldine.

Schutz, A.
1970 Reflections on the Problem of Relevance. R. M. Zaner (ed.). New Haven: Yale University Press.

Selby, H.
1974 Zapotec Deviance: The Convergence of Folk and Modern Sociology. Austin: University of Texas Press.

Shweder, R. A.
1977a Illusory Correlation and the M.M.P.I. Controversy. Journal of Consulting and Clinical Psychology 45:917–924.
1977b Likeness and Likelihood in Everyday Thought: Magical Thinking in Judgments About Personality. Current Anthropology 18:637–648.

Shweder, R. A. and R. D'Andrade
1980 The Systematic Distortion Hypothesis. In New Directions for Methodology of Behavioral Science: Fallible Judgment in Behavioral Research. R. Shweder (ed.). San Fransisco: Jossey-Bass.

Simon, B.
1978 Mind and Madness in Ancient Greece: The Classical Roots of Modern Psychiatry. Ithaca: Cornell University Press.

Simons, R. C.
1980 The Resolution of the Latah Paradox. Journal of Nervous and Mental Disease 168:195–206.

Singer, K.
1975 Depressive Disorders from a Transcultural Perspective. Social Science and Medicine 9:289–301.

Townsend, J. M.
1978 Cultural Conceptions and Mental Illness: A Comparison of Germany and America. Chicago: University of Chicago Press.
1979 Stereotypes and Mental Illness: A Comparison with Ethnic Stereotypes. Culture, Medicine and Psychiatry 3:205–230.

Tseng, W.
1975 The Nature of Somatic Complaints Among Psychiatric Patients: The Chinese Case. Comprehensive Psychiatry 16:237–245.

Turner, V.
1964 An Ndembu Doctor in Practice. In Magic, Faith and Healing. A. Kiev, (ed.). New York: Free Press.

Tversky, A. and D. Kahneman
1974 Judgment Under Uncertainty: Heuristics and Biases. Science 185:1124–1131.
1981 The Framing of Decisions and the Psychology of Choice. Science 211:453–458.

Waxler, N. E.
1974 Culture and Mental Illness: A Social Labeling Perspective. Journal of Nervous and Mental Disease 159:379–395.
1979 Is Outcome for Schizophrenia Better in Traditional Societies? The Case of Sri Lanka. Journal of Nervous and Mental Disease 167:144–158.

Westermeyer, J., ed.
1976 Anthropology and Mental Health. The Hague: Mouton.

Westermeyer, J. and R. Wintrob
1979 "Folk" Criteria for the Diagnosis of Mental Illness in Rural Laos: On Being Insane in Sane Places. The American Journal of Psychiatry 136:755–761.

White G. M.
  1978 Ambiguity and Ambivalence in A'ara Personality Descriptors. American Ethnologist 5:334–360.
  1980 Conceptual Universals in Interpersonal Language. American Anthropologist 82:759–781.
  1982 The Role of Cultural Explanations in "Psychologization" and "Somatization". *Social Science and Medicine* 16:1519–1530.
Wiggins, J.
  1980 Circumplex Models of Interpersonal Behavior. *In* Review of Personality and Social Psychology. Vol. 1. L. Wheeler (ed.). Beverly Hills: Sage.
Wing, J. K., J. E. Cooper, and N. Sartorius
  1974 Measurement and Classification of Psychiatric Symptoms. Cambridge: Cambridge University Press.
Witkin, H., H. Lewis, and E. Weil
  1968 Affective Reactions and Patient-Therapist Interactions Among More Differentiated and Less Differentiated Patients Early in Therapy. Journal of Nervous and Mental Disease 146:193–208.
World Health Organization (WHO)
  1973 Report of the International Pilot Study of Schizophrenia. Vol. 1. Geneva: World Health Organization.
Young, A.
  1976 Some Implications of Medical Beliefs and Practices for Social Anthropology. American Anthropologist. 78:5–24.
Young, J.
  1979 A Model of Illness Treatment Decisions in a Tarascan Town. American Ethnologist 7:106–131.
Zola, I. K.
  1966 Culture and Symptoms: An Analysis of Patients' Presenting Complaints. American Sociological Review 31:615–630.

HORACIO FABREGA JR.

2. CULTURE AND PSYCHIATRIC ILLNESS: BIOMEDICAL AND ETHNOMEDICAL ASPECTS

INTRODUCTION

In this paper I will look at psychiatric illness from a biomedical as well as from an ethnomedical perspective. Several themes will be emphasized throughout the discussion. In thinking about medical problems generally, and psychiatric ones specifically, I have found it useful to distinguish between purely physical (i.e., neurophysiologic, neurochemical) factors as opposed to symbolic factors, namely psychological and social factors consisting of behaviors, feelings, etc. of the person. I have employed the terms *disease* and *illness* to designate these two sets of factors respectively. I will posit that *psychiatric illness* is a psychosocial "entity" which is extended in time and space. This means (1) that the domain of personal experience (e.g., self definition, attitudes toward others, emotions, etc.) and that of social activity (e.g., role functioning, social relations) together form the substance of psychiatric illness and (2) that the illness duration in time and space is critically influenced by these social-psychological factors. Furhermore, I have assumed that an individual's theory of illness and of self, which impact on one another and are complementary, strongly influence how an underlying psychiatric disease condition expresses itself psychosocially or in psychiatric illness generally. This means that (1) an individual's representation or attributions about illness, illness causes, mental functioning, body functioning, symptoms, etc. together with (2) an individual's representation or attributions regarding personhood (e.g., volition, self-control, boundaries of the self, social responsibility, etc.) play a critical role in how the underlying psychiatric disease process is expressed in behavior, how it unfolds, how it is handled, how long it lasts, and indeed how it is shunted about in the social system. The person who is psychiatrically ill is thus held to behave and function in ways which reflect his or her theory of illness-self. Moreover, his or her readiness to seek and accept care of a certain type will be influenced by this theory. To the extent that significant others share the individual's representation and attributions regarding the "illness", to that extent harmony and support are generated and this promotes and/or sustains social and psychological functioning as the afflicted individual and significant others see it. Similarly, to the extent that the individual's representation or attributions of illness overlap with that of care providers, to that extent they will seek orthodox psychiatric care, comply with medical regimen and be influenced positively by medicines and procedures which such providers have available to them.

From a general anthropological point of view, a medical problem or illness may be defined as a disvalued change in the adaptation-functioning of an individual

39

A. J. Marsella and G. M. White (eds.), Cultural Conceptions of Mental Health and Therapy, 39–68.

which gives rise to a need for corrective action. The idea of illness, like the idea of person or self — to which it has an important relation — is very likely a universal in human societies. I like to think of illness as having a manifest appearance or form. In other words, the term "illness" seems to be used with reference to a concrete individual who is somehow changed from the way he was when he was not ill; moreover, he is changed in a certain or special way. Certainly there exist many types of disvalued changes which affect individuals which are not judged as "illness". Although one could argue that what a people will call illness will depend entirely on cultural conventions, empirically it appears to be the case that there may exist universal or generic indicators of illness. Bodily symptoms-changes and/or an impairment in the ability to carry out expected tasks are integral properties of illness. Some of the defining characteristics of this concept (e.g., medical problem, illness) which set it apart from related concepts (e.g., handicap) have been outlined previously (Fabrega 1972, 1975, 1979).

Culturally specific conventions are clearly operative in the way a people explain illness, orient to it socially and psychologically, and handle it concretely as a "problem". The part of a people's symbolic system in terms of which they explain and handle illness can be termed its theory of illness. A theory of illness, like the idea of illness itself, is probably universal in human societies. People differ in terms of how elaborately they go into the explanation of illness; that is, how probing is their account of a particular occurrence of illness. One obvious factor that influences how an illness is explained is the nature of the theory of illness which a people have developed. Characteristics of the theories of illness of different people have been described (Fabrega 1976). Another factor influencing how illness is explained involves the concrete properties of the illness itself. Trivial changes in the functioning of a person may hardly be gone into at all, whereas more profound changes are invariably viewed as threatening and dangerous and occasion significant inquiry. The basic issue is that an individual is now "medically" changed or ill in some determinate way and the symbolic task is to make sense of this change. One fundamental question that seems to be asked is: Why is this person now ill? One could call this the question of causation. Another question that seems to be asked is: How is this person ill? One could call this the question of mechanics. It is likely that these types of questions are interrelated and that both influence the kind of explanation that is arrived at as a course of action for dealing with the illness. That arriving at a "course of action" or treatment response *vis-à-vis* an occurrence of illness is exquisitely a social and cultural affair is well established in social science (Fabrega 1974; Parsons 1951; Young 1976).

There are now two basic approaches that one can adopt if one intends to study the medical problems of illnesses of various people of the world. One can attempt to understand how illness is construed and handled by the people themselves. This, of course, is quintessentially a social science task, most closely linked to the discipline of cultural anthropology. In fact, the generalizations I have presented above flow out of this approach to the study of illness. One could term this approach "ethnomedical". In this instance, one is handling a group or society as a distinct social unit or system and examining its view and approach to illness from a symbolic as well as from a social point of view. By "symbolic" I mean that one is attempting to arrive at the meanings behind the actions people take in anticipation, association and/or response to illness, including, of course, the person who is ill, his friends and kinfolk as well as helpers or practitioners. By "social" I mean that one is examining medically relevant actions from a social relationships point of view as well as from the standpoint of the way existing (more or less differentiated) social institutions operate. I believe that there is a close interrelation between the social and the symbolic. The aim of the ethnomedical scientist could be said to be to arrive at an understanding of how a group or society's system of medicine functions, to delineate different types of systems of medicine, and ultimately to derive theories which explain how different systems of medicine operate and change.

One can also undertake the comparative study of illness from what can be termed a biomedical approach. In this instance one is beginning a study with a fairly clear picture of what illness "is" for one is relying on Western biomedical scientific knowledge as the basis for defining and explaining illness. One who studies illness comparatively from a biomedical standpoint assumes that the biomedical sciences offer a coherent set of ideas, methods and principles for understanding medical problems. A dominating emphasis of a biomedical scientist involves the physical (i.e., chemical, anatomical, physiological, etc.) changes in the individual which can lead to or correlate with a condition of illness. Factors which can produce physical disorders in the individual's body, which in turn lead to overt illness, are a principal concern of the biomedical scientist. These factors are well known and include such diverse things as genes, diet, enzymes, physiologic systems, organs, microorganisms, climate-altitude and social stressors. Earlier I indicated that the concern of the ethnomedical scientist involves mainly the (overt and covert) social actions of a people that are prompted by illness considered as a concrete or possible social occurrence. In this light, it is useful to conceptualize the concern of the biomedical scientists as involving mainly the underlying physical substrates of illness, whether these be in the individual's own body, in his physical and social environment, or in his family or social history. In other words, it is the effects of these and related factors on the structure and functioning of the body viewed as a physical system which is crucial. It is disturbances in this physical system which lead to illness.

It should be clear by now that from an ethnomedical standpoint, a biomedical scientist is approaching the study of medical problems using his own biomedical theory of illness as guide. What one terms the biomedical sciences in other words are clusters of related theories which have evolved in Western literate societies to explain, account for, and deal with concrete illness problems. Put differently, to an ethnomedical scientist, the meanings of the symbols which a biomedical scientist uses to study illness relate to the person considered as physical structure or machine.

PSYCHIATRIC ILLNESS IN BIOMEDICAL THEORY

Illness has been defined as a disvalued state or condition of the whole individual and in a concrete sense is manifest in the sphere of behavioral adaptation. The cultural orientations of the person who is ill and of the group to which he or she belongs play a critical role in how illness will be enacted, interpreted, explained, responded to, dealt with and given meaning. An illness does not contain these latter parameters; rather its meaning is assigned via symbolic conventions. Among some people, for example, a distinction is made between illness of the self or "of the whole me" as opposed to illness of my leg or of my joint. These conceptualizations are handled differently. One must also keep in mind that a "part" of a person is both an anatomical fact and also a social or symbolic fact. Anatomically, all people have brains, livers, hearts, and nerves. In a social symbolic sense, however, Western people are distinguished by having minds, brains, and nerves. Features of their knowledge base lead them to make these distinctions. A person who is ill in our culture can state that his liver is bad, that his nerves are overactive, or that he has a brain tumor. In another culture, these complaints may not be possible since these concepts are not part of their knowledge of the body. Instead, other peoples when ill will report pain due to a coldness, or to an object which has "entered" the body; weakness will be explained by a supernatural "robbing" of the spirit. The explanation of the *cause* and mechanics of the symptom will influence behavior and actions of the person, and so, of course, will the symptom itself, viewed in a strict biophysiologic sense.

A key premise in biomedical theory is that illness manifestations result from disease changes in the body. All people, of course, have what one could term "disease-like" explanations of how and why illness occurs. Their concepts which resemble our notions of disease do not necessarily involve physical things, but can include life forces, energies, heat, etc. Another premise of our biomedical theory is that the domain of the body contrasts with that of the mind. Hence, we are able to speak of bodily and mental illness and bodily and mental health. From a general anthropologic point of view, one can say that if a person starts to act differently and to say strange things, (i.e., he seems to "lose" his individuality) and also begins to function poorly or erratically in a social sense, the question of illness may arise. Based on one's theory of illness, one could say that the illness is due to influence of the devil; he has an illness of his "mind" (i.e., the locus or essence of his will and volition is ill and disturbed) or, the physical part or organ which regulates and/or which accounts for his behavior, that is, his brain, is physically diseased. Each proposition flows from a different theory of illness. In biomedical theory, a psychiatric illness is currently explained as the outcome of distinctive kinds of disease processes which produce neurotransmitter changes in subcortical centers of the hemispheres of the brain and/or lead to asymmetries in hemispheric control mechanisms. Such changes are held to physically alter the regulation and control of behaviors subserving cognition, action, affect, and/or attention. However, as I shall suggest later, from a social and psychologic point of view, the behaviors of illness need to be seen as partly an outcome of distinctive cultural conventions.

Modern, Western-influenced societies and theories of illness allow the making of a basic distinction between mental illness and physical illness. One must appreciate the great value of this (cultural) distinction between the mental and the physical. The distinction has helped channel and focus medical research and has promoted the development of the biological sciences, general physiology, neurophysiology, and psychophysiology. It is, of course, no accident that mainly modern, Western societies have a highly structured medical practice system with disciplines such as psychiatry, medicine, and neurology, that is disciplines whose areas of focus follow our theory of personhood and illness. Cultural assumptions are obviously mirrored in social institutions. In other cultures, persons are not believed to possess minds as opposed to bodies, nor are their bodies held to have respiratory and genitourinary "systems". Humans are judged more wholistically, and practitioners have a more unified theory of "disease" and illness. Since there exists a wholistic conception of mankind, one does not find neurologists, psychiatrists, and internists, that is, disciplines reflecting a physical segmentation of the person.

It should be noted that in this and previous sections I have made a distinction between (1) our theory of illness as one cultural theory among many others of the world, all of which serve as a basis for explaining (and rationalizing the treatment of) illness; (2) our theory viewed as one (also of many) system of meanings which individuals of a society learn and internalize and which then comes to influence how they themselves behave and how they (and others of their group) explain their own behavior while ill; and (3) our theory of illness viewed as a scientific (i.e., "correct") interpretation of disease and illness. Each of these is a key epistemological distinction (science as a cultural system, as a system for explaining human action, and as a basis for explaining the way the world operates).

PSYCHIATRIC ILLNESS AND THE ETHNOMEDICAL APPROACH

To one who studies medicine from a comparative standpoint, the contemporary view that certain mental, behavioral, and emotional disturbances constitute a special type of illness is obviously arbitrary and conventional. A review of literature in anthropology discloses that in small-scale societies, body-centered ailments and disturbances in physiologic functions are invariably dealt with informally as medical problems or illness. When these conditions fail to improve, worsen, and/or reach crisis proportions, there is a shift in the level of concern and in the strategy of resort: the person is ill and significant co-members take

special formal actions which involve seeking practitioners. Very often, there is
a redefinition of the nature of the illness. Madness or bizarre behavior which
includes an inability to care for self is among the kinds of medical problems
dealt with formally in small scale societies. However, in the system of medicine
of Western societies, a number of additional behavior problems (i.e., besides
madness, insanity) are classified as (psychiatric) illness and distinctive attitudes
and social responses are linked to this. Specific social, historical and cultural
factors have led to the evolution of this Western contemporary view of psychiatric illness as a distinctive type of illness.

From a strict logical point of view, because the idea of a psychiatric illness
is quintessentially a Western idea, one is being ethnocentric when inquiring how
such conditions are dealt with in other societies where the idea is not used and,
hence, where some persons showing "mental and emotional disturbances" may
not be defined as ill and if they are, may not necessarily be handled in a different
way from other ill persons as is the case in Western societies. (To avoid awkward-
ness, I will often use quotation marks and speak of "psychiatric illness" when
referring to how other peoples handle analagous conditions.) As is well known,
disturbances in social and psychological behavior analagous to those which today
we term hysteria, depression, schizophrenia and dementia, were present in earlier
epochs of Western history and some could be universal in human societies
(Ackerknecht 1959; Veith 1965; Klibansky et al. 1964; Wing 1978 and Torrey
1979). However, whether these disturbances of behavior are necessarily handled
as illness in small-scale societies has been controversial and the idea of a psychiatric illness itself has had its ups and downs in Western European history.

An explanation of why and how the idea of a psychiatric illness developed
in Western European societies is a complex undertaking. Such an explanation
would emphasize a variety of topics such as (1) the development of the idea
of an inner entity or force "behind" human action, termed mind, psyche, etc.
as opposed to the body; (2) the emphasis of the Greeks (especially Plato) on the
rational and irrational, and the equating of the latter with "disease"; (3) the
Hippocratic emphasis on natural causes of disease, and in general, the heavy
somatic emphasis of Graeco-Roman medicine (i.e., that so-called mental illnesses
or symptoms were caused by physical disorders) and (4) the creation of administrative structures that empowered individuals to represent others who were
(mentally) disabled in a court of law. Factors such as these seem to at least
partially explain the observations of Neugebauer regarding how the insane
person was dealt with in Medieval times (Neugebauer 1978, 1979). His observations, based on historical documents of the times, paint a picture of a society
endorsing the idea that diseases accounted for the disabilities of the insane or
lunatic (i.e., underlying "naturalistic" or organic factors).

Contemporary approaches to psychiatric illness are an outcome of important
social consequences that the idea of psychiatric illness had in Western societies.
Among these the following can be singled out (1) the social stigma attached
to madness and insanity; (2) the handling of the mentally ill as a separate class,

needing formal protection or hospitalization; (3) the various reforms in the kinds of treatment given the hospitalized insane, culminating in humane and medical treatment; (4) the slow evolution of separate medical disciplines dealing with mental-brain disorders, eventually the creation of neurology and psychiatry; (5) the development of psychoanalysis and the increased emphasis given to the unconscious and irrational and (6) the growth in the understanding-explanation of human social behavior leading to a blurring of the line between normal-healthy vs. abnormal-ill.

A number of tenets drawn from the contemporary structure of psychiatric theory and practice could be examined in a comparative medical frame of reference. Only a few will be mentioned here. A first one is the equating of a set of *highly* disordered social (and psychological) behavior changes (e.g., psychosis, madness, insanity) with the idea of illness or disease as has been the case in Western societies. A key question is how such conditions are handled in small scale societies. A second tenet from biomedicine that one could examine cross-culturally involves the cultural meaning or identity of "madness" (or insanity, psychosis). Thus, in the event these conditions are handled as illness, are they handled as a separate and distinct category of illness having a different meaning when compared to other illnesses in the native system of medicine? A third tenet involves how "psychiatric illnesses" are handled and specifically whether ("psychiatrically ill") individuals to whom the label of illness is applied, are stigmatized. Another tenet involves the question of the way other "psychiatric illness" (i.e., other than madness-insanity) are viewed and handled. I am referring to "illnesses" such as the neuroses, anorexia nervosa, the personality disturbances and the substance abuse problems (e.g., alcoholism). Generally speaking, there is very little literature on the comparative medicine of small-scale societies that deals with these types of "psychiatric illness". It is possible that some of these "psychiatric illnesses" could be limited to modern complex societies or conversely, that only in the modern biomedical system of medicine are they identified as illness. A related topic is that of culture bound syndromes; disorders labeled as illness that appear to be peculiar or unique to specific societies or regions of the world, and that appear not to be prevalent in Western modern nations. Finally, one could raise the question of the nature of the manifestations of insanity and of other "psychiatric illnesses" which might set them apart from other illnesses and "normal" behavior in a society's system of medicine, and whether these manifestations are universal or merely culturally specific. The two latter tenets are controversial and raise the question of culture and brain behavior relations. Before turning to them, I would like to discuss briefly the other tenets, since this will provide a background for the substance of the chapter.

The terms madness and insanity are social in character and carry negative symbolic associations in Western societies. The term "psychiatric illness" is biomedical and grows out of the history of Western medicine. Obviously, there is overlap in reference between these two terms and symbolic connotations of the one attach to the other. I will use the term madness and insanity purely to refer to a subset of (serious, major, more pronounced, etc.) types of psychiatric illness and not in the valuational sense.

The literature in comparative medicine provides evidence that mad and/or insane persons are frequently judged as ill in small-scale societies (Murphy 1976; Westermeyer and Wintrob 1979; Edgerton 1966, 1969, 1980; Fabrega 1970, Leighton et al. 1963). However, there is also evidence that in some societies, seriously ill persons are abandoned and most likely this would apply in some instances to those classified as insane or mad and those who are retarded and unable to care for themselves (Woodburn 1979; Holmberg 1950). Moreover, in small-scale societies, not all persons who would qualify as mad or insane by biomedical criteria are necessarily seen as ill (Fabrega 1970, Leighton et al. 1963). One key factor appears to be the relative ability of the person to care for him or herself; that is, whether social functioning is preserved. Another is the form or content which the madness or insanity has in the society and, inseparable from this, how the behavior of "madness and insanity" is labeled and judged. To the extent that mad or insane persons have social support, can be controlled, are not threatening and their behavior conforms to models or stereotypes of illness, to that extent medical labels are likely to be applied.

A long standing question in anthropology has been the putative mental health of shamans, there being indications that many of these would be judged as mad or insane on Western criteria yet function adaptively in the society (Fabrega 1974). The existence of individuals "normal" on native criteria and "abnormal" on Western criteria, has most pointedly raised the question of cultural conventions regarding the nature of illness. This question is much less controversial now. Most recently, the work of Murphy and Westermeyer and Wintrob has indicated that mad or insane persons, showing highly disordered social and psychological behaviors, are regarded as ill in native rural communities of Alaska and Laos (Murphy 1976; Westermeyer 1979). The work of Edgerton in Africa clearly supports these observations and provides additional details about native criteria of madness (Edgerton 1966, 1969, 1980). A large number of works in anthropology and related disciplines support these generalizations and, hence, one is led to entertain the notion that a significant portion of persons who are unable to care for themselves and who show very disordered social-psychological behaviors are consistently classified as ill by peoples of the world. This generalization underscores the social character of illness and the fact that human need and caring are integral to it. However, it is important to re-emphasize that many instances of madness or insanity are not handled as illness. Moreover, in the event that the idea of illness is invoked, responses to many "mad" persons are highly socialized and politicized. It is not always clear why persons showing socially disordered behaviors are labelled as "ill" as opposed to other social categories available to the people. To explain this, the behavior and status of the person and his family in the group needs to be taken into account as well as the social circumstances surrounding the labeling of illness. As social critics have clearly pointed out, a similar medical vs. social-political equivocation in the handling of disordered social behaviors has been characteristic in Western European history (Szasz 1961). Additional factors related to this generalization are discussed later in the section dealing with the major psychiatric disorders.

The idea that insane or mad persons who are labeled ill on native criteria are also judged to have a special type of illness in the native system of medicine (as is the case in the Western system), is difficult to answer. That the manifestations and social implications of these "illnesses" differ from those of others is obviously recognized and handled accordingly (see below). In this sense, distinguishing featues of these illnesses are recognized. One aspect of the question of whether psychiatrically-ill persons are judged to be ill in a categorically different way would seem to involve the cause which is invoked to explain these illnesses.

In Graeco-Roman medicine there was no significant theoretical separation of mental-psychiatric illnesses (i.e., insanity) from other medical illnesses (Ackerknecht 1959; Simon, 1978). Thus, the ethnophysiologic ideas used to explain common medical illnesses generally prevailed in cases of insanity and other "psychiatric illnesses". Conversely, even during Renaissance times, at the height of the tendency to equate insanity with witchcraft and demonological notions, these latter explanations were also entertained for other illnesses, physical handicaps and human aberrations more generally (Neugebauer 1978, 1979; Kroll 1973, Thomas 1973, Webster 1975). Throughout most of European history, explanations of the causes of illness have ranged over a number of categories variously classified as humoral, chemical, natural, supernatural, etc. and these have been posited for all varieties of illness. This generalization appears to hold up for certain literate civilizations, such as Hindu and Chinese (Obeyesekere 1977; Tseng 1973). The literature involving small-scale societies clearly supports this generalization involving the native causes of "psychiatric illness" or of insanity-madness. There does not appear to be a difference in the way insanity as opposed to other "medical" illnesses are accounted for causally in the theories of illness which have been described among egalitarian and ranked societies.

The singling out of insanity as a special category of illness would appear to be based on the idea of mechanism; that is, how these types of illnesses are produced. Since the content or appearance of this category of illness is quite different from other illnesses, indeed basic elements of sociality are compromised and explained through it (see below), it is understandable that an account of how the illness is produced tends to draw on special ideas (when compared to how other illness manifestations are explained). In Western history, explanations of insanity have been linked to explanations of the bases of rationality, culminating in understanding of the functions of the central nervous system. The literature in comparative medicine contains numerous references to the effect that insanity is due to physical disorders of the brain, but it is difficult to determine the sources of this idea or the meanings which it has had. It is frequently the case that madness, insanity or other types of "psychiatric illnesses" are linked to ideas of possession, and it is possible that this latter idea operates as an explanation of both cause and mechanism in some non-Western and non-literate societies. It would appear that insanity can be judged more or less as a separate category of illness (based on notions of mechanism) in other literate systems of medicine. In fact, the explanations about the nature of "mental illness" held in Ayurvedic and Chinese medicine clearly invoke ideas about the nature of man, human action and consciousness; and especially how disorders of the body can disturb basic human faculties (e.g., competence, cognitions, etc.) (Obeyesekere 1977; Tseng 1973). One can conclude, tentatively, that "insanity" is not set apart on the basis of causation, but that what sets it apart is explanations invoking how these illnesses are produced. At issue is the task of socially rationalizing disordered social behavior and frequently this will require the using of special ideas about human rationality. Ideas about the mechanisms of illness (medical and psychiatric) seem to be more elaborate in literate traditions of medicine, but this may be an artifact of the focus of ethnographers.

Although insanity and madness are, generally speaking, not singled out causally in other societies, but in terms of how their manifestations are produced (i.e., ethnopsychophysiologic notions), it is very clear that they are dealt with differently from other "medical" illnesses when one compares the way systems of medicine operate. These differences, however, are trivial in that they are obvious consequences of the special manifestations of these illnesses. A hallmark of illness is that corrective action is deemed relevant and individuals are offered various kinds of treatment. The nature of the manifestations of illness, the energy and well-being of the person, and indeed his cooperation and expressed need for treatment are obvious factors influencing when treatment is instituted and the conditions under which this takes place. The "psychiatric illnesses" we have been designating as insanity-madness consist of manifestations that are different from other illnesses in that social behaviors of a highly disordered and disruptive kind (and also threatening) are prominent. A dominating if not criterial feature is that these individuals are unable to care for themselves. All of these factors compel others to intervene in treatment and that the individual who is labelled as ill often be coerced into treatment and indeed physically restrained if necessary. This could be said to stand as a generalization about this category of illness. Moreover, given that this type of illness can be persistent if not permanent, the social group is forced to care for these individuals on a long-term basis and does so in a variety of ways — ranging from informal support, offering of meals, shelter, and protection, to confinement in homes or hospitals.

The question of how "psychiatric illnesses" other than madness-insanity (e.g., neurosis, somatoform disorders) are viewed and handled in small-scale societies is very complex and difficult to discuss. Little in the way of empirical information is available regarding the prevalence and mode of handling of many types of behavior changes singled out as psychiatric illness in biomedicine. Illnesses such as anorexia nervosa have not been described in small-scale societies. Many psychiatric illnesses, such as problems related to substance abuse, are uncommon and if present seem not to have been qualified as illness (Waddel and Everett 1980). Moreover, many psychiatric illnesses involve body symptoms as well as significant impairment in social functioning and as implied, it is very likely that these will be labelled as illness. What exactly is a criterion of a psychiatric illness (as opposed to a non-psychiatric illness) is far from clear and the theory and practice of psychiatry are changing and evolving. The use of "psychiatric" in an etiological sense to denote illnesses produced by social and psychological conflicts (functional illnesses) is debatable since biological factors are also influential. The question of what "psychiatric illness" means also touches on distinctive cultural, historical, social, economic, and political factors and discussion of these is beyond the scope of this chapter. A related topic, that of culture bound syndromes, is discussed later in the chapter.

The question of the social consequences produced by the label of illness (for psychiatric disorders) and indeed the implications of this label in different societies is highly complex. The literature involving the labeling perspective and stigmatization in Western society is relevant to this topic and no attempt will be made to review it here (Szasz 1961; Foucault 1965). In small-scale societies, the labeling of someone as being ill is a precondition for effective social action (Edgerton 1966, 1969, 1980). The literature involving egalitarian and ranked systems of medicine leads one to a generalization that medical intervention has constructive consequences for the person ill and for the social group. The literature involving culture-bound syndromes (see below) offers strong support for this generalization as well, since these syndromes seem to have evolved special forms of treatment (Newman 1964). The long-term consequences of labeling in those instances of madness-insanity are far from clear. As Murphy and Westermeyer and Wintrob indicated, some penalties accrue to those singled out as "insane" but the penalties or burdens were judged as not significant in light of the caring and support which were offered (Murphy 1976; Westermeyer and Wintrob 1979). Waxler (1979) indicated that in Sri Lanka, differences in social labeling account for the shortened course of psychiatric illness. Indeed, this question of the social responses to the labeling of psychiatric illness in other societies is under active investigation in psychiatric epidemiology.

CULTURE AND THE MANIFESTATIONS OF PSYCHIATRIC ILLNESS

Statement of the Problem

The characteristics of insanity-madness as these have been studied cross-culturally, are very general and also quintessentially *social* in that behaviors disvalued or theatening to others (and, of course, to the property of others) are prominent features. An additional *social factor* is, of course, the concern of others for the well-being of the person for it is this which often leads them to intervene. An indicated earlier, altruistic attitudes of others toward the ill person (involving protection, care, etc.) seem intrinsic to the way illnesses (not just those termed here madness-insanity) are handled ethnomedically. The matter of the social characteristics of insanity-madness (where commonalities seem to obtain) is only partly related to the question of the possible universality in psychological manifestations of this type of illness. Two separate issues bearing on this question need to be distinguished. The first is a trivial one and involves what one can term the content of the ill person's behavior (e.g., what the ill person does or thinks) and here it is obvious that differences will obtain across societies and historical epochs. The other is whether the manifestations of insane-mad persons can be equated with defining properties of distinct types of Western psychiatric illnesses; and as a corollary to this, in instances when this can be done, whether the form or *structure* of the behaviors and manifestations are similar. It is this latter issue which is controversial and which will be dealt with presently.

A long-standing question in psychiatry concerns that of possible cross cultural differences in the manifestations of psychiatric illness. There is little doubt that insofar as people differ with regard to such things as language spoken, values and beliefs, as an example, they will show different concerns and preoccupations when ill. A critical issue is the significance which such seemingly "superficial" or content issues have, and also whether in a more basic structural sense, the manifestations of the psychiatric illness are still the same cross-culturally. To a large extent, this problem has in the past been analyzed and studied using descriptive methods of procedures. More recently, controlled studies based on structured questionnaires involving psychiatric symptoms have been used (Edgerton 1966, 1969, 1980; Fabrega 1970; Leighton et al. 1963; Woodburn 1979; Holmberg 1950).

One way to classify the claims and apparent assumptions of those studying the question of possible cultural differences in the manifestations of psychiatric illness is to describe them as universalists versus relativists depending on whether they believe the manifestations of such illnesses to be uniform or different across societies. Although universalists and relativists tend to view the problem which divides them as essentially empirical, we believe that basic theoretical issues about the nature of psychiatric illness are also involved. Moreover, although previous studies have concentrated largely on psychological phenomena, in particular the phenomenology of psychiatric illness, we believe that the question of possible cultural differences in psychiatric illness manifestations raises basic issues in brain behavior relations.

The question of whether the manifestations of psychiatric illness differ across cultural groups is basic to an understanding of such illnesses and not esoteric and restricted in its implications. The issues behind this question are important for at least three reasons. First of all, how culture might differentially affect the manifestations of psychiatric illness is integral to the whole question of how culture might differentially affect perception, cognition and behavioral organization more generally. Whereas general psychologic notions based on psychoanalytic theory and the Sapir-Whorf hypothesis have, in the past, dominated thinking in this general area, the subdisciplines of linguistic, biological and experimental anthropology now exert greater influence. Research in neuropsychology has broached the topic of possible cultural differences in behavior. Some of the findings in this field bear on the question of psychiatric illness and its manifestations. The preceding body of knowledge was reviewed in an earlier (Fabrega 1979b) publication and its possible relevance for understanding the question of possible cultural differences in the manifestations of psychiatric illness will be discussed briefly in this paper.

The question of culture and the manifestations of psychiatric illness is also important because it is so often misunderstood and trivialized. For example, that culture significantly colors the manifestations of psychiatric illness is taken to support the claims of some labeling theorists that such illnesses are not only culturally specific, but also fictive and specious entities altogether (Murphy 1976). The latter claims are unwarranted and indeed inconsistent with our view that psychiatric illness may reflect underlying organic disease processes in the central nervous system that are universal among *homo sapiens*. It is important that extremist claims of labeling theorists be separated from the claim that cultural and social factors necessarily play a role in both manifestations and social responses to psychiatric illness for this has theoretical and practical implications for psychiatry. This leads directly to the third factor accounting for the importance of the question of culture and the manifestations of psychiatric illness: namely, its possible bearing on the social responses to psychiatric illness and the general issue of the role of social and cultural factors on the duration and course of psychiatric illness. There exist reports suggesting that cultural factors significantly affect course of major psychiatric illness (Waxler 1979; Murphy and Raman 1971; Sartorius et al. 1973). The reasons or mechanisms for this effect are not entirely clear presently. I believe that findings involving the course of psychiatric illness bear on the question of how culture influences its manifestations.

As indicated earlier, the manifestations of major psychiatric illnesses (like schizophrenia and depression) are currently held to result from physical disturbances in the functioning of brain structures. These structures regulate arousal, attention, sensory inhibition, motivation, and mood and disturbances in them produce widespread behavioral effects which include activation of the motor programs for speech-cognition. Psychiatric epidemiologists appear to handle key manifestations of these illnesses as though they constituted special *signs* of nueropsychiatric *disease* (i.e., direct expressions of brain changes). The term sensori-motor behaviors can be used to refer to behaviors from which symbolic factors were factored out (e.g., muscular tone, involuntary movements, etc.). The behavior changes seen in aphasia, apraxia, agnosia, amnestic disorders and the disconnection syndromes can be classified as sensorimotor in nature and constitute signs of neuropsychiatric diseases. That is, the behaviors follow directly from a physical disorder in the brain and symbolic aspects are relatively unimportant. It would appear that many psychiatrists think of the behavioral changes of depression (e.g., sadness-despondency, psychomotor retardation, sleep disturbance) and schizophrenia (e.g., first rank symptoms) as sensorimotor in nature.

Culture Bound or Culture Specific Disorders

For well over the last half-century, anthropologists and then psychiatrists have been interested in the nature of certain behavior disturbances which were seen in specific societies and regions of the world. Most of these disturbances (variously called culture-bound syndromes or disorders) are familiar, and include *bena bena, amok, koro, susto*, Windigo psychosis and arctic hysteria. Some of the properties of these syndromes include (1) abrupt onset, (2) relatively short duration (i.e., days, seldom weeks – though information here is notoriously weak) and (3) absence of what psychiatrists term a formal thought disturbance. In some instances, persons afflicted show unusual mental changes and hyperactivity and although behavior can appear to us bizarre, it must be judged as reasonably organized. In fact, it is the coherence and pattern inherent in the manifestations of these disturbances that render them interesting and important. Some of the disturbances are characterized by mental symptoms, the content of which is highly specific (*Koro*, fear of the penis disappearing) and in some instances symbolic (Windigo – possession by a mythologically important spirit leading to a craving for human flesh, eventually cannibalism).

In many respects it is not surprising that "culture bound syndromes" should differ so dramatically with respect to global psychosocial behavior-symptoms. This is so because the manifestations of illness involve the meanings and implications of beliefs about self, other, nature, social action, individual purpose, agencies of control, etc. all of which are known to differ widely cross-culturally. In other words, the content of the beliefs and of the reasons for the behaviors seen in these disturbances deal with themes that are important in the group. It is true that why these disturbances occur (i.e., their etiology) is far from clear. There is a very large body of literature dealing with the question of etiology (Bourguignon 1979; LeVine 1973; Wallace 1961; Yap 1974; Leighton and Murphy 1965; Langness 1965). Personality and child rearing factors as well as environmental and biological ones have been invoked as explanations. Very frequently, the marginal status of the individual in the group and intercurrent stressors of various types have been invoked. However, the question of why the various manifestations take on the content that they do is not, generally speaking, problematic. A review of literature of cross-cultural psychology suggests that many commonalities are found regarding what languages/cultures single out in nature and in social life, whereas differences are found in what signficance these are given and how they enter into behavior and action. Thus, that culture-bound syndromes should involve strange beliefs and actions is not surprising given that the syndromes are described with reference to cultural themes. In brief, atypical or culture bound syndromes are described in terms of global psychological and social parameters (i.e., attitudes, behaviors, beliefs) and not in terms of what one could term the "substructure" of social action and personal experience (i.e., underlying perceptual-cognitive categories and or processes, attention, memory, experiences involving the body) where the presence of cultural differences would be far more significant and controversial.

An additional problem posed by culture-bound disturbances is their nosologic identity or status within the Western system of psychiatry. These disorders are usually classified as functional psychoses, atypical psychoses and/or hysterical psychoses. In Western societies, one frequently observes dramatic clinical pictures and the explanation of these (as well as nosology) is controversial (e.g., anorexia nervosa, Ganser syndrome). There is a tendency now towards rigorous criteria of diagnosis favoring the major psychiatric disorders. Unusual clinical pictures which do not conform to the strict criteria oulined are usually given a provisional status and the significance of these is under investigation.

In summary, a dominating opinion about culture bound syndromes seems to be that they are in some way "reactive" to sociocultural circumstances and that they are atypical variations of "psychogenic" disturbances which are felt to have a very wide distribution in human populations anyway. The words "reactive" and "psychogenic" have significance and utility in culture-personality theory and in psychological anthropology. However, these words pose problems for one who tries to formulate an understanding of culture and psychiatric illness in neurobiologic terms; the words, as it were, block out the nervous system. That the nervous system is grossly affected in varieties and instances of culture bound disturbances is very clear for persons afflicted sometimes show features of a toxic or confusional psychosis with an impairment in the level of consciousness which is followed by amnesia. In other instances, a phobic or obsessive hyper-alerted state without impaired consciousness is found. There is little more that can be said about the neurobiologic aspects of culture bound syndromes. One must emphasize the poverty of information which exists about phenomenology and behavioral manifestations of these disturbances. A recent critical review of the literature dealing with the concept, supporting evidence for, and validity of the so-called atypical psychoses has concluded that problems of methodology, sampling and diagnosis preclude firm generalizations about the nature of these psychoses. The reviewers included in their analysis so-called culture bound syndromes (Manschreck and Petri 1978).

Major Psychiatric Disorders

1. *Schizophrenia*. There exists a large literature in anthropology and psychiatry dealing with the role of culture on the manifestations of the major psychiatric disorders (Newman 1964; Waxler 1979; Odejide 1979; Gharagozlou 1979; Marsella 1980; Katz 1978; Morice 1978; Orley 1979; Leff 1973; Wallace 1961;

Yap 1974; Leighton and Murphy 1965; Langness 1965; Manschreck and Petri 1978; Kleinman 1977; Prince 1968; Fabrega 1974). As implied earlier, a dominating perspective has been that behaviors which in one culture are viewed as pathological may be viewed as entirely normal in another. This persepctive seemed totally to deny the possibility that psychiatric disorders possessed any universal aspects. A related perspective was that cultural factors could mask the manifestations of psychosis and even protect certain individuals (such as shamans) who suffered from specific psychiatric disorders. While not denying possible universal aspects of psychosis, the perspective also argued for a relativistic emphasis regarding manifestations. In recent years, thsee old relativistic perspectives have been severely undermined. Two lines of attack have been prominent: one stemming from an increasing appreciation of the neurobiological aspects of psychosis (e.g., schizophrenia) and the other from a scrutiny of data from cross-cultural field studies dealing with the social interpretations of psychiatric disorders (Murphy 1976; Westermeyer and Wintrob 1979; Edgerton 1966, 1969, 1980; Waxler 1979).

Murphy's article, in particular, seems to suggest that the neurobiologic changes of schizophrenia produce changes in behavior which will inevitably be judged as illness (and not deviance, or shamanism, or eccentricity, etc.) (Murphy 1976). It is important to keep in mind that the presentation of Murphy is directed at the extremist claims of a few labeling theorists who, in emphasizing the importance of social responses, argue for the "specious", "fictive" and "culture boundedness" of schizophrenia. Moreover, the material reviewed in her article is based largely on judgments about severe, chronic and deteriorated forms of schizophrenia, conditions better labeled as madness, insanity, lunacy, etc. (see discussion in previous section). In brief, as Edgerton has implied, it is in no way inconsistent to judge that schizophrenia has a neurobiological basis, that severe and chronic forms of schizophrenia (and other forms of insanity-madness) are consistently judged as illness across societies and historical epochs, and that social cultural factors are critically important in affecting both the psychosocial manifestations of and social responses to psychiatric disorders (Edgerton 1969).

Cultural factors are operative during socialization as individuals come to acquire adult behaviors. One could also say that cultural influences are operative during the period of brain maturation. Persons and selves are thus partially constructed in a cultural context and this process of "construction" embraces all levels of the nervous system. Schizophrenia also is realized in (an alteration of) the nervous system and will be manifest in the different spheres of behavior which this system regulates. It may be that important loci of schizophrenia are the neostriatum and limbic striatum, but given their roles in brain-behavior regulation, effects are likely to be general and widespread indeed. As an example, it is said that (limbic system) behaviors "released" during schizophrenia are relatively insenstive to ordinary neocortical regulation (Stevens 1973). Yet, such behaviors don't simply occur as physical phenomena, but are enacted and expressed in terms of prevailing ideas and cognitions. The important point is that, given the view of culture endorsed here, to some extent the physical changes of schizophrenia take place in different types of nervous systems. In other words, the neurophysiologic and neurochemical changes of schizophrenia affect behaviors whose neurologic substrates are themselves affected by culture.

One needs to focus on an important implication of the unique tie which neuropsychiatric diseases like schizophrenia have with cultural factors. Since these diseases, when fully played out in social and psychological illness behaviors, are connected in special ways with cultural symbols, one is forced to ask: to what extent are the form and content of the neuropsychiatric entities, as we now understand them, an outgrowth of our own natural language system and scientific culture? Or, to what extent might we be promulgating a deviant or atypical view of what these diseases look like and have looked like in human history?

To develop and make this point clearly, one needs to keep separate two different aspects about science and the perspective of man which it necessarily fosters. On the one hand, this perspective is instrumentally useful and, at least in a practical sense, is "correct". Science occupies an obviously dominating position in contemporary society, and it may some day unquestionably become the main governing principle in the species. Science and the scientific perspective with which it is associated have allowed the species unparalleled success in its quest for persistence and maintenance in the planet. It has allowed man to control the environment, to make and verify predictions, to achieve a greater understanding about nature and about life and about human origins. From this standpoint, then, science constitutes a powerful method, procedure and body of knowledge about the world.

Viewed from another point of view, however, science also constitutes a cultural perspective that man has about himself and about the world and in this sense it is simply one of many such perspectives which have existed in the species. Science, in other words, constitutes an ideology or perspective about the world which man, as part of his culture, internalizes and passes on to his descendants. This perspective, moreover, importantly shapes his own behavior. It is necessary to emphasize the comparative newness and indeed atypicality of this scientific perspective of man. It is associated with a view about man far different from the ones he has had across millenia. Men are now seen as having brains, composed of any number of structures such as speech "centers" and verbal memory "centers". Man is now said to have free will, to be his own agent, and to live in a world which houses only naturalistic forces or causes and not preternatural ones. This general scientific perspective is clear enough and need not be developed further. What must be emphasized is how different it is from the perspective common in nonliterate societies and, by implication, from the perspective which man has had during by far the longest portion of his existence. Thus, when viewed across human history, the contemporary scientific cultural perspective contains any number of new and indeed "atypical" assumptions about man and behavior. These views are products of science and although undeniably "correct" and useful nonetheless are still simply cultural premises which go into shaping how man himself behaves and conceives of himself.

It follows, then, that contemporary realizations of neuropsychiatric entities like schizophrenia reflect the peculiar cultural environment in which man himself gets shaped. One is thus forced to ask questions such as the following: To what extent are the descriptors of schizophrenia peculiar to our own cultural assumptions about the world and about ourselves? By "descriptors" I mean the set of social and psychological behaviors which are believed to realize the "lesion" of schizophrenia.

To illustrate the importance of language and cultural factors in the definition of schizophrenia one can take the so-called first rank symptoms of schizophrenia which many believe constitute sufficient conditions which enable one to diag- nose the "disease" in Western nations. These symptoms include having audible thoughts; experiencing one's thoughts being withdrawn or inserted in one's mind by others; experiencing the diffusion or broadcasting of thoughts; experi- encing one's feelings, impulses, or actual actions as somehow alien or externally controlled; and finally having a delusional mood and/or a delusional perception. These psychological experiences, it is claimed, constitute the fundamental symptoms of schizophrenia. Level of social functioning is not an explicit com- ponent of these systems though it is implied that this is likely to be impaired. Koehler has recently discussed first rank symptoms as embracing three types of continua (Koehler 1979). Specifically, he posits a delusional continuum, a passivity continuum, and a sense deception continuum. Rather than con- stituting basic indications of schizophrenia *per se*, one can view phenomena described by Koehler as implicating basic Western assumptions about human action and social reality. It may very well be the case that among Western people the neurobiologic changes of schizophrenia produce manifestations which include, phenomenologically, the eroding or blurring of these particular assumptions.

In other words, a working assumption can be that the first rank symptoms of schizophrenia are partly based on our cultural conventions about the self. These symptoms imply that to a large extent persons are independent beings whose bodies and minds are separated from each other and function auton- omously. In particular, they imply that under ordinary conditions external influences do not operate on and influence an individual: that thoughts, are recurring inner happenings that the self "has"; that thoughts, feelings, and actions are separable sorts of things which together account for self identity; that thoughts and feelings are silent and exquisitely private; that one's body is independent of what one feels or thinks; and finally that one's body, feelings and impulses have a purely naturalistic basis and cannot be modified by outside "supernatural" agents. In brief, contemporary Western psychology articulates a highly differentiated mentalistic self which is highly individuated and which looks out on an objective, impersonal, and naturalistic world; and it is based on this psychology (i.e., a Western cultural perspective) that schizophrenic symptoms have been articulated.

All of the assumptions which underlie the first rank symptoms – which provide a rationale for their "pathological" nature – seem linked to Western notions about human psychology and causality. Any careful ethnography of the way non-Western peoples explain phenomena, account for human action, and delineate personal identity will point to ethnocentric components in these assumptions. Many such people believe in the constant interconnection between the natural and preternatural, between the "bodily" and the "mental" and between the various dimensions and contents of human awareness which are arbitrarily set apart in Western psychology. If, in fact, people already believe themselves affected by external influences, if they sense and experience these influences constantly and accommodate themselves in various ways to the necessary connection which they judge holds between feeling, thinking, bodily activity and external control – then how will the "basic lesion" of schizophrenia show itself behaviorally? In short, which of the behavioral descriptors of schizo-phrenia is one likely to see; and which one is one likely to see different versions of, in the event that the assumptive world of the person who has the basic lesion rests on highly different premises about self, behavior, and causality? It should be clear that the claim here is not that unusual psychological experiences or social behaviors are not part of "schizophrenia" but rather that the form and meaning which they take in European culture are partly an outcome of the way "selves" are constructed there.

In summary, rather than constituting universal "indicators" of schizophrenia *per se*, one can view phenomena described by Koehler as implicating basic Western assumptions about personal identity, human action, and social reality. A basic question is the level of behavior at which the continua of Koehler operate. Do the so-called first rank symptoms-behaviors of schizophrenia implicate, for example, assumptions involving the meaning of self, other, the world and social action? Or, do they instead implicate basic perceptual-cognitive processes that enable one to think and maintain elemental boundaries between self and units of nature (with culture merely adding content and meaning)? These questions are similar to those raised above, *vis-à-vis* culture-bound syndromes. In brief, do the assumptions behind the various continua of Koehler constitute conditions for meaningful psychosocial and interpersonal behaviors among Westerners (i.e., do they operate at a level at which, it seems, cross-cultural differences exist) or do the assumptions and continua instead involve what was termed the substructure of social action (i.e., level at which persons identify and refer to basic units, entitles and/or categories of nature – a level at which, it seems, some commonalities are observed across cultures/languages)?

2. *Depression*. A recent review of the literature on manifestations of depression (Marsella 1980) has pointed to cultural differences, a finding consistent with the writings of other culturally-oriented psychiatrists (Kleinman 1977; Prince

1968; Fabrega 1974). The review encompassed literature involving clinical observations, culture specific disorders, symptoms among patients matched by diagnosis and sample, international surveys, and factor analytic studies. Of special importance is that psychological aspects of depression (e.g., depressed mood, guilt, feelings of self deprecation, purposelessness, etc.) seen in the Western world are oftentimes absent in non-Western societies. Somatic aspects were noted quite frequently, regardless of culture. Oftentimes it is only when non-Westerners become Westernized that the anticipated psychological aspects of depression emerge. Depressed somatic functioning "vegetative depression" — thus appeared not to have the corresponding depressed mental experience seen in the West. Whether a retardation in psychological processes was found was not reported. If the quality of mental experience associated with occurrence of depression is influential in how a depressed individual behaves, then different types of psychosocial manifestations and social responses can be anticipated across societies.

One could use the conclusions of this review of empirical studies to argue for a uniform disease entity termed depression which affects subcortical structures of the brain (i.e., the similarity in vegetative phenomena). On the other hand, differences in the psychological and social behaviors of depressive illness would imply differences in the organization and function of cortical substrates which subserve language, thought, and experience.

Related to this question of the character of psychosocial behavior changes in depressive illness in different cultures, is the study by Leff (1973). He used reliable information collected (by means of the Present State Examination) on patients hospitalized in different psychiatric centers. Psychiatrists' ratings of patients' verbal reports and social behavior thus constituted the data base. Scores on three emotion variables were correlated: anxiety and depression, depression and irritability, and anxiety and irritability. Leff compared the correlations of emotions across a number of social cultural groups of patients which he classified as belonging to developed and developing nations. In using correlations between emotion scores, Leff posited that a correlation of +1 between two emotions represented the least possible discrimination between the two emotions. On the other hand, a correlation of −1 represented the greatest possible discrimination between the two emotions. One could, of course, say that both types of emotions could, in fact, be present, but implicit in Leff's reasoning is that a similar level of overlap of symptoms probably existed in these centers and that the size of the correlations reflected the degree of discrimination of the subjects. His results showed an interesting pattern of differences. As an example, China and Nigeria subjects showed the highest intercorrelations. As predicted patients from developing countries showed significantly higher correlations in all three pairs of emotions when compared to patients from developed countries. Leff concluded that groups (cultures) differ in ease of differentiation between emotional states and that this was due to the relative availability of linguistic categories for the description of subjective states.

Understanding the role of culture on the manifestations of depression is facilitated if one distinguishes between emotion as a basic category of human experience and emotion as a symbolic domain which is lexically coded — which languages "capture" in a direct and explicit way. All indications are that emotions are probably universal and that the structure of affective experience also has universal features (Ekman 1972, 1973). However, the prevalence of linguistic labels for emotions may vary in frequency across societies. By means of lexically-encoded emotion terms, one is able to speak and think more precisely and elaborately about internal subjective states. In a fundamental way, the domain of emotion and that of the self impact on each other semantically. Besides serving as a means for qualifying the state of the self, emotion words can also be used to qualify other types of phenomena such as social situations and bodily states. This appears to be the case with emotion in our culture, with the effect that social relations, bodily experience, and the self are linked semantically and in an elaborate way through emotion and related mentalistic terms. Such a symbolic dimension of emotion can be expected to affect the psychosocial manifestations of and social responses to psychiatric illness.

What needs emphasis here can be equated with the term "biocultural", namely the connectedness which exists between things we describe as neurological or biological as opposed to cultural-linguistic. In Western populations, the psychiatric illness we term depression and conditions of social disarticulation appear to be elaborated in mentalistic and emotional terms. It is very likely that this is partly a consequence of what anthropologists term the *psychic unity* of man. This is to say that all people, regardless of culture, are likely to feel "down" and "bad" when things go away for them either socially or physically. However, to a certain extent, the similarity which these conditions show is also partly a consequence of the fact that the psychic sphere, considered now as a linguistic — especially semantic — domain, is richly encoded and symbolically important in Western cultures. The fact that our lay, cultural theories of illness and of personhood draw heavily on emotion and related mentalistic premises serves to further ambiguate the appearance of these conditions.

If one wishes to conduct a comparative analysis of the psychiatric illness of depression and/or to assess its general significance across human populations, a number of factors already alluded to need to be analytically separated. Some of the factors which need to be distinguished are summarized in Figure 1. In this contingency table conditions of individuals (i.e., A=Depression; B=Social Disarticulation) are set against parameters of the social system. Each of the conditions of individuals can be assumed to be correlated with three sets of changes, namely, subjective states of awareness (in principle, held to be unmeasurable), changes in behavior and physical states of the body which can be measured biomedically. The complexities which can be created by factors listed in Figure 1 can be illustrated by considering conditions of individuals singly and in relation to parameters of the social system. Thus, if the two conditions could be measured unproblematically, then it would be possible to arrive at their frequency in different societies. It should be clear that (1) condition A requires a biomedical metric which could be applied to all societies (2) condition B requires a social metric which would require consideration of specific language/cultural factors and (3) that only by the use of both could a true prevalence for these two conditions be estimated (column 1).

		SOCIAL SYSTEM			
		True Prevalence	Behavioral Appearance	Social Significance	Institutional Location
PERSONAL SYSTEM	A Neuropsychiatric Depression				
	B Social Disarticulation				

Fig. 1. Interrelation of Personal system and social system.

These points suggest that measuring the true cross-cultural prevalence of depression is a complex enterprise which will require the application of both biological and cultural modes of analysis. In the table, the columns marked behavioral appearance, social significance and institutional location draw attention to areas where cultural factors may prove especially influential in the way these two conditions distribute in a society. The table could be used to study other societies or different social groups within our own society. Thus, it is probably the case that the cells of the table would be occupied by different parameters where men and women of our society to be compared.

In summary, a review of the literature suggests cultural differences in the manifestations of depression. Psychological and mental symtoms appear to be less prominent (and/or less differentiated) in certain non-Western societies. One way of explaining those differences is to point to the influence of our (culturally dominant) psychologic perspective which is heavily mentalistic and which elaborates semantically on "emotion" as a descriptor of the self. In my view, it is not strictly correct to say that depression is different in other cultures; one should say that depression is different in *our* culture. When thinking of the major psychiatric illnesses (like schizophrenia and depression) we need to realize that at issue are psychological and social (i.e., illness) behaviors which necessarily are colored by cultural factors. This means that our view of these illnesses is to an indeterminate extent ethnocentric.

The basic point is that from a biomedical standpoint, depression and schizophrenia (considered earlier) imply universal changes in the functioning of the brain which, it is assumed, produce or are associated with equally universal changes in behavior. Moreover, in our society, these behavior changes are, in fact, labeled illness. The behaviors found in these psychiatric disturbances, however, are partly social and psychological in nature and hence, necessarily cultural. The latter sphere is by definition not universal: symbolic conventions pertaining to self, and natural order and "supernatural" agencies necessarily color social behavior and psychological experience. The work of Ohnuki-Tierney (1977) and Lewis (1977) has underscored the importance of considering how symbolic conventions affect the manifestations and responses tied to bodily disease changes. Such conventions are no less likely to affect the behavioral manifestations linked to the brain changes of depression and schizophrenia. Finally, the behaviors linked to depression and schizophrenia — whatever these might be — may not necessarily be labeled as illness cross-culturally although advanced and deteriorated forms of these disorders appear to be so labeled (see earlier discussion on madness and insanity). Symbolic conventions of a people that bear on the question of psychiatric illness cross-culturally are thus of three different, but no doubt related, types: conventions underlying social behavior and psychological experience, conventions underlying the definition of illness, and conventions underlying the social responses to deviance and illness. In Western societies, conventions about the self, about emotion, and about the nature of human action and purpose, seem intertwined in the definition, measurement, and responses to depression and schizophrenia, conditions which are thought of as universal in nature. What is at issue is the question of what is the focus of a biomedical fact as opposed to a social fact, a question I return to below.

On the Epistemologies of Psychiatric Illness

The influence of the culture on the manifestations of psychiatric illness is a controversial topic in psychiatry. That key manifestations may differ cross-culturally is contested. The increasing emphasis on organic factors in psychiatry has tended to weaken the claims of social scientists who speak of cultural differences. However, the problem of how the role of culture is to be understood is critical for an understanding of psychiatric illness. Culture is here defined as a system of symbols and its meanings which are shared by a people and which guide and give significance to social behavior. From the standpoint of an individual, culture is usually handled as an environmental or "external" variable. However, since an individual is born without culture, learns it from co-members of a group, and eventually reflects it in his overt behavior, culture is therefore internalized. This means that culture has a representation in the brain. It follows that the role of culture on the manifestations of psychiatric illness needs to be conceptualized from a neurobiologic standpoint. This forces consideration of the question of the neurologic substrates of culture within the biomedical perspective.

Neuropsychologists speak of the engram as the physical brain substrate of memory. Although not often mentioned explicitly, it is very likely that part of what social scientists have in mind when speaking of "culture" and "symbolic" can be equated with the engrams of the semantic memory system. As described by Tulving (1972) and illustrated by Warrington (1975), it is this system which presumably embodies the repository of knowledge and beliefs that an individual acquires as he learns his culture. Information of the semantic memory system may be judged to embrace such overlearned things as role prescriptions, attitudes, values and beliefs, all of which constitute the data of social scientists.

Another brain analogue of culture (and also not explicitly mentioned as such in the literature) can be equated with what neuroscientists mean when they speak of "motor programs". That is, physical changes (again involving molecular arrangements, patterns of synaptic transmission, neural nets, etc.) in the brain which mediate and/or serve to organize sequences of coordinated skeletal and visceral muscle movements. Motor programs are posited so as to account for the execution of organized human action, including neuromuscular activity, nonverbal communication, the expression of affect, emotion, and speech, all of which are linked to internal bodily states. Speech is an example, par excellence, of a form of human motor activity which is dominated and coordinated by thought processes (McNeill 1979). Complex motor actions like those involving speech are generally thought of as coordinated by hierarchical structures, the uppermost or executive structure of which has little or no direct control over actual motor output. The executives in charge of speech are defined as sensorimotor ideas or concepts. These are outgrowths of sensorimotor action schemas which in infants serve to generate movement and constitute the earliest forms of cognitive activity. Thus, at an early stage of development, sensorimotor ideas are viewed as simultaneously part of action and meaning, serving as the basis of sensorimotor behavior and cognition. These ideas and schemas are viewed as the earliest templates for speech and as providing a motor base for thought and awareness.

When neurologically-oriented researchers explicitly invoke "cultural factors" they seem to refer to such things as patterns of cerebral asymmetry and/or relative amounts of brain tissue of a certain type which might be required (for cultural reasons) to carry out specific psychologic functions (Albert and Obler 1978; Rogers et al. 1977; Scott et al. 1979). A basic assumption, in other words, is that the brain is like a vector of connected centers and processes, each of which is organized and functions in a uniform way across the species. This "vector" is judged as a potential that social experiences can draw on. Cultural influences are equated with the way entries in this vector are used, i.e., over-emphasized or underemphasized. Neurologically, then, culture seems to be implicated when neurobiologists speak of the uses to which specific brain regions are put, and to the overall pattern and arrangement which results from such differential uses.

A neuroscientist intent on demonstrating cultural influences on brain-behavior relations needs first to show that an association exists between a culturally relevant situation or stimulus and a brain event; and/or an association between a stimulus or situation and a behavior known to be an outcome of a specific brain event. Each of the three classes of phenomena (i.e., stimulus, brain event and behavior) obviously needs to be clearly specified and measured. Given this, it would be necessary for the neuroscientists to show that there exist differences on the relevant measures across groups of individuals who belong to different language and cultural communities. It should be obvious that to show associations between culture and brain-behavior relations, the neuroscientist is forced to reduce observations to very discrete phenomena. The logic just reviewed is also essentially that of the cognitive psychologist intent on demonstrating that cultural groups differ in ways of perceiving, making decisions, remembering, discriminating, or problem-solving. The psychologist is required to make his test understandable, and appropriate to the subject so as to motivate and engage equivalent cognitive processes. Moreover, he must assure that responses of his subjects are discrete and unambiguous so that they can be reliably measured. Key elements in the strategy of the neuroscientists or cognitive psychologist are thus those of *abstraction* and *specificity*.

A neurologically oriented psychiatrist who is pursuing the question of possible cultural differences in psychiatric illness can adopt the strategy of the neuroscientists or cognitive psychologist and concentrate on highly discrete phenomena. If he or she found differences on measures of psychiatric illness which could be related to brain events or functions, this would allow claiming that the brains of the persons with the disease-illness were different across cultural groups, and/or that the disease-illness itself was different in the groups.

Phenomena ordinarily studied by culturally oriented psychiatrists are at a very far different level of abstraction than that studied by neurologically oriented ones. Thus, such things as "mental" symptoms and social adjustment changes are far removed from the discrete and abstract items engaging the neural scientist and/or cognitive psychologist. A culturally oriented psychiatrist is interested in demonstrating differences in the configuration of psychiatric illness as a whole; the logic or psychosocial rationale inherent in illness, viewed as an experiential and whole behavioral structure, claims his or her interests. Such a psychiatrist seeks to demonstrate that the illness, viewed either in terms of the person ill or in terms of group co-members, "makes sense" only when semantic aspects (i.e., its context or meaning) are taken into consideration. A useful way to capture these differences in orientation is to say that culturally-oriented psychiatrists are principally drawn to features of illness (i.e., psychosocial behavior changes) whereas neuroscientifically-oriented ones are drawn to features of disease (i.e., physical changes in the brain).

SUMMARY

The preceding theory of illness-self conceptualization as it applies to psychiatric disorders bears an obvious relationship to contemporary trends in multiaxial diagnosis and social psychiatric research more generally. In a fundamental sense, the emphasis on a multiaxial approach to psychiatric disorders reflects the growing appreciation that the nature of such disorders is complex and multifactorial genetic, etc.). This in essence means that the identity of a disorder, its manifestations, its duration and course, and its responsiveness to treatment are all influenced by a number of different factors. It follows from these considerations that an investigator's ability to predict the time course of a disorder is enhanced should he or she employ a multiaxial approach. I am, in essence, positing that the "axis" which describes how the individual defines his own condition of illness and well-being and, indeed, his view of his self and behavior, all influence key parameters of a psychiatric disorder.

A number of social psychological factors which appear to influence the duration and course of psychiatric disorder bear a relation to the "theory of illness-self" conceptualization presented above. Some of these factors are already included as separate axes in various multiaxial systems or models. Several examples can be suggested. First, the tendency for multiaxial systems to incorporate background social information, such as age, education, marital status and work participation-history, reflects an appreciation that an individual's social competence and "connectedness" in the social system affect the duration and course of psychiatric disorder. Related to this is the axis involving number and quality of social relations. Social variables such as these have long been known to bear a relation to course and duration of disorder. The emotional environment that the patient returns to has recently been shown to be important in influencing course of schizophrenia. Finally, the extent to which an individual accepts diagnosis and complies with treatment can be expected to influence duration and course.

All of these psychologic factors might be expected to bear a relation to an individual's theory of illness. Thus, the more socially competent and educated an individual is, the more likely he or she is to embrace the dominant "scientific" model of psychiatric disorder of health providers. Similarly, given that they share the traditional view of psychiatric disorder, socially competent and "connected" individuals when ill are more likely to behave in conformance with social expectations of how mentally ill persons behave. Such persons are thus more likely to receive support and encouragement, show "typical" symptoms of psychiatric disorder, seek orthodox psychiatric treatment, and respond to medication and treatment procedures along the lines anticipated by health providers.

In the belief of sick persons and in the expectations others hold about him, one is likely to find embedded key notions about the theory of illness that is prevalent in the group and here one is likely to find differences across societies. Theories of illness and theories of personhood, which interrelate, help shape the content and perhaps the structure of psychiatric illness. This type of illness is quintesentially a cultural as well as biologic entity; both its manifestations and social responses can be expected to reflect culture and biology. An important question involves the content of the theory and the extent to which patient and significant others share basic postulates of it. In general, since social psychologic factors have been shown to help predict outcome and duration of disorder, I anticipate that a refined measurement of the axis of "theory of illness-self" which I believe partially influences them, will help explain additional variance pertaining to ourcome and duration.

REFERENCES

Ackerknecht, E. H.
1959 A Short History of Psychiatry. New York: Hafner Publishing Co.
Albert, M. K. and L. K. Obler
1978 The Bilingual Brain. New York: Academic Press.
Andersen, E. S.
1977 Lexical Universals of Body-Part Terminology. In Language Universals, Volume III, Word Structure. J. Greenberg, et al. (eds.). Atlantic Highlands, N. J.: Humanities Press.
Bourguignon, E.
1979 Psychological Anthropology: An Introduction to Human Nature and Cultural Differences. New York: Harper and Row.
Edgerton, R. B.
1966 Conceptions of Psychosis in Four African Societies. American Anthropology 2: 408–425.
1969 On the "Recognition" of Mental Illness. In Changing Perspectives in Mental Illness. S. C. Plog and R. B. Edgerton (eds.). New York: Holt, Rinehart and Winston, Inc.
1980 Traditional Treatment for Mental Illness in Africa: A Review. Culture, Medicine and Psychiatry 4:164–189.
Ekman, K.
1972 Universals and Cultural Differences in Facial Expressions of Emotions. In Nebraska Symposium on Motivation. J. K. Cole (ed.). Lincoln: University of Nebraska Press.
1973 Cross-Cultural Studies of Facial Expression. In Darwin and Facial Expression: A Century of Research in Review. P. Ekman (ed.). New York: Academic Press.
Fabrega, H. Jr.
1970 Psychiatric Implications of Health and Illness in a Maya Indian Group: A Preliminary Statement. Social Science and Medicine. 3:609–626.
1972 Concepts of Disease: Logical Features and Social Implications. Perspectives in Biology and Medicine 15:583–616.
1974a Problems Implicit in the Cultural and Social Study of Depression. Psychosomatic Medicine 36(5):377–398.
1974b Disease and Social Behavior: An interdisciplinary Perspective. Cambridge, Mass. and London: MIT Press.
1975 The Need for Ethnomedical Science. Science 189:969–975.
1976 The Biological Significance of Taxonomies of Disease. Journal of Theoretical Biology 63:191–216.
1979a The Scientific Usefulness of the Idea of Illness. Perspectives in Biology and Medicine 22(4):554–558.
1979b Neurobiology, Culture, and Behavior Disturbances. Journal of Nervous and Mental Disorders 167:467–474.
Fabrega, H. Jr. and S. Tyma
1976 Culture, Language and the Shaping of Illness: An Illustration Based on Pain. Journal of Psychosomatic Research 20:323–337.

Foucault, M.
    1965   Madness and Civilization. New York: Random House.
Gharagozlou, H. and M. T. Behin
    1979   Diagnostic Evaluation of Schneider First Rank Symptoms of Schizophrenia
           among Three Groups of Iranians. Comprehensive Psychiatry 20:242–245.
Holmberg, A. R.
    1950   Nomads of the Long Bow: The Siriono of Eastern Bolivia. Smithsonian Institu-
           tion Publications of the Institute of Social Anthropology No. 10.
Katz, M. M., et al.
    1978   Ethnic Studies in Hawaii: On Psychopathology and Social Deviance. *In* The
           Nature of Schizophrenia. L. Wynne, et al. (eds.). New York: John Wiley and Sons.
Kleinman, A. M.
    1977   Depression, Somatization and the "New Cross-Cultural Psychiatry". Social Science
           and Medicine 11:3–9.
Klibansky, R., E. Panefsky, and F. Saxl
    1964   Saturn and Melancholy: Studies in the History of Natural Philosophy, Religion
           and Art. London: T. Nelson and Sons.
Koehler, H.
    1979   First Rank Syndromes of Schizophrenia: Questions Concerning Clinical Bound-
           aries. British Journal of Psychiatry 134:236–248.
Kroll, J.
    1973   A Reappraisal of Psychiatry in the Middle Ages. Archives of General Psychiatry
           29:276–283.
Langness, L. L.
    1965   Hysterical Psychosis in the New Guinea Highlands: A Bena Bena Example. Psy-
           chiatry 28:258–277.
Leff, J. P.
    1973   Culture and the Differentiation of Emotional States. British Journal of Psychiatry
           123:299–306.
Leighton, A. H. and J. M. Murphy
    1965   Approaches to Cross-Cultural Psychiatry. Ithaca: Cornell University Press.
Leighton, A. H., et al.
    1963   The Psychiatric Disorder Among the Yoruba. Ithaca: Cornell University Press.
LeVine, R. A.
    1973   Culture, Behavior and Personality: An Introduction to the Comparative Study of
           Psychosocial Adaptation. Chicago: Aldine Publishing Co.
Lewis, G.
    1977   Knowledge of Illness in a Sepik Society. London: The Athlone Press.
Manschreck, T. C. and M. Petri
    1978   The Atypical Psychoses. Culture, Medicine and Psychiatry 2:233–268.
Marsella, A. J.
    1980   Depressive Experience and Disorder Across Cultures. *In* Handbook of Cross-
           Cultural Psychology, Volume 5: Culture and Psychopathology. Draguns and H.
           Triandis (eds.). Boston: Allyn and Bacon
McNeill, D.
    1979   The Conceptual Basis of Language. Hillsdale, N. J.: Erlbaum Publishing Co.
Morice, R.
    1978   Psychiatric Diagnosis in a Transcultural Setting – the Importance of Lexical
           Categories. British Journal of Psychiatry 132:87–95.
Murphy, J. B. M. and A. C. Raman
    1971   The Chronicity of Schizophrenia in Indigenous Tropical Peoples – Results of a
           Twelve-Year Follow-Up Survey in Mauritius. British Journal of Psychiatry 118–
           497.

Murphy, J. M.
    1976 Psychiatric Labeling in Cross-Cultural Perspective. Science 191:1019–1028.
Neugebauer, R.
    1978 Treatment of the Mentally Ill in Medieval and Early Modern England: A Reappraisal. Journal of the History of Behavioral Sciences 14:158–169.
    1979 Medieval and Early Modern Theories of Mental Illness. Archives of General Psychiatry 36:477–483.
Newman, P. L.
    1964 "Wild Man" Behavior in a New Guinea Highlands Community. American Anthropologist 66:1–19.
Obeyesekere, G.
    1977 The Theory and Practice of Psychological Medicine in the Ayurvedi Tradition. Culture, Medicine and Psychiatry 1:155–181.
Odejide, A. O.
    1979 Cross-Cultural Psychiatry: A Myth or Reality. Comprehensive Psychiatry 20(2): 103–109.
Ohnuki-Tierney, E.
    1977a The Classification of the 'Habitual Illnesses' of the Sakhalin Ainu. Arctic Anthropology 14(2):9–34.
    1977b An Octopus Headache? A Lamprey Boil? Multisensory Perception of 'Habitual Illness' and World View of the Ainu. Journal of Anthropological Research 33(3): 245–257.
Orley, J. and J. L. Wing
    1979 Psychiatric Disorders in Two African Villages. Archives of General Psychiatry 29:177–189.
Parsons, T.
    1951 The Social System. New York: Free Press.
Prince, R.
    1968 The Changing Picture of Depressive Syndromes in Africa: Is it Fact or Diagnostic Fashion. Canadian Journal of African Studies 1:177–192.
Rogers, L., et al.
    1977 Hemispheric specialization of Language: An EEG Study of Bilingual Hopi Indian Children. International Journal of Neuroscience 8:1–6.
Sartorius, N., A. Jablensky, and R. Shapiro
    1973 Cross-Cultural Differences in the Short-Term Prognosis of Schizophrenia by Psychoses. Schizophrenia Bulletin: 102–113.
Scott, S., et al.
    1979 Cerebral Speech Lateralization in the Native Navajo. Neuropsychologia 17:89–92.
Simon, B.
    1978 Mind and Madness in Ancient Greece. The Classical Roots of Modern Psychiatry. Ithaca: Cornell University Press.
Stevens, J.
    1973 An Anatomy of Schizophrenia? Archives of General Psychiatry 29:177–189.
Szasz, T.
    1961 The Myth of Mental Illness — Foundations for a Theory of Personal Conduct. New York: Hoeber-Harper.
Thomas, K.
    1973 Religion and the Decline of Magic. Middlesex, England: Penguin Books.
Torrey, E. F.
    1979 Schizophrenia and Civilization. New York: Aronson Publishing Co.
Tseng, W. S.
    1973 The Development of Psychiatric Concepts in Traditional Chinese Medicine. Archives of General Psychiatry 29:569–575.

Tulving, E.
    1972 Episodic and Semantic Memory. *In* Organization of Memory. E. Tulving and W.
          Donaldson, (eds.). New York: Academic Press.
Veith, I.
    1965 Hysteria: The History of a Disease. Chicago: University of Chicago Press.
Waddell, K. P. and M. W. Everett
    1980 Drinking Behavior Among Southwestern Indians: An Anthropological Perspective.
          Tucson: University of Arizona Press.
Wallace, A. F. C.
    1961 Mental Illness, Biology, and Culture. *In* Psychological Anthropology. F. L. K. Hsu
          (ed.). Homewood, Ill.: Dorsey Press.
Warrington, E. K.
    1975 The Selective Impairment of Semantic Memory. Quarterly Journal of Experi-
          mental Psychology 27:635—657.
Waxler, N. E.
    1974 Culture and Mental Illness — A Social Labeling Perspective. The Journal of
          Nervous and Mental Disease 159:379—395.
    1979 Is Outcome for Schizophrenia Better in Traditional Societies?: The Case of Sri
          Lanka. The Journal of Nervous and Mental Disease 167:144—158.
Webster, C.
    1975 The Great Instauration — Science, Medicine and Reform — 1626—1660. New
          York: Holmes Y. Meier Publishers.
Westermeyer, J. and R. Wintrob
    1979 "Folk" Criteria for the Diagnosis of Mental Illness in Rural Laos: On Being Insane
          in Sane Places. American Journal of Psychiatry 136:755—761.
Wing, J. K.
    1978 Reasoning About Madness. New York: Oxford University Press.
Woodburn, J.
    1979 Hunters and Gatherers Today in the Reconstruction of the Past. *In* Soviet
          and Western Anthropology. E. Gellner (ed.). London: Gerald Duckworth and
          Company.
Yap, P. M.
    1974 Comparative Psychiatry: A Theoretical Framework. *In* M. P. Lau and A. B. Stokes
          (eds.). Toronto: University of Toronto Press.
Young, A.
    1976 Some Implications of Medical Beliefs and Practices for Social Anthropology.
          American Anthropologist 78:5—24.

GEOFFREY M. WHITE

3. THE ETHNOGRAPHIC STUDY OF CULTURAL KNOWLEDGE OF "MENTAL DISORDER"

INTRODUCTION

Illness and medicine are among a limited number of topical domains which cross-cultural researchers have for some time described as organized bodies of cultural knowledge (e.g., Clements 1932; and see Conklin 1972:363–392 for a bibliography). One reason for this is that illness is viewed universally as an intrusive disruption of body, person and community which requires explanation and corrective action (Fabrega 1974) and thus gives rise to some form of folk theory as a basis for interpreting or making sense of that experience. While particular definitions of illness may vary widely, concern with illness as an area of problematic human experience (and as a topic for folk theories) is commonly expressed in ordinary conversation across cultures. Thus, interpretations of illness events are an important focus for comparative research on social, cultural and cognitive questions generally, as well as for the investigation of medical issues. Just as cultural understandings about social organization may be most visible during conflict situations in which normative, desirable relations are discussed more openly or deliberately, so cultural understandings about personhood and social behavior may be brought closer to the surface of natural discourse by illness events which evoke interpretations of personal dysfunction or deviations from social norms. The ethnographic study of cultural knowledge of illness attempts to discover and represent conceptual models which underly the construction of meaningful interpretations of illness. As discussed below, this enterprise must venture well beyond the narrow confines of illness and medicine.

Although this paper is concerned particularly with research on cultural knowledge of "mental disorder" and its analogs across cultures, much of the research on illness beliefs generally is also directly relevant to the study of cultural knowledge of mental disorder. The notion of "mental health" derives from a particular tradition of medical research and practice which does not provide a neutral stance from which to analyze or represent the way "other cultures" conceptualize disorders of the person and social behavior. To begin with, the boundary between disorders of the mind (the province of psychiatry and neurology) and of the body (the province of internal medicine) is itself a cultural construction which underlies the segmentation of a class of illnesses we refer to as "mental". The potential for variation in how this boundary is drawn is well illustrated by many of the papers in this book describing systems of medical belief in Asian societies.

The relation of cultural conceptions of "mental disorder" to cultural definitions of "illness" or to "social deviance," etc. are empirical questions to be

A. J. Marsella and G. M. White (eds.), Cultural Conceptions of Mental Health and Therapy, 69–95.

answered by ethnographic research. Questions such as these require an investigation of ethnopsychological understandings about personhood and normal social behavior. These more general ethnopsychological constructs form some of the basic premises of folk theories used to interpret departures from normative, ideal or desirable states of the person or social interaction. For example, cultural understandings about 'responsibility' or 'culpability' are important definitional components of illness in Western folk theories (Young 1976), and also play an important role in distinguishing mental illness from other forms of social deviance, particularly criminal behavior. An ethnographic description of these understandings requires an account of notions such as 'causality', 'control' and 'intentionality' in social action, and of the ways these constructs are used in common sense reasoning about behavior.

In Western societies where common sense notions of "mental health" pervade popular culture (Nunnally 1961; Townsend 1978), similarities between professional and lay conceptions of mental disorder are due in part to implicit understandings about the nature of persons and social behavior which influence both formal and informal theories of illness (Lazare 1973; Gaines, this volume). However, psychiatric nosology is built upon a medical model of illness made up of explicit propositions about the interconnection of overt symptoms and underlying causes of disorder located primarily in individual minds, brains and personalities. In contrast, common sense theories are formulated in terms of persons as social beings who "feel bad", "get sick" and decide what to do about illness based on its personal, social and moral implications (Eisenberg 1977). Thus, much of folk knowledge of mental disorder is shaped by cultural definitions of personhood, social identities and role expectations which can be investigated in ways similar to the study of social cognition generally (see e.g., Carroll and Payne 1976; Townsend 1979; Horowitz et al. 1981; Clement, this volume).

This paper reviews developments in methodological approaches to the study of cultural knowledge about illness and social behavior, particularly symbolic and cognitive studies which have made conceptual description a primary goal. On the one hand, a considerable amount of research has examined directly the cognitive organization of common-sense understandings about illness. These approaches (termed "ethnoscience" at an earlier stage) have generally used formal methods to explore systematically the organization of abstract conceptual models which structure cultural understandings about illness — frequently by eliciting individual judgments about the meanings of indigenous terms and their appropriate use in describing illness. On the other hand, a substantial amount of research has focused on actual or reported illness episodes and recorded the ways common-sense interpretations of illness are expressed and negotiated in actual social situations. These studies have attempted to "distill" indirectly representations of the symbolic organization of cultural beliefs about illness from behavioral observations.

The former style of cognitive research has led to an increasing awareness that it is not the "diagnostic features" of illness categories, but their personal and social implications which are the most salient aspects of cultural knowledge about specific illnesses. As a result, researchers have recognized the limitations of lexical methods used to examine the meanings of illness categories in terms of the contrast and variation of category labels in terminological sets.

The latter style of "symbolic" research, associated more recently with "hermeneutic" analysis which assumes that texts and natural discourse express multiple overlapping meanings (see Rabinow and Sullivan 1979; Good and Good, this volume), has shown the importance of social context in determining what kinds of interpretations of illness are expressed and accepted. Although Geertz (1973) has placed these two styles of research in opposition to one another, they are in many ways extensively complementary. Whereas cognitive models represent the range of inferences which constitute culturally appropriate or plausible interpretations of illness; hermeneutic analysis attempts to specify the social and cultural processes whereby alternative interpretations are posed and selected in social interaction. While cognitive models are likely to be insensitive to the social and contextual forces which impinge on interpretive processes, hermeneutic analyses usually do not specify how "semantic" models are constructed or could be validated.

This review focuses primarily on research which has attempted to represent abstract conceptual models which organize cultural knowledge of illness. However, it should be noted that this concern with semantic and cognitive structures is but one piece of a larger picture. The process of interpretation of natural discourse about illness is usually an interactive process which is influenced by a great many contextual variables, including the nature of social institutions, relations among interactants, and rules of communication, both verbal and nonverbal. The hermeneutic focus on the *interactive* construction of meaningful interpretations (see W. Lebra, this volume), as well as current research in sociolinguistics (e.g., Labov and Fanshel 1977) and ethnomethodology which analyze the performative aspects of speech and nonverbal cues in conversation, are not included within the purview of the present paper.

CULTURAL MODELS OF MENTAL DISORDER: COMPARATIVE RESEARCH

Although cultural variation in beliefs about mental disorder has been studied almost as much as mental disorder itself, research in this field has not produced an accumulation of findings or a convergence of methodological approaches which could prove useful to clinical researchers or practitioners. While this failure is not unique to the domain of illness knowledge, the lack of convergence in ethnographic approaches to mental health constructs is due in part to the small number of studies in which *conceptual* description has been the primary goal of research, rather than ancillary to more broad ethnographic or clinical concerns.

Comparative psychiatric studies generally rely on fixed, standardized elicitation techniques and rarely focus explicitly on the cognitive organization of cultural constructs. For example, a number of cross-cultural psychiatric studies have addressed cultural beliefs about disorder by way of interpreting variation in epidemiological data. Researchers have used factor analysis to explore the interrelation of psychiatric constructs within non-Western societies; and have noted culturally distinctive patterns in the structure of responses to health inventories (Marsella et al. 1973; Binitie 1975). However, this research does not address cultural conceptions directly, and it is unclear whether the findings of cross-cultural variation indicate differences in the manifestation of disorder or differences in the interpretation of questions on symptom checklists. Furthermore, epidemiological research is usually based on standardized, prestructured questionnaires which may not be relevant to indigenous interpretations of symptomatology (although in some cases researchers have attempted to incorporate culture-specific constructs in the inventory of questions used to elicit symptom complaints (e.g., Beiser et al. 1976).

In contrast to the above, ethnographic studies of medical beliefs tend to present rich descriptions of particular cases or illness episodes with limited comparative significance. In only a few cases have researchers attempted to use systematic procedures or report them so that they could be applied by other researchers working elsewhere. Data are generally derived from interviews or behavioral observations organized according to the interests of the researcher, and presented in a form which is difficult to generalize or compare cross-culturally. While psychiatric and epidemiological data are usually impoverished with regard to cultural meaning, ethnographic accounts of illness beliefs are generally neither testable nor easily replicated cross-culturally.

Given the amount of ethnographic research on illness beliefs and behavior that has now been carried out, it is perhaps surprising that there is so little consensus on such fundamental issues as the recognition of particular forms of psychiatric disorder in folk knowledge across cultures. Existing research suggests that major psychoses may be viewed in substantially similar ways cross-culturally, and that the degree of similarity in conceptions of mental disorder across cultures increases with the severity of the disorder (Edgerton 1966; Murphy 1976). However, there has been little attempt to subject such an eminently testable hypothesis to experimental scrutiny. Jane Murphy (1976) has argued that, contrary to the predictions of social labeling theory (Scheff 1966; Waxler 1974), her observations in several societies, especially Eskimo and Yoruba, indicate that "similar kinds of disturbed behavior appear to be labeled abnormal in diverse cultures". Furthermore, she claims that the recurrent pattern of recognized symptoms resembles what is called schizophrenia in Western psychiatry. This conclusion is presented largely on the basis of the author's familiarity with the cultures involved, with no clear specification of procedures by which her observations were recorded or could be repeated. Murphy states that "explicit labels for insanity exist in these cultures (which) refer to beliefs, feelings, and actions that are thought to emanate from the mind or inner state of an individual and to be essentially beyond his control"; and that, "the labels of insanity refer not to single, specific attributes but to a pattern of several interlinked phenomena" (1976: 1027). However, no account of how this essentially semantic analysis was conducted is given. The veracity of these fundamental issues is left open to question and the possibilities for repeating this research in other societies are limited.

The lack of consensus on such fundamental issues as the similarity of conceptions of schizophrenia or of depression (see Singer 1975; Kleinman 1977; Marsella 1978) across cultures reflects the lack of adequate methods for the ethnographic description of cultural knowledge of illness. Few studies have focused explicitly on the linguistic and cognitive processes which underlie ordinary cultural interpretations of mental disorder and social deviance. As one author noted in his review of aboriginal American beliefs about mental disorder,

These observations on the foundations and organization of aboriginal psychiatric beliefs themselves suffer from lack of systematic approach and are not generally based on explicit, comparative methodology (Hahn 1978:51).

Fabrega has suggested that one of the first problem areas for ethnomedical research is, "The symbolic characteristics of beliefs about illness, non-illness and medical treatment" (1977:221), a view also expressed by Kleinman (1977) in his call for a "new transcultural psychiatry" which would attend explicitly to cultural definitions of illness and medicine as an essential component in clinical research and practice. Although there is general agreement that an adequate ethnography of cultural knowledge of mental disorder must begin with close attention to culture-specific modes of conceptualizing and talking about illness, there is far less agreement about the appropriate methodology for accomplishing this objective, or even about the feasibility of developing an analytic framework for genuinely comparative research.

Some of the major developments in ethnographic approaches to medical knowledge have come from paying close attention to the language used to describe and talk about illness. It is an important insight of cultural research that much of our implicit everyday knowledge about the world is reflected in ordinary language which encodes and expresses that knowledge. However, in the case of medical knowledge where linguistic terms serve an important function in designating categories used in diagnosis, the study of cultural knowledge has often been reduced to the study of lexical categories (e.g., Morice 1978). This preoccupation with lexical classification has led to a good deal of misplaced concreteness and reification of disease concepts by treating disease terms as if they were names attached to their denotata like gummed labels. Good (1977; this volume) discusses this emphasis on the "ostensive" functions of disease terminology and notes parallels between a model of illness as biomedical disease and a view of medical language as labels referring to biologically-based symptoms and diseases. There has been a tendency in the cross-cultural psychiatric literature to make casual ethnographic generalizations about mental health concepts on the basis of the presence or absence of words for particular mental disorders. The fact that a disease term may be a good indicator of under-lying folk concepts does not justify the inference that the lack of a particular term indicates the absence of a corresponding concept. Even such "object"-ified domains as botany present evidence that well-formed folk concepts may go unlabeled (Berlin et al. 1966).

THE TAXONOMY MODEL: CLASSIFICATION AND DIAGNOSIS

The first significant attempts to give systematic accounts of medical knowledge on the basis of linguistic data were based on close analysis of disease terminology as a well-structured vocabulary. One of the best examples of this genre is the study by Frake (1961) of the "diagnosis of disease" among the Subanun.

As noted above, the focus of ethnographic research on categories of illness and their structural interrelation appears to be connected with the prominent role of disease terms in diagnosis. In the medical domain, the cognitive activity of *classification* serves the social and clinical function of *diagnosis*. As a result, folk classification of illness is a much more explicit and deliberate enterprise than is classification in other areas of daily life. The "distinctive features" which define one category in contrast with another are, in the medical domain, "diagnostic criteria" which distinguish one type of illness from another (such as the "degree of penetration" which differentiates Subanun categories for different types of ulcers). Lexical or "ethnosemantic" studies attempted to discover the structure of indigenous illness categories by analyzing the referential meaning of disease terminology. This approach was based on the view, stated by Frake (1961:131), that,

Conceptually the disease world, like the plant world, exhaustively divides into a set of mutually exclusive categories. Ideally every illness either fits into one category or is describ-able as a conjunction of several categories.

One of the most important modifications of the above-stated view comes from the findings of recent research in cognitive psychology which demonstrates that folk categorization is generally neither discrete nor exclusive. Unlike classical set theory which requires that any given object either *is* or *is not* a member of a given category, the categories of ordinary language admit *degrees* of membership (Zadeh 1965: Rosch 1975; Kempton 1978). So, for example, one type of object (e.g., 'robin') may be a good example ("prototype") of a certain category ('bird'), while other members of that category (e.g., 'penguin') may only be "sort of" like that category. This type of typicality structure appears to be extremely common in the internal organization of folk categories. Psychological research is showing that differences in judgements about degrees of member-ship are often highly predictable, based on the extent of overlapping or inter-secting semantic features (Tversky 1977). Models of categories as "fuzzy" sets or as "prototypes" provide a more adequate way of representing diagnostic judg- ments which are likely to be probabilistic assessments of a cluster of symptoms as possible examples of one or more diseases with varying degrees of likelihood (Szolovits and Pauker 1978).

Far from being inconsistent with lexical studies of classification, prototype models offer more of a refinement than an alternative to the study of folk knowledge in terms of categorical structures. Basic categorical structures continue to be analyzed in terms of relations of contrast and inclusion, although these relations may be "fuzzy" rather than discrete. It is relations of inclusion of more specific categories within more general categories which give classification schemes their *taxonomic* character. Disease categories, like many other termino- logical domains, contrast with one another at successive levels of generality, forming taxonomic hierarchies in which two or more categories which contrast with one another at one level are included in a single category at a higher level (e.g., 'depression' and 'anxiety' are both 'affective disorders'). One of the appeals of the taxonomy model is that it describes a conceptual structure defined in terms of set-theoretical relations of subset and superset which exhibit highly regular logical properties. Taxonomic relations provide an economical structure for the organization, storage and retrieval of complex knowledge from memory which people use to discriminate and talk about a multitude of types of illness. As a result, taxonomic structures have been a persuasive model in ethnographic accounts of disease concepts. The seeming logical properties of illness categories have also fueled attempts to specify formal models of medical diagnosis based on classical, syllogistic types of reasoning (Fabrega 1972; Feinstein 1973; Miller 1975; Levin 1976).

Initial ethnographic studies which carried out systematic analyses of illness categories as defined by diagnostic features and organized into hierarchical structures noted specific shortcomings of the taxonomy model. The authors of one of the few genuinely comparative studies in this area wrote that,

Our early attempts to discover how diseases are categorized were based mainly on analytic models developed to describe domains of kin terms and plant names ... Attempts to construct taxonomies resulted in shallow, nonexhaustive and cross-cutting structures ... Informant responses tended to be idiosyncratic, and individuals frequently changed their responses from one session to another (D'Andrade et al. 1972:10).

A taxonomic model is most useful in analyzing the use of words for *classifica- tion* and diagnosis. This orientation is consistent with methodological approaches subsumed under the rubric of "ethnoscience" — a term which implies that people act as intuitive "scientists" in classifying the natural world. Although classifica- tion is a fundamental and universal cognitive process, it is but one of the cognitive tasks which people undertake in thinking and talking about illness. As D'Andrade observed (1976:159—160)

... the characteristics that our informants discussed in the informal interview sessions and which formed the core of the different belief clusters appeared to be consequences and preconditions of the illnesses rather than the features used to *define* them.

For example, salient aspects of Americans' beliefs about, say, tuberculosis, may include knowledge that it is contagious and serious, (see also Sontag 1978), but only minimal understandings about the bacterial pathogens which distinguish it from other forms of infection. Unconstrained discourse about the meaning of illness terms often does not refer to diagnostic features such as organic symptoms. Fabrega and Silver noted that, " ... to a Zinacanteco an illness, regardless of its specific bodily correlates, 'is' or 'means' what it connotes, mostly in terms of its severity and its socio-moral implications" (1973:112). Observations such as these have led to a progressive broadening of the range of cultural propositions examined as relevant to the conceptual organization of illness knowledge.

PROPOSITIONAL MODELS: STRUCTURE AND PROCESS

In their attempts to discover the culturally relevant aspects of illness concepts, ethnographers have broadened their analytic net to include whatever salient propositions their informants state about illness (Colson 1971; D'Andrade et al. 1972; Fabrega and Silver 1973; Clement 1974; Micklin et al. 1974; Good 1977; Young 1978). In other words, researchers have expanded their focus from a study of the linguistic meaning of illness terms to one of the social and cultural meaning of illness concepts. From this perspective, the study of illness concepts is not so much a matter of specifying the way words designate categories, as the way cognitive constructs interrelate to form coherent systems of cultural knowledge. It is in this broadened notion of cutural meaning that Good has developed the notion of "semantic network" to describe the interconnected propositions which are frequently associated with specific, key types of illness (1977, this volume).

Unlike Good who has derived models of "semantic networks" from data collected in a survey of actual cases of illness, other researchers have examined the cultural organization of illness beliefs by eliciting directly informants' judgments about salient propositions associated with specific types of illness. This has been done by deriving a set of short statements regarded as culturally relevant attributes of illness, ranging from statements about causality ('is caused by germs'), symptomatology ('gives you a runny nose'), treatment ('cures itself'), consequence ('is usually fatal') or type of victim ('afflicts children'). These propositions are then "mapped" onto various types of illness by asking a sample of informants to judge which propositions are characteristic of which diseases. This approach produces a matrix showing which propositions are associated culturally with which illnesses, as in the schematic drawing in Figure 1.

This type of data matrix may be used not only to analyze the relation of propositions to illness categories, but also to analyze relations among propositions or relations among different types of illness. So, for example, the conceptual structure of illness propositions may be examined on the basis of their relevance for various kinds of illnesses. The extent to which any two propositions are predicated of the same illnesses provides a measure of implicit similarity between them which may be derived from the analysis of two-by-two tables such as that shown in Figure 2.

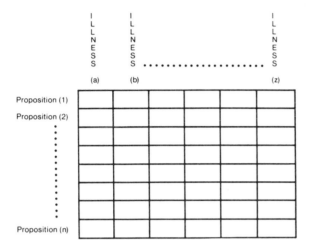

Fig. 1. Matrix of cultural propositions and illness categories.

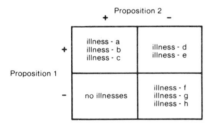

Fig. 2. Relation of two propositions based on their relevance for illness categories.

The measured similarities among all pairs of propositions reflect the cultural organization of folk knowledge about illness. The overall structure of similarities among propositions may be represented in visual models with multivariate techniques, such as hierarchical clustering and multidimensional scaling (D'Andrade et al. 1972; Clement 1974; Young 1978). Figure 3 is an example of the kind of representation of conceptual similarities among a set of illness propositions produced by combined use of multidimensional scaling and cluster analysis (from D'Andrade et al. 1972:33). The diagram depicted in Figure 3 is a two-dimensional model which represents similarity relations among propositions in terms of distance in space, and in terms of clusters which encircle propositions relatively more similar to one another. The arrangement of illness propositions in a spatial configuration can be used as a heuristic device to interpret the cultural significance or meaning of the conceptual organization of folk understandings of illness. The configuration in Figure 3 reflects two major dimensions of cultural knowledge about illness, "contagion" and "seriousness," which do seem to fit American intuitions about salient aspects of illness.

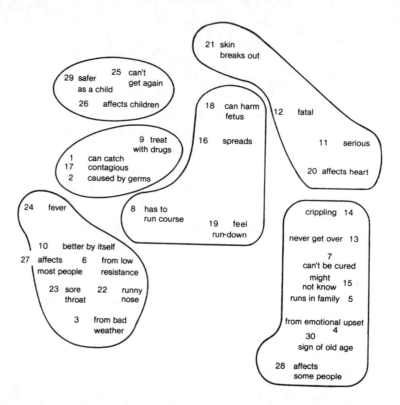

Fig. 3 Similarity relations among American propositions about illness represented by multi-dimensional scaling and hierarchical clustering (from D'Andrade et al. 1972:33).

The implicit similarities among illness types may be analyzed on the basis of shared attributes using the same procedures as those discussed above. Combining these analyses can provide a representation of the "mapping" of salient attributes onto illness types (D'Andrade et al. 1972:41). In addition to examining the similarities among illness-types or propositions, it is possible to analyze a matrix of propositional judgments in terms of the pattern of agreement and disagreement among *respondents*. This form of analysis can provide information about the social distribution of medical knowledge in a given population (e.g., Clement 1974; Mitchell and Mitchell 1980). Quantitative analysis of the distribution of cultural knowledge about illness can be used to examine specific hypotheses, such as the degree to which medical knowledge is shared by healing specialists and lay persons (Fabrega and Silver 1973: Ch. 7; Young 1979).

Ethnographic data in the form of propositional matrices are especially useful for comparative research on the variation of illness knowledge within as well as between cultures. However, there are also limitations in the adequacy of this approach for the purpose of discovering the ways in which people think and talk about illness in ordinary contexts. The type of conceptual model which can be constructed from standardized propositional judgments is constrained by the nature of procedures used to elicit judgments from informants. Among the limitations imposed by this kind of task are: (1) the use of a fixed set of illness categories and propositional frames which is usually obtained from only a few individuals, and (2) the elicitation of judgments about the attributes of illness categories in a one-at-a-time fashion which excludes the kind of social and contextual contingencies which normally influence everyday thinking about illness.

The use of a fixed set of illness categories and propositional frames has the virtue of standardization which has considerable advantages in comparative research. However, any model of the conceptual organization of illness categories will be a product of the particular items which are chosen, and would be changed in possibly unforeseen ways by the deletion or addition of further categories. Studies which have taken a more open-ended approach and simply asked informants for synonyms or word-associations to illness terms demonstrate the wide variety of potential propositions which may be obtained (Micklin et al. 1974; Tanaka-Matsumi and Marsella 1976). However, such free-response studies generally rely to a greater extent on post-hoc categorizations of responses in order to interpret their findings.

It is also likely that the self-conscious procedure by which illness categories and propositional frames are obtained in an interview setting will lead to certain kinds of items being over-represented and others being left out. One example of this situational skewing is given by Clement (this volume) in her discussion of Samoan explanations of mental disorder which avoid references to possession by 'spirits' which may be deemed unacceptable by church representatives or Europeans generally. In another example of elicitation difficulties, Sheila Cosminsky (1977) has documented that informants tend to describe the causes of illness differently depending on whether they are answering survey-type questions, or are discussing illness in extended case studies. She found that external conditions of weather, emotions and witchcraft were more often mentioned as causes of illness in case studies, which also included more statements about multiple causes than were obtained in the survey approach.

The elicitation of propositional judgments about illness in a one-at-a-time fashion extracts judgments about symptoms, causes or consequences from normal contexts in which multiple factors impinge upon the process of interpreting illness. Data in this form reflect the early focus of ethnoscience on classification, which tended to treat "questions and responses as chunks of verbiage

isolated from their settings and speakers" (Frake 1977:2) in order to derive
abstract, formal models of indigenous categorizations of illness (see also Frake
1980). This approach may omit significant information about the social contexts
and purposes which influence everyday thinking about illness.

ILLNESS AND INFERENCE

The propositional approach aims at discovering the interrelation of illness
constructs in the form of overall similarities among propositions, as in Figure 3.
However, the similarity relations depicted in Figure 3 embody a static structure
of illness propositions which fails to represent the dynamic quality of cultural
knowledge which may be used in complex ways to interpret a seemingly infinite
variety of illness events. In order to look more closely at the various ways in
which illness propositions may be combined in American common sense reasoning about illness, D'Andrade (1976) developed a procedure to specify what
logical relations, such as implication (A *implies* B), exclusion (A *contrasts with*
B) or equivalence (A *equals* B), hold between different propositions. Essentially,
this procedure determines the existence of logical relations between any two
propositions by using 2 × 2 tables such as that shown in Figure 2 to compare
systematically their associations with various types of illness. So, for example, the
absence of any illnesses associated with proposition-2 but not with proposition-1
(as indicated by "no illnesses" in the lower left-hand cell of Figure 2) indicates
that if proposition-2 is predicated of a certain kind of illness, then by *implication*
proposition-1 is also true. The kind of implicational relations obtained from
applying this procedure to illness judgments made by American college students
is shown in Figure 4 which represents a number of chains of inference which
are a subset of the overall relational analysis described above (see D'Andrade
1976 for more details).

The implicational structure shown in Figure 4 depicts reasoning processes
by which U.S. Americans, given some information about illness, might infer
additional properties, causes or consequences of that illness. In other words, it is
a *generative* model which specifies a much broader range of cognitive processes
than just the definition of illness categories in terms of diagnostic features. The
diagram represents culturally appropriate ("grammatical") paths in common
sense reasoning used to construct meaningful interpretations of illness. However,
the model suggests that a meaningful interpretation is constituted by thought
processes which go well beyond the identification or categorization of symptomatology (diagnosis). Also relevant are inferences about what type of person
is likely to be affected; what are the causes; what behavioral consequences may
result; what are appropriate treatments; and a host of other aspects of illness
experience. It is important to note that a model such as that in Figure 4 is far
from deterministic, but rather represents a range of possible inferences which
would be regarded as plausible or sensible in the framework of folk knowledge.
The potential complexity of necessary, contingent and sufficient causes of

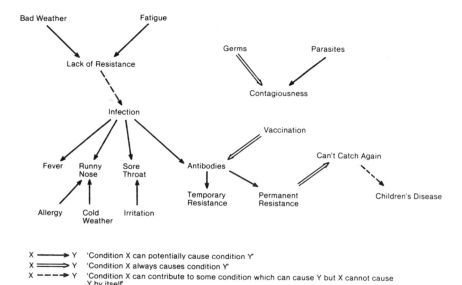

Fig. 4. Inferences in American beliefs about illness (from D'Andrade 1976:175).

illness represented in the diagram reflect the multiple, interacting conditions which impinge upon common-sense interpretations.

One of the most important types of inference to emerge from the implicational analysis of American common sense theories about illness is that of *causal* reasoning. This also proved to be the case in Good's "semantic network" analysis of the Iranian concept of "heart distress" which produced an entire clustering of folk etiological constructs. The recognition that causal inferences are a fundamental, indeed universal, aspect of folk knowledge of illness provides a framework for the comparative analysis of common-sense reasoning about illness. White (1982) used a query about 'causality' to elicit open-ended explanations of several symptom complaints from both American and Hong Kong Chinese in order to explore and compare causal inferences in the two cultures. The use of a known, relevant inferential relation ('causality') as an elicitation device, produced responses which are not constrained by a predetermined, fixed list of propositions. However, inferences elicited in this way must be further coded for relevant elements of meaning if the data are to be used for quantitative or direct, comparative analysis. In the study by White (1982), this approach revealed areas of similarity and contrast in cultural explanations obtained from Americans and Chinese for a range of 30 problem statements, some of which tended to confirm ethnographic characterizations of Chinese as more "situational" in their explanations than Americans who make greater use of psychological and affective constructs (See Kleinman 1980). An example of the format used to represent the results of comparative analysis of causal constructs associated with four types of problem statements (symptom complaints) is shown in Figure 5. The problem statements are listed in the center, with causal constructs used frequently by each cultural group shown on either side (dotted lines indicate a statistically significant contrast in the fequency with which one cultural group used a given construct in comparison with the other).

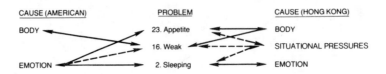

Fig. 5. Comparison of causal inferences about illness complaints among Americans and Hong Kong Chinese (dotted lines indicate $p < .05$, Fisher's Exact Test)(from White 1982).

Causal inferences have long been described as the "backbone" of folk theories of illness. The greatest emphasis in the ethnographic literature on medical beliefs has been the description of indigenous explanations of illness. Although this focus may over-emphasize the rational orientation of cognition (just as did the ethnoscience emphasis on classification), it points to a universal preoccupation with making sense, or giving meaning to illness events. As Fabrega (1974) has written, people in many different (all?) societies see occurrences of illness as behavioral discontinuities or disruptions in people's lives. A study involving interviews with both healthy and sick people in the U.S. revealed that they saw health as an

expected, normative, 'natural' property of human existence ... In contrast, illness was regarded as an intrusion, an external imposition that renders the person passive and power-less (Herzlich 1973, cited in Haan 1979:118).

Illness, it seems, induces attempts to explain it; and folk theories of illness provide the symbolic means by which to accomplish that task. Yet we know very little about how different cultures organize explanations of illness *as a conceptual task*. Most studies of cultural explanations of illness have given either fragmentary or overly abstract typologies (e.g., Foster 1976) which specify neither (1) the structuring of multiple causal factors, nor (2) the significance of causal constructs for other aspects of reasoning about illness, such as the recognition of behavioral consequences (but see Fabrega and Hunter 1979) or health-seeking decisions (see Young 1980). Promising exceptions to this state of affairs include Kleinman's (1974, 1980) formulation of a series of interrelated questions often posed by folk "explanatory models"; Young's (1976:16–17) discrimination of a least four types of etiological information evident in explanations of illness cross-culturally; D'Andrade's (1976) differentiation of 'potential', 'sufficient' and 'contributory' causal relations diagrammed in Figure 4; and

Fabrega's (this volume) distinction between 'why' ("causal") questions and 'how' ("mechanism") questions in cultural explanations.

One of the few instances of an attempt to explore the internal organization of causal reasoning and construct an explicit model of the structure of indigenous explanations of illness is given by Colson (1971a:29). The model, based on Malay data obtained through a large number of interviews, is shown in Figure 5. The value of such a model is that it makes explicit the culturally-appropriate ("allowable") inferences about the causes of illness in a way which can be checked and revised as additional interpretations of illness episodes are recorded. This form of representation also entails a certain generative capacity, in that it describes 717 possible (culturally appropriate) explanations of illness (Colson 1971a:35). The model describes several varieties of both "immediate" and "ultimate" cause which constitute four major types: "natural", "supernatural", "unethical behavior", and "inappropriate behavior"; and represents the inter-relations among the various causal constructs. However, it purposefully excludes any connections between these constructs and additional conceptual factors such as types of symptom, illness or treatment choice. Although Colson writes that, "An illness label is a summary of symptoms . . . (which) can be the result of numerous different 'causes'"; and claims further that, "the 'labeling' of a disorder does not specify or even imply an etiology" (1971a:28), it would be surprising if his Malay informants normally ponder the full range of 717 possible causal sequences in explaining a given pattern of symptoms.

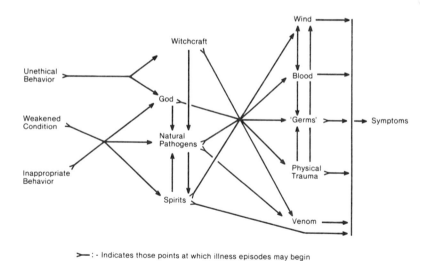

: - Indicates those points at which illness episodes may begin

Fig. 6. Malaysian theories of illness causation (from Colson 1971:29).

It is difficult to evaluate the above statement about the relation of etiology and "labeling" without examples of actual medical discourse which illustrate the process of reasoning about illness and selecting among potential causal explanations. Compare Colson's statement above to Clement's claim that "Samoan categories of mental illness are largely based upon knowledge of cause rather than classification of symptoms ... the cause is implied in the diagnosis or classification of the problem" (1974:253). Is this a matter of cultural difference, or an artifact of different ethnographic procedures? How are we to decide?

In addition to implicational relationships between type of *illness* and *causation*, a number of studies have suggested that inferences about *causation* may provide a basis for choice of *treatment*. For example, Fabrega and Silver observed that,

... the distinctions made among illnesses on the basis of cause seem to correspond to methods of curing ... The correspondence ... is salient enough to reinforce other indications that concepts of cause and cure are intimately bound up with one another in Zinacanteco medical beliefs (1973:230).

Their statement has been echoed by many ethnographic studies, including Gaines' description of decision-making by psychiatrists who " ... define problems (diagnose) in terms of their notions of etiology and from these notions come their ideas about what to do about such problems so conceived" (1979: 410). Similar inferential relations described for widely different cultures suggest that there are cross-cultural regularities in the cognitive *processes* which underlie interpretations of illness. For example, in writing about Kongo medical diagnosis, Janzen (1978:189) notes that, despite marked differences in the definition of illness,

The syllogism used is the same as in Western medicine: If symptom (or disease) A is not cured by medicines W or X, then the affliction must be disease B, for which medicines Y and Z are appropriate.

These cross-cultural similarities are echoed in Feinstein's (1973:212) argument that there are *historical* regularities in the form of diagnosis in Western medicine:

During the past century both ends of the diagnostic process [i.e., "input" (what counts as evidence) and "output" (known disease entities)] have received many alterations, but the internal rational pathway that connects input to output has retained the same general purpose and format (Brackets added).

Ethnographic accounts suggest that cultural beliefs about the association of *cause* and *cure* may be quite impervious to change on the basis of contradictory evidence (Lieban 1976). For example, the fact that a Solomon Islands' priest may not cure a particular instance of 'spirit attack' does not mean that one believes less in the efficacy of priestly cures for 'spirit attacks'. Rather, his failure implies either that the treatment process was flawed or that the diagnosis of 'spirit attack' is mistaken. Such inference-chains linking symptomatic expressions of illness, causes and treatments appear to be extremely common cross-culturally.

Just as the "health-seeking process" (Chrisman 1977) consists of goal-oriented social behavior aimed at obtaining relief from illness, the "health-inferencing process" is a sequence of cognitive operations through which existing information about illness is used to pose relevant questions and fill in missing information for a particular purpose, such as explaining a symptom-pattern, deciding about appropriate treatment, or controlling negative consequences. This cognitive process proceeds according to cultural beliefs about meaningful event structures. (See Schank and Abelson (1977) for a more general discussion about the episodic organization of common sense knowledge.) Narrative descriptions of illness episodes as well as medical "cases", the unit of professional discourse, exhibit a definite processual structure with abundant evidence about the conceptual relations which organize perceptions of health and illness. Just as actual cases of illness have an episodic structure in which symptoms may change and multiple treatments are pursued, the interpretation of illness is an active process which may be revised repeatedly on the basis of social context, new information about symptoms, or the success of a particular treatment. It is cultural beliefs about "what goes with what", "what causes what", "what cures what", etc. which make some inferences or interpretations more plausible than others. Studies which have constructed models of the sequential organization of "paths" in cultural interpretations and treatments of illness (e.g., Lewis 1975:250; Young 1976:16; Amarasingham 1980) indicate that processual models are a useful format for representing the contingent, branching structures characteristic of folk theories of illness.

THE CASE OF THE MISSING DOMAIN

The conclusion that everyday thinking about illness ranges far beyond diagnostic characteristics of disease is especially relevant for conceptions of mental disorder, where the subject-matter is more explicitly behavioral and social. Ordinary definitions of mental disorder are informed by cultural understandings about personal, social and supernatural worlds. Ethnographic investigations of conceptions of mental disorder cannot be bounded by a-priori definitions of what is symptomatic of a problem, or what counts as a possible cause or cure. The cross-cultural researcher may rightly ask, "What is 'mental' about 'mental health'?"

It is the job of ethnographic research to discover the nature of the "tasks" people are engaged in when they think and talk about mental illness. A recent review of cognitive anthropology stated that, " . . . the ethnographer's question, 'What is going on here?' is not different from the psychologist's question, 'What thought processes are involved in this task?' ", and went on to argue that theoretical debates about cultural beliefs have at times turned on the point of what people are attempting to *do* in a given context involving everyday thinking (Laboratory of Comparative Human Cognition 1978:66).

One of the major debates in psychiatry involves just such a question of task-definition. "Social-labeling" theorists such as Szasz (1961), Scheff (1966) and Rosenhan (1973) have argued that interpretations of mental disorder by lay people and psychiatrists alike are primarily a form of social control which operates through culturally shared definitions of deviant behavior. This position contrasts with the psychiatric model of mental illness which views the same interpretive process as the diagnosis of an essentially medical disorder through reasonably objective procedures. Of course, these differing views of mental illness do not necessarily contradict one another, and one needn't choose between them. However, the issue of what definitions of mental disorder are all about needn't be left to armchair theorizing. Close attention to what people are saying and doing when they talk about psychosocial problems can show to what extent people are making evaluative, moral statements and to what extent people are problem-solving in the sense of attempting to explain and cope with perceived illness.

There is abundant evidence to suggest that ordinary discourse about mental disorder, at least in clinical settings, involves both sorts of "task". Analysis of conversations between practitioner and client in diagnostic and therapeutic situations indicates that much of what a client says is an attempt to define a role for himself in relation to the practitioner or others outside the clinical setting (Labov and Fanshel 1977; Caughey 1978). In contrast, Kleinman (1980: 105) suggests that individuals afflicted with illness commonly seek answers to five types of questions which range from "etiology" to "treatment". These questions all presuppose that implicit "explanatory models" resemble closely the medical process of diagnosing and treating disease. As Kleinman also observes, this type of illness-oriented problem solving is undoubtedly integrated closely with clients' social and moral preoccupations. Claims that one "task" or the other, social control or medical treatment, predominates in cultural interpretations of mental disorder have generally rested on thin ethnographic ice. J. K. Wing has written that, " ... the two concepts of 'illness' — disease theory and social attribution — exist side by side" (1978:19). One can only agree, except to note that these "concepts" are by no means distinct or compartmentalized in common sense knowledge of illness.

One of the most promising areas of comparative research is the interconnection of these two aspects of common sense thinking about illness: implicit "theories" of disease, and ethnopsychological "theories" of social behavior. Conceptions of mental disorder must articulate with cultural conceptions of the person and social reality. It is, universally, people who become ill or disturbed. How this is viewed within a cultural community depends as much on ideas about persons and social behavior as on ideas about disease (Hallowell 1967; Levy 1973; Selby 1974; Strauss 1977).

Comparative research on cultural conceptions of the person suggests that Western views of the person as a "bounded, unique, more or less integrated motivational and cognitive universe" are by no means universal (Geertz 1973; Shweder and Bourne, this volume). The seemingly obvious notion that a person acts on the basis of a bundle of feelings, motives and intentions, housed within the individual is, in fact, specific to a particular cultural way of looking at the social world. Although it is risky to invoke the stereotype of Western society as "individualistic", this seems an apt characterization of cultural themes which organize American beliefs about persons and behaviors, in contrast with certain non-Western cultures as argued by Shweder and Bourne (this volume) and Murase (this volume). In the English-speaking world, the interpretation of illness and social behavior is often "psychologized" by describing or explaining it in terms of person-centric constructs like "mind", "personality" and "emotion". This was a finding of the study by White (1982) mentioned earlier, in which Americans made greater use of emotive constructs in explaining somatic complaints than did Hong Kong Chinese (see Figure 5). It is important to note that the "psychologization" of concepts of illness and social behavior is by no means uniform in Western cultures (see Gaines, this volume). A number of studies suggest that personal distress is expressed more frequently with psychological constructs by White, educated and upper-middle class individuals (Derogatis et al. 1971). Members of these populations are more frequently judged "suitable for psychotherapy", *even when diagnosis is held constant* (Meltzer 1978).

Psychotherapy, especially psychoanalysis, which is embedded in Western cultural traditions, attempts to treat mental disorder and alter deviant behavior by probing the individual as a storehouse of past experiences, more or less in isolation from his social environment (Pande 1968). Even when emotive constructs are employed in non-Western psychotherapies, they may only mediate physical and environmental factors which are regarded as the root sources of disorder (Wu, this volume). A recent study examining the type of interpersonal problems expressed in psychotherapy chose to identify problem-statements on the basis of sentences in the general form "I can't . . . (do something)" (Horowitz 1979). The use of these sorts of person-centric constructs in this study makes a clear statement about the way in which even interpersonal problems are phrased in an idiom focused on the individual as a unitary, active agent.

Comparative research is beginning to highlight some of the implicit characteristics of Western concepts of personhood and social behavior which guide theory building in both social science and psychiatry. Among the characteristics of Western person-concepts which seem to influence cultural definitions of mental disorder, is the primacy given to internal, mentalistic constructs (such as 'minds' and 'personalities') in explaining social events and psychiatric disorder. This type of causal inference segregates the individual conceptually from perceived influences in the external environment, both social and supernatural. Just how different this person-centered mode may be in contrast to non-Western beliefs is discussed by many of the authors in this volume, especially Shweder and Bourne. Fabrega and Silver noted that " . . . systematic ideas about the structure and function of the body are not important in Zinacanteco medical knowledge. What are important are concepts of causality . . . " (1973:87); and "To some extent, Zinacantecos also lack the concept of self that is internally housed, autonomous, and separate from the selves of other "objects", i.e., persons, things, deities, or animals" (90). Similar observations have been made in a wide range of ethnographic studies. For example, Janzen writes, "Kongo etiology consistently draws the effective boundary of the person differently, more expansively, than classical Western medicine, philosophy and religion" (1978: 189).

These fundamental characteristics of social perception may have pervasive influences on the nature of cultural interpretations of mental illness. Given an explanatory system not defined on the basis of autonomous individuals, it is understandable that folk healing may focus more on relationships (with other people, or with supernatural entities) than with processes internal to the individual. This orientation is evident in the cultural form of certain kinds of "therapy" in Santa Isabel, Solomon Islands. Both illness and social conflict are "treated" with a ritualistic form of verbal and social interaction known as 'disentangling'. A 'disentangling' session may focus on the ailments of one individual, or on social strains evident in the community. In either case, 'disentangling' sessions provide a context for the public discussion of conflicted relations within a particular group (usually kinship), in order to locate the social and interpersonal causes of illness. Close attention to the nature of conversation in such 'disentangling' sessions indicates that discussion of 'emotion' is aimed more at correcting "entangled" social relations than at describing the internal states of individuals (White 1979, 1980; see also Ito 1978).

In global perspective, this sort of causal reasoning which looks for social interdependencies in constructing accounts of illness or behavior, seems more prevalent than the type of person-centric explanations typical of American culture. The underlying logic or cultural rationale of 'disentangling'' sessions in Santa Isabel is evident in a great many ethnographic accounts which have noted expanded definitions of personhood which seem to encompass various significant others, such that actions of one person (especially moral transgressions) may have direct consequences (such as illness or misfortune) for other, related persons. In these systems of belief, ill-health is one of the most potent symbols of social conflict and moral transgression (see also Turner 1964).

It is important to note that such notions as conceptions of "the person" are at least as susceptible to reification as conceptions of illness. There is a growing amount of evidence that the way in which cultures define personal and social worlds can have a definite impact on the course and outcome of serious mental disorders, such as schizophrenia (IPSS 1973, Waxler 1979). However, these observed differences in the outcome of treatment for schizophrenia are "explained" on the basis of cultural constructs which have so far not received a convincing, satisfactory account in ethnographic research. We have almost no framework for conducting comparative investigations of social perception in explicit linguistic or cognitive terms which would bring such complex notions as "the self" or "the person" into the realm of ethnographic and experimental scrutiny. The study by White (1982) suggests that both *within-culture* coherence and *between-culture* contrasts in folk explanations of illness are linked to more fundamental assumptions about personhood and social behavior. And the research reported by Shweder and Bourne (this volume) indicates that it is possible to identify specific features of social cognition which correspond with cultural variations in person concepts. In their analysis, the use of personality trait words in contrast to situation-specific vocabulary in explanations of social events, provides a reliable indication of cultural differences in conceptions of the social universe. Continued development of our ability to give adequate ethnographic accounts of social cognition may increase the role of cultural variables in future mental health research.

CONCLUSION

This paper began by alluding to the influence of implicit cultural models on the interpretation of mental disorder by lay persons and professionals alike. Cultural knowledge structures people's responses to those disruptive intrusions which are labeled "illness" or "craziness" and which evoke attempts at explanation. Although it is largely cross-cultural research which has produced an awareness of the role of cultural models in illness behavior and mental health services, the significance of such implicit models is by no means confined to "exotic" or plural populations. Cultural beliefs about illness and social behavior are an important ingredient in ordinary, everyday explanations of disorder as well as in clinical judgments in mental health research and practice. It is through the discovery and description of such cultural constructs that we may gain explicit understanding of the cognitive and social processes which organize interpretations of and responses to illness events.

A review of methodological issues in the study of cultural models of mental disorders shows that there have been few studies aimed primarily at describing the conceptual organization of folk knowledge about illness, especially "mental disorder". Formal analyses of illness constructs have shown that it is possible to study systematically the distribution of medical knowledge in specific populations. In addition, procedures have been devised to represent cognitive processes which structure cultural reasoning about illness. However, formal models of illness beliefs have often produced overly static and narrowly "medical" descriptions of folk knowledge. Recent ethnographic approaches to the study of everyday thinking about illness have included a progressively wider range of cultural constructs which appear relevant to the kinds of inferences people make about physical or behavioral disturbance. Comparative research suggests that perceptions of mental disorder are informed by basic cultural assumptions about the nature of personhood and social behavior. Further studies of the linkages between specific types of illness beliefs and socio-moral constructs may yield significant generalizations about mental disorder across cultures.

ACKNOWLEDGMENTS

This paper has profited from helpful comments by Dorothy Clement Holland and Arthur Kleinman. I would also like to acknowledge the support of the Social Science Research Council Foreign Area Program and the Wenner-Gren Foundation for Anthropological Research for fieldwork carried out in the Solomon Islands between 1974 and 1976.

REFERENCES

Amarasingham, L. R.
   1980 Movement Among Healers in Sri Lanka: A Case Study of a Sinhalese Patient. Culture, Medicine and Psychiatry 4: 71–92.
Beiser, M., et al.
   1976 Measuring Psychoneurotic Behavior in Cross-Cultural Surveys. The Journal of Nervous and Mental Disease 163:10–23.
Berlin, B., D. E. Breedlove, and P. H. Raven
   1968 Covert Categories and Folk Taxonomies. American Anthropologist 70:290–299.
Binitie, A.
   1975 A Factor-Analytic Study of Depression Across Cultures (African and European). British Journal of Psychiatry 127:559–563.
Carroll, J. S. and J. W. Payne
   1976 Cognition and Social Behavior. New York: Wiley.
Caughey, J.
   1978 Identity Struggles in the Mental Status Examination. Paper presented at the 77th Annual Meetings of the American Anthropological Association. Los Angeles, California.
Chrisman, N. J.
   1977 The Health Seeking Process: An Approach to the Natural History of Illness. Culture, Medicine and Psychiatry 1:351–377.
Clement, D.
   1974 Samoan Concepts of Mental Illness and Treatment. Unpublished Ph.D. dissertation. University of California, Irvine.
Clements, F. E.
   1932 Primitive Concepts of Disease. University of California: Publications in American Archeology and Ethnology 32:185–252.
Colson, A. C.
   1971a The Prevention of Illness in a Malay Village: An Analysis of Concepts and Behavior. Winston Salem: Wake Forest University Developing Nations Monograph Series.
   1971b The Perception of Abnormality in a Malay Village. In Psychological Problems and Treatment in Malaysia. N. Wagner and E. Tan (eds.). pp. 88–101. Kuala Lumpur: University of Malaya Press.
Conklin, H. C.
   1972 Folk Classification. New Haven: Yale University Department of Anthropology.
Cosminsky, S.
   1977 The Impact of Illness Concepts in a Guatamalan Community. Social Science and Medicine 11:325–332.

D'Andrade, R. G.
   1976 A Propositional Analysis of U.S. American Beliefs About Disease. *In* Meaning in Anthropology. K. Basso and H. Selby (eds.). Albuquerque: University of New Mexico Press.
D'Andrade, R. G., N. Quinn, S. Nerlove, and K. Romney
   1972 Categories of Disease in American-English and Mexican-Spanish. *In* Multidimensional Scaling: Theory and Applications in the Behavioral Sciences, Volume 2, Applications. A. Romney, R. Shephard, and S. Nerlove (eds.). pp. 9–54. New York: Seminar Press, Inc.
Derogatis, L., et al.
   1971 Social Class and Race as Mediator Variables in Neurotic Symptomology. Archives of General Psychiatry 24:454–464.
Edgerton, R. B.
   1966 Conceptions of Psychosis in Four East African Societies. American Anthropologist 68:408–425.
Eisenberg, L.
   1977 Disease and Illness: Distinctions Between Professional and Popular Ideas of Sickness. Culture, Medicine and Psychiatry 1:9–23.
Elstein, A. S.
   1976 Clinical Judgment: Psychological Research and Medical Practice. Science 194:696–700.
Fabrega, H.
   1972 Concepts of Disease: Logical Features and Social Implications. Perspectives in Biology and Medicine 15:583–616.
   1974 Disease and Social Behavior. Cambridge: MIT Press.
   1977 The Scope of Ethnomedical Science. Culture, Medicine and Psychiatry 1:221–228.
Fabrega, H. and J. Hunter
   1979 Beliefs About the Behavioral Effects of Disease: A Mathematical Analysis. Ethnology 18:271–290.
Fabrega, H. and D. B. Silver
   1973 Illness and Shamanistic Curing in Zinacantan: An Ethnomedical Analysis. Stanford: Stanford University Press.
Feinstein, A. R.
   1973 An Analysis of Diagnostic Reasoning. Yale Journal of Biology and Medicine 46:212–232.
Foster, G. M.
   1976 Disease Etiologies in Non-Western Medical Systems. American Anthropologist 78:773–782.
Frake, C. O.
   1961 The Diagnosis of Disease Among the Subanun of Mindanao. American Anthropologist 63:113–132.
   1977 Plying Frames Can Be Dangerous: Some Reflections on Methodology in Cognitive Anthropology. The Quarterly Newsletter of the Institute for Comparative Human Development 1(3):1–7.
   1980 Interpretations of Illness: An Ethnographic Perspective on Events and Their Causes. *In* Language and Cultural Description. C. P. Frake (ed.). Stanford: Stanford University Press.
Gaines, A. D.
   1979 Definitions and Diagnoses: Cultural Implications of Psychiatric Help-Seeking and Psychiatrists' Definitions of the Situation in Psychiatric Emergencies. Culture, Medicine and Psychiatry 3:381–418.

Geertz, C.
  1973 Person, Time and Conduct in Bali. *In* The Interpretation of Cultures. C. Geertz (ed.). pp. 360–411. New York: Basic Books.
Good, B. J.
  1977 The Heart of What's the Matter: The Semantics of Illness in Iran. Culture, Medicine and Psychiatry 1:25–58.
Haan, N. G.
  1979 Psychosocial Meanings of Unfavorable Medical Forecasts. *In* Health Psychology. G. Stone, F. Cohen, and N. Adler (eds.). pp. 113–140. San Francisco: Jossey Bass.
Hahn, R. A.
  1978 Aboriginal American Psychiatric Theories. Transcultural Psychiatric Research Review 15:29–58.
Hallowell, A. I.
  1960 Ojibwa Ontology, Behavior and World View. *In* Culture in History. S. Diamond (ed.). New York: Columbia University Press.
  1967 The Self and Its Behavioral Environment. *In* Culture and Experience. A. I. Hallowell (ed.). New York: Schocken Books.
Herzlich, C.
  1973 Health and Illness: A Social-Psychological Analysis. New York: Academic Press.
Horowitz, L. M.
  1979 On the Cognitive Structure of Interpersonal Problems Treated in Psychotheray. Journal of Consulting and Clinical Psychology 47:5–15.
Horowitz, L. M., R. S. French, and C. Anderson
  1981 The Prototype of a Lonely Person. *In* Loneliness: A Sourcebook of Current Theory, Research and Therapy. L. Peplau and D. Perlman (eds.). New York: Wiley-Interscience.
International Pilot Study of Schizophrenia
  1973 Report of the International Pilot Study of Schizophrenia, 1. Geneva: World Health Organization.
Ito, K.
  1978 Symbolic Conscience: Illness Retribution Among Urban Hawaiian Women. Unpublished Ph.D. Dissertation, University of California, Los Angeles.
Janzen, J. M.
  1978 The Quest for Therapy in Lower Zaire. Berkeley: University of California Press.
Katz, M. M., J. O. Cole, and H. A. Lowrey
  1969 Studies of the Diagnostic Process: The Influence of Symptom Perception, Past Experience, and Ethnic Background on Diagnostic Decisions. American Journal of Psychiatry 125:109–119.
Kay, P.
  1971 Taxonomy and Semantic Contrast. Language 47:866–877.
Kempton, W.
  1978 Cateogry Grading and Taxonomic Relations: A Mug is a Sort of a Cup. American Ethnologist 5:44–65.
Kleinman, A.
  1974 The Use of "Explanatory Models" as a Conceptual Frame for Comparative Cross-Cultural Research on Illness Experiences and the Basic Tasks of Clinical Care Amongst Chinese and Other Populations. *In* Medicine in Chinese Cultures. A. Kleinman et al. (eds.). pp. 645–658. Washington, D.C.: U.S. Government Printing Office.
  1977 Depression, Somatization and the "New Cross-Cultural Psychiatry". Social Science and Medicine 11:3–10.
  1980 Patients and Healers in the Context of Culture: An Exploration of the Borderland

Between Anthropology, Medicine and Psychiatry. Berkeley: University of California Press.

Laboratory of Comparative Human Cognition.
1978 Cognition As A Residual Category in Anthropology. Annual Review of Anthropology 7:51–69.

Labov, W. and D. Fanshel
1977 Therapeutic Discourse: Psychotherapy As Conversation. New York: Academic Press.

Lazare, A.
1973 Hidden Conceptual Models in Clinical Psychiatry. The New England Journal of Medicine 288:345–351.

Leff, J. P.
1973 Culture and the Differentiation of Emotional States. British Journal of Psychiatry 123:299–306.

Levin, J.
1976 Proteus: An Activation Framework for Cognitive Process Models. Unpublished Ph.D. dissertation. University of California, San Diego.

Levy, R. I.
1973 The Tahitians: Mind and Experience in the Society Islands. Chicago: Chicago University Press.

Lewis, G.
1975 Knowledge of Illness in a Sepik Society. London: The Athlone Press.

Lieban, R. W.
1976 Traditional Medical Beliefs and the Choice of Practitioners in a Philippine City. Social Science and Medicine 10:289–296.

Marsella, A. J.
1978 Thoughts on Cross-Cultural Studies of the Epidemology of Depression. Culture, Medicine and Psychiatry 2:343–357.

Marsella, A. J., D. Kinzie, and P. Gordon
1973 Ethnic Variations in the Expression of Depression. Journal of Cross-Cultural Psychology 4:435–458.

Meltzer, J. D.
1978 A Semiotic Approach to Suitability for Psychotherapy. Psychiatry 41:360–376.

Micklin, M., M. Durbin, and C. Leon
1974 The Lexicon for Madness in a Colombian City: An Exploration in Semantic Space. American Ethnologist 1:143–156.

Miller, P. B.
1975 Strategy Selection in Medical Diagnosis. Cambridge: MIT Technical Report #153.

Mitchell, H. F. and J. C. Mitchell
1980 Social Factors in the Perception of the Causes of Disease. In Numerical Techniques in Social Anthropology. J. C. Mitchell (ed.). Philadelphia: Institute for the Study of Human Issues.

Morice, R.
1978 Psychiatric Diagnosis in a Transcultural Setting: The Importance of Lexical Categories. British Journal of Psychiatry 132:87–95.

Murphy, J. M.
1976 Psychiatric Labeling in Cross-Cultural Perspective. Science 191:1019–1028.

Nunnally, J. C.
1961 Popular Conceptions of Mental Health. New York: Holt, Rinehart and Winston, Inc.

Pande, S. K.
1968 The Mystique of "Western" Psychotherapy: An Eastern Interpretation. Journal of Nervous and Mental Disease 146:425–432.

Rabinow, P. and W. Sullivan, eds.
   1979 Interpretive Social Science. Berkeley: University of California Press.
Rosch, E.
   1975 Universals and Culture Specifics in Human Categorization. *In* Cross-Cultural
         Perspectives on Learning. R. W. Brislin, S. Bochner, W. J. Lonner (eds.). pp.
         177–206. New York: Wiley.
Rosenhan, D.
   1973 On Being Sane in Insane Places. Science 179:250–258.
Scheff, T.
   1966 Being Mentally Ill: A Sociological Theory. Chicago: Aldine.
Selby, H.
   1974 Zapotec Deviance: The Convergence of Folk and Modern Sociology. Austin:
         University of Texas Press.
Schank, R. and R. Abelson
   1977 Scripts, Plans, Goals and Understanding: An Inquiry Into Human Knowledge
         Structures. Hillsdale, NJ: Lawrence Erlbaum Associates.
Shweder, R. A.
   1977a Illusory Correlation and the M.M.P.I. Controversy. Journal of Consulting and
         Clinical Psychology 45:917–924.
   1977b Likeness and Likelihood in Everyday Thought: Magical Thinking in Judgments
         About Personality. Current Anthropology 18:637–648.
Shweder, R. A. and R. G. D'Andrade.
   1980 The Systematic Distortion Hypothesis. *In* New Directions for Methodology of
         Behavioral Science: Fallible Judgment in Behavioral Research. R. Shweder (ed.).
         San Francisco: Jossey-Bass.
Singer, K.
   1975 Depressive Disorders From a Transcultural Perspective. Social Science and Medi-
         cine 9:289–301.
Sontag, S.
   1978 Illness as Metaphor. New York: Farrar, Straus and Giroux.
Strauss, A. D.
   1977 Northern Cheyenne Ethnopsychology. Ethos 5:326–357.
Szasz, T. S.
   1961 The Myth of Mental Illness: Foundations of a Theory of Personal Conduct. New
         York: Harper.
Szolovits, P. and S. G. Pauker
   1978 Categorical and Probabilistic Reasoning in Medical Diagnosis. Artificial Intelligence
         11:115–144.
Tanaka-Matsumi, J. and A. J. Marsella
   1976 Cross-Cultural Variations in the Phenomenological Experience of Depression:
         Word Association. Journal of Cross-Cultural Psychology 7:379–396.
Townsend, J. M.
   1978 Cultural Conceptions and Mental Illness: A Comparison of Germany and America.
         Chicago: University of Chicago Press.
   1979 Stereotypes and Mental Illness: A Comparison With Ethnic Stereotypes. Culture,
         Medicine and Psychiatry 3:205–230.
Turner, V.
   1964 An Ndembu Doctor in Practice. *In* Magic, Faith and Healing. A. Kiev (ed.). pp.
         230–263. New York: Free Press.
Tversky, A.
   1977 Features of Similarity. Psychological Review 84:327–352.

Waxler, N. E.
  1974 Culture and Mental Illness: A Social Labeling Perspective. Journal of Nervous
        and Mental Disease 159:379–395.
  1979 Is Outcome for Schizophrenia Better in Traditional Societies? The Case of Sri
        Lanka. Journal of Nervous and Mental Disease 167:144–158.
White, G. M.
  1979 Some Social Uses of Emotion Language: A Melanesian Example. Paper presented
        at the 78th annual meetings of the American Anthropological Association. Cincin-
        nati, Ohio. November 28–December 1, 1979.
  1980 Conceptual Universals in Interpersonal Language. American Anthropologist 82:
        759–781.
  1982 The Role of Cultural Explanations in "Psychologization" and "Somatization".
        Social Science and Medicine 16:1519–1530.
Wing, J. K.
  1978 Reasoning About Madness. Oxford: Oxford University Press.
Young, A.
  1976 Some Implications of Medical Beliefs and Practices for Social Anthropology.
        American Anthropologist 78:5–24.
Young, J. C.
  1978 Illness Categories and Action Strategies in a Tarascan Town. American Ethno-
        logist 5:81–97.
  1979 Variation in a Mexican Folk Medical Belief System. Paper presented at the 14th
        Annual Meeting of the Southern Anthropological Society. Memphis, Tennessee,
        February 21–24, 1979.
  1980 A Model of Illness Treatment Decisions in a Tarascan Town. American Ethno-
        logist 7:106–131.
Zadeh, L. A.
  1965 Fuzzy Sets. Information and Control 8:33–353.

RICHARD A. SHWEDER AND EDMUND J. BOURNE

DOES THE CONCEPT OF THE PERSON VARY
CROSS-CULTURALLY?

INTRODUCTION

Our concern in this essay is with other people's conceptions of the person and ideas about the self. Our aim is to interpret a widespread mode of social thought often referred to as concrete, undifferentiated, context-specific, or occasion-bound thinking, a mode of social thought culminating in the view that specific situations determine the moral character of a particular action, that the individual person *per se* is neither an object of importance nor inherently worthy of respect, that the individual as moral agent ought not be distinguished from the social status s(he) occupies; a view that, indeed, the individual as an abstract *ethical* and *normative* category is not to be acknowledged.

Our aim, we wish to emphasize, is to interpret an alien mode of social thought. Thus, before we look at the person concepts of such peoples as the Oriya, Gahuku-Gama, and Balinese we feel obliged to consider a more fundamental question: In what terms should we understand the understandings of other peoples and compare those understandings with our own?

For over 100 years anthropologists have tried to make sense of alien idea systems. For over 100 years anthropologists have been confronted with all sorts of incredible and often unbelievable beliefs, as well as all sorts of incredible and often unbelievable accounts of other people's beliefs. A review of the history of the anthropological attempt to translate the meaning of oracles and witchcraft, wandering and reincarnated souls, magical "therapies", unusual ideas about procreation, and all the other exotic ideational formations that have come their way would reveal, we believe, a tendency to rely on one of three interpretive models for rendering intelligible the apparent diversity of human understandings. These three interpretive models can be referred to as *universalism*, *evolutionism*, and *relativism*.

There is a fourth model; perhaps it should be named *confusion(ism)*. Confusion(ism) calls for the honest confession that one fails to comprehend the ideas of another. We will not have much to say about confusion(ism) in this essay. We would, however, like to confess, right here, that not infrequently we are left in a muddled condition, especially when we are told, without exegesis, such incredible things as, e.g., the Bongo-Bongo believe that their sorcerers are bushcats, their minds are located in their knees, and their father is a tree, or when we read, e.g., that the Guki-Gama cannot distinguish between the products of their imagination and the objects of their perceptions.

Many anthropological accounts lack intelligibility. One does not know what to make of them; whether to treat them as accurate reports about the confused

97

A. J. Marsella and G. M. White (eds.), Cultural Conceptions of Mental Health and Therapy,
97–137.

and/or erroneous beliefs of others or dismiss them as bad translations; whether to search for common understandings hidden behind superficial idiomatic differences; or whether, alternatively to generously assume that the ideas of the other form a coherent system derived from premises, or related to purposes, that the anthropologist has failed to appreciate. Although we will not have much to say about confusion(ism) we would like to discuss, however briefly, the three other deeply entrenched models of anthropological interpretation: *universalism, evolutionism*, and *relativism*.

Universalists are committed to the view that intellectual diversity is more apparent than real, that exotic idea systems, alien at first blush, are really more like our own than they initially appear.

Evolutionists are committed to the view that alien idea systems not only are truly different from our own, but are different in a special way; viz., other people's systems of ideas are really incipient and less adequate stages in the development of our own understandings.

Relativists, in contrast, are committed to the view that alien idea systems, while fundamentally different from our own, display an internal coherency which, on the one hand, can be understood but, on the other hand, cannot be judged.

The universalist opts for homogeneity. "Apparently different but really the same" is his slogan. Diversity is sacrificed to equality; equal because not different! The evolutionist, however, opts for hierarchy. Diversity is not only tolerated, it is expected, *and it is ranked*. "Different but unequal" is the slogan of the evolutionist. The relativist, in contrast, is a pluralist. "Different but equal" is his slogan; equality *and* diversity his "democratic" aspiration.

UNIVERSALISM, EVOLUTIONISM, AND RELATIVISM: INTERPRETIVE RULES OF THUMB

Universalists, evolutionists, and relativists all try to process information about alien idea systems following rules of thumb peculiar to their interpretive model of choice. Indeed, the universalist, evolutionist and relativist each has his way of processing data to help him arrive at his desired interpretation.

Universalism

Confronted with the apparent diversity of human understandings, there are two powerful ways to discover universals in one's data: (a) emphasize general likenesses and overlook specific differences ("the higher-order generality rule"): and/or (b) examine only a subset of the evidence ("the data attenuation rule").

1. *The higher-order generality rule*. Osgood's (1964) investigations of universals in connotative meaning illustrate the application of the "higher-order generality rule". Emphasizing the way things are alike, and ignoring the ways they are

different, Osgood discovers that all peoples appraise objects and events in terms of three universal dimensions, viz. good vs. bad (evaluation), strong vs. weak (potency), and fast vs. slow (activity). The universals are discovered, in part, by moving to a level of discourse so general that "God" and "Ice Cream" are descriptively equivalent; both are perceived as good, strong, and active.

The tendency to overlook specific difference and emphasize general likeness is ubiquitous among universalists. In Levi-Strauss' mind (1963, 1966, 1969a, b), for example, the distinction between, e.g., voiced/unvoiced (in phonetics), raw/cooked (in the culinary arts), sexual reproduction/asexual reproduction (in the Oedipus Myth), and exogamy/endogamy (in marriage systems) are all rendered equivalent, each an example of a purported human tendency to think in terms of binary oppositions [Is this a trivially true logical claim, or a false empirical claim?]. For ethologists and sociobiologists it is "conversation" (in human primates) and "barking" (e.g., in canine folk) that are voiced in the same breath, each an example of a universal "signaling" function of communication systems [What does a cow say? Moo! What does a sheep say? Baa! What does a person say?], while for others it is "marriage" and "pair-bonding" whose general affinities are made much of at the expense of potentially significant grounds for divorce [what ever happened to the "sanctity" of marriage?].

2. *The data attenuation rule.* Not infrequently, the discovery of a universal is the product of a sophisticated process of data restriction and data attenuation. Berlin and Kay (1969), for example, discover universal prototypes for the definition of color categories, and a universal sequence for the emergence of a color lexicon. Their study begins with two applications of the data attenuation rule. First, "color" classification is equated with the task of partitioning a perceptual space, pre-defined in terms of hue, saturation and intensity (thus, attenuating the referential range of the "color" concept as understood by, at least, some cultures (Conklin 1955). Secondly, all color categories whose linguistic expression fails to meet certain formal criteria (e.g., superordination, monolexemic unity) are eliminated from consideration. The consequence of the application of these two data attentuation rules is that 95% of the world's expressions for color and most of the world's color categories are dropped from the investigation.

A second illustration of the data attenuation rule can be found in Nerlove and Romney's (1967) work on universal cognitive processes underlying the formation of "sibling" terminological systems. A major finding of their study is the universal disinclination of the human mind to process disjunctive categories (e.g., it is rare to have the same "sibling" term apply distinctively to both a younger sister and an older brother). Yet Nerlove and Romney consider only one portion of the referential range of "sibling terms" (nuclear family referents). Secure in the conviction that nuclear family referents are expandable prototypes, they decide not to examine the application in many cultures of "sibling" terms to such (disjunctive?) kin types as "cousins" etc.

3. *Universalism's benefits and costs.* There are benefits and costs to the adoption of a universalist stance. A major benefit is the thrill of recognition[My God! They're just like me after all!] that comes with the identification of a significant point of resemblance. An Azande consults the chicken oracle (see Evans-Pritchard 1937). "Will I be killed on my journey to Z?" The chicken is administered a magical "poison". If the chicken dies it means "Yes"; if it lives, "No". The chicken lives. A second chicken is consulted. This time the chicken's survival is taken as a caution to stay at home. But, the chicken dies. Reassured, our Azande goes on the journey to Z. He is murdered en route! Do the Azande doubt the veracity of their oracle? No! Instead they explain away the event in one of two ways. Counter-witchcraft was being practiced at the time of consultation, or perhaps women, standing too close, had polluted the consultation grounds. Should one fail to notice within these practices some of the methodological concepts of the Western applied scientist (?), viz., reliability checks (double consultations), interfering background variables (counter-witchcraft), and measurement error (pollution). The idioms differ, but they are easily overlooked in the light of the recognition that the Azande's search for truth relies on principles not unlike our own.

Universalism, however, has its difficulties. All too often the pursuit after a "higher-order generality" is like searching for the "real" artichoke by divesting it of its leaves (Wittgenstein 1958, paragraph 164). The "higher-order" sphere is all too often a higher-order of vacuity, the air gets very thin.

Consider, for example, the concept of "justice" ("fairness" or "equity"). Stated as a higher-order generality ("treat like cases alike and different cases differently") "justice" is a universal concept. Appreciate, however, the laundered emptiness of this higher-order formulation. As Hart (1961:155) remarks: the abstract concept of justice

cannot afford any determinate guide to conduct ... This is so because any set of human beings will resemble each other in some respects and differ from each other in others and, until it is established what resemblances and differences are relevant, 'treat like cases alike' must remain an empty form.

For example, Americans deny 10 year olds the right to vote, enter into contracts, etc. This exclusion, however, does not violate our abstract concept of justice. Quite the contrary, it indicates that we subscribe to the belief that in certain crucial respects, children are different from adults (e.g., they lack the information and judgement to make informed decisions, etc.). From a cross-cultural and historical perspective there have been many places in the world where, given received wisdom and without relinquishing the "higher-order" concept of justice, the difference between male and female, Jew and Christian, Brahman and untouchable, Black and White, has seemed as obvious to others as the difference between an adult and a child seems to us. Unfortunately, all these concrete, culture-rich ("thick" if you will; see Geertz 1973) variations in the way people treat each other get bleached out of focus in the "higher-order" description of "justice" as an abstract universal. Universality of agreement wanes as we move from higher-order abstract principles to substantive cases.

Application of the "data attenuation rule" has its costs, as well. These costs are clearly understood by Berlin and Kay (1969:160) who note:

... it has been argued, to our minds convincingly, that to appreciate the full cultural signif-icance of color words it is necessary to appreciate the full range of meanings, both referential and connotative, and not restrict oneself arbitrarily to hue, saturation, and brightness. We thus make no claim — in fact we specifically deny — that our treatment of the various color terminologies presented here is an ethnographically revealing one.

The path traveled by the universalist is rarely the one that leads to ethnographic illumination; only occasionally does it lead to a powerful, context-rich universal generalization. However, when it does it should not be scorned.

Evolutionism

Confronted with the apparent diversity of human understandings, evolutionists rely on a powerful three-stage rule of thumb for ordering that variety into a sequence of lower to higher (primitive to advanced, incipient to elaborated) forms; viz., (a) locate a normative model (e.g., the canons of propositional calculus, Bayes' rules of statistical inference, Newton's laws of motion, Rawl's theory of justice, Mill's rules for experimental reasoning, etc.); (b) treat the normative model as the endpoint of development; (c) Describe diverse beliefs and understandings as steps on an ideational Jacob's ladder progressively moving in the direction of the normative endpoint (see e.g., Piaget 1966; Kohlberg 1969, 1971).

The normative model *defines* what it is to have an adequate understanding (e.g., given that $P \rightarrow Q$ it is more adequate to conclude $\sim Q \rightarrow \sim P$ than to con-clude $\sim P \rightarrow \sim Q$). Variations in thought are ranked in terms of their degree of approximation to the endpoint. The image is one of subsumption, progress, and hierarchical inclusion. Some forms of understanding are described as though they were incipient forms of other understandings, and those other forms of understanding are described as though they can do everything the incipient forms can do plus more (see Figure 1a); post-Copernican astronomy replaces pre-Copernican astronomy — experimental logic (Mill's laws of agreement and difference) replaces magical thinking (Frazer's laws of contagion and similarity). If the subsumed, less adequate form of understanding can also be time-dated, i.e., linked to early periods in history and/or childhood, so much the better.

Evolutionism has its appeal. For one thing, it permits the existence of variety. Instead of searching for "higher-order" equivalences it takes variety and dif-ference at its face-value (and tries to assign it a rank). Secondly, it does provide a yardstick (the normative model) for talking about *progress*. The vocabulary of the primitive vs. modern, adequate vs. inept, better vs. worse, adaptive vs. maladaptive, is highly "developed" in the evolutionist literature.

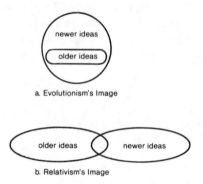

a. Evolutionism's Image

b. Relativism's Image

Fig. 1. Evolutionism's and relativism's image of relationship between historically sequenced ideas (adapted from Feyerabend 1975:177–178).

Evolutionism, however, has its pitfalls. There is no normative model for many domains of social thought — no way of saying whether one form of understanding is better or worse than another. Which is better? A kinship system where older and younger brothers are terminological distinguished, or one where the distinction is not encoded? The mind boggles at the evolutionary presumption of the question. Which is better? A policy for allocating resources based on the principle "to each equal amounts" or one based on the principle "to each according to his work (or "to each according to his needs"). There seems to be no *general* answer (see Perelman 1963).

There is a second difficulty with the evolutionary model, viz., the problem of "presentism". "Presentism" is the tendency to perceive the ideas of others through the filter of one's own current concerns. This pattern of perception is diagrammed in Figure 1b (see Feyerabend 1975). It is all too easy to unwittingly rewrite (and distort) the historical and ontogenetic record on others' ideas, dropping out or overlooking those problems, ideas and principles which are no longer of contemporary concern. This is especially true when one's search through the ideas of others is guided by a contemporary normative model. But, consider the possibility that our ideas have succeeded the ideas of others, not through a process of subsumption, betterment and advance, but rather, merely by "giving up" on the problems, principles and concepts of our ancestors (see the hatched in area of Figure 1b). "Presentism" obscures the historical record, making it appear our ideas can do everything the ideas of our predecessors could do, plus more, when all we may have done is shifted our field of interest, and *altered the questions* to be answered.

Relativism

Confronted with the apparent diversity of human understandings, relativists seek to preserve the integrity of the differences and establish the co-equality of the variegated "forms of life". Relativists typically process evidence according to two rules of thumb: (a) The "contextualization rule"; and (b) The "principle of arbitrariness".

1. *The contextualization rule.* A primary goal of the relativist is to seek, and display, more and more information about the details of other peoples' objectives, premises, presuppositions, standards, knowledge, meanings, etc. [the famous "native's point of view"]; so much detail that the ideas and conduct of others come to make sense *given* the "context" (premises, standards, etc.). Thus, for example, Benedict (1946), in her classic analysis of Japanese culture, takes bits and pieces of Japanese conduct in World War II, their lack of respect for national sovereignty (e.g., the invasion of China and attack on Pearl Harbor), the suicide bombings, the "mistreatment" of American prisoners of war, etc., and places them in a conceptual framework (the Japanese understanding of the advantages and necessity of "taking one's proper place" in a domestic, national and international hierarchy of individuals, groups and nations), a conceptual framework *within which* "militaristic expansionism" is redescribed as an obvious remedy for international anarchy, and the "atrocities" of the camps redescribed as a valorous contempt for materialism and scorn of "damaged goods".

2. *The principle of arbitrariness.* A closely related goal of the relativist is to show that equally rational folk can look out on the "same" world and yet arrive at different understandings; the relativist must find a way for reason to leave us a free choice. To the extent that no rule of logic and no law of nature dictates what is proper or necessary for us to believe or value, that is, to the extent there is an element of "arbitrariness" or "free-choice" in our understandings, to that extent reason is consistent with relativism. Socrates may be right that the concept of "truth" implies "one" not many, but there are many points in a cognitive structure where questions of truth and falsity, validity, error etc., are simply beside the point.

Hence, the passionate interest among relativists in the types of ideas underlying *non*-rational action, ideas that fall beyond the scope of scientific evaluation, for example, *constitutive presuppositions* (Collingwood 1972) (e.g., "all behavior is motivated by a desire to maximize pleasure and minimize pain"; what could possibly count as a disproof?), *performative utterances* (Austin 1962) (e.g., "You're fired", "I dub thee ... "; in such cases the problem of getting one's words to correspond to, or match, reality does not seem to arise) and other *declarative speech acts* (Searle 1979) (e.g., various acts of "definition"), *categorical judgments of value* (e.g., Hempel 1965) (e.g., "Killing is evil" and other avowals or expressions of a commitment to a norm of conduct) and, of course, Pareto's *"sentiments"* (1935).

Hence, the rejection among relativists of both the "innocent eye" (i.e., "we classify things as we do because that's the way things are") and the "absolute given" (i.e., "we classify things the way we do because that's the way people are") (Goodman 1968; quoted phrases from Volney Stefflre: personal communication). For the relativist, knowledge, at its limits, is without foundation; what is of value and importance is a matter of consensus; social "facts" are created not discovered. The world of the relativists is a world where objects and events are not classified together because they are more alike than other things; quite the contrary, the relativist argues, objects and events seem to be alike because they have been classified together (Goodman 1972). And why have those folk classified things together in that way? That, the relativist will retort, "depends on their purposes". And, why do those folk pursue the purposes they pursue? That, the relativist will say, is a question for the historian.

3. *Relativism's benefits and costs*. Relativism, like universalism and evolutionism, has its distinctive benefits and costs. Relativism is consistent with a kind of pluralism or cognitive egalitarianism, a definite benefit, at least for some observers. Relativists provide us with a charitable rendition of the ideas of others, placing those ideas in a framework that makes it easier to credit others, not with confusion, error or ignorance, but rather with an alternative vision of the possibilities of social life.

Relativism, however, has its problems. Despite its egalitarian intentions, relativism ironically lends support to a world based on intellectual domination and power assertion. The relativist views the understandings of others as self-contained, incommensurate, ideational universes (i.e., "paradigms"): *across* these universes there is no comparability, no common standard for rational criticism (see, e.g., Rorty 1979). Consequently, if people change ideational worlds (as they do) it can only be explained, by the relativist, in terms of domination, force, or non-rational conversion. And, if two or more peoples should disagree, as they often do, the only means of adjudication is "force of arms" – there is nothing to discuss. When "consensus" is the final arbiter of what's real, numbers count, and the powerful and/or the masses have their way.

Kurt Vonnegut, in his novel *Slaughterhouse Five*, points to relativism's second bane. Says Vonnegut:

I think of my education sometimes. I went to the University of Chicago for a while after the Second World War. I was a student in the department of anthropology. They taught me that nobody was ridiculous or bad or disgusting. Shortly before my father died he said to me – "You know you never wrote a story with a villain in it." I told him that was one of the things I learned in school after the war.

AN ALTERNATIVE CONCEPT OF THE PERSON: THE PHENOMENON

Any observer of an apparently alien concept, belief, or value must address the question: in what terms shall this understanding be understood? How shall this idea be translated? In this section we describe an apparently alien concept of the person – we introduce the phenomenon of interest. In the next section we discuss universalist, evolutionary, and relativist interpretations of the phenomenon.

Many Western observers of *some* non-Western peoples have made note of a distinctive apperceptive style or mode of social thought; it goes under a variety of cognate descriptions — concrete, non-abstractive, non-generalizing, occasion-bound, context-specific, undifferentiated, situational.

Levy (1973:24) illustrates this "concrete style" of social thinking by reference to one of his Tahitian informants, Poria. Poria is asked to define the word *hoa* which Levy glosses abstractly as "friend". Poria, however, responds by enumerating a list of restricted, context-dependent conditions:

A hoa — we love each other — I come and get you to go to my house so that we may eat together. Sometimes we go and stroll together on the path. Sometimes I go to your house to eat. Sometimes I want you to help me with my work. Sometimes I go to help you. Sometimes we joke with the girls.

Levy notes that "much of village behavior having to do with personal and social description" is marked by an emphasis on "contexts and cases" (262), and is "oriented to richness of detail . . . " (268). He believes that Poria's thinking and the thinking of most Tahitian villagers involves "a calculus in which terms are understood on the basis of a large number of contextual factors" (262). Numerous other observers in Africa, Central America, New Guinea and Central Asia (e.g., Werner and Kaplan 1956; Bruner et al. 1966; Piaget 1966; Horton 1967; Greenfield 1972; Luria 1976) concur in the observation that certain cultures perceive things (e.g., "an apple found in a store" and "an apple found on the ground") in terms of unique contextual features (e.g., time, place, coterminous objects, co-occurent events, etc.) while failing to generalize across cases or equate things in terms of cross-contextual invariances (e.g., they're both "applies"; see Price-Williams (1975:28) for an illuminating discussion of concrete thinking). Informants either respond to questions about how things are alike by enumerating the ways in which things are different, or else emphasize the way objects and events fit together in functional complexes or action sequences, without abstracting a common likeness.

This same style of concrete, contextualized, non-abstractive, apparently undifferentiated thinking is found in various cross-cultural reports about the concept of the "person". What is noted is a tendency to *not* abstract out a concept of the inviolate personality free of social role and social relationship — a tendency to not separate out, or distinguish, the individual from the social context.

Geertz (1975:48), for example, asserts that

the Western conception of the person as a bounded, unique, more or less integrated motivational and cognitive universe, a dynamic center of awareness, emotion, judgment, and action organized into a distinctive whole and set contrastively both against other such wholes and against a social and natural background is, however incorrigible it may seem to us, a rather peculiar idea within the context of the world's cultures.

There is, he notes, in Bali

... a persistent and systematic attempt to stylize all aspects of personal expression to the point where anything idiosyncratic, anything characteristic of the individual merely because he is who he is physically, psychologically or biographically, is muted in favor of his assigned place in the continuing, and, so it is thought, never-changing pageant that is Balinese life. It is dramatis personae, not actors, that endure; indeed it is dramatis personae, not actors, that in the proper sense really exist. Physically men come and go — mere incidents in a happen-stance history of no genuine importance, even to themselves. But the masks they wear, the stage they occupy, the parts they play, and most important, the spectacle they mount remain and constitute not the facade but the substance of things, not least the self (Geertz 1975:50).

Twenty years earlier, in a brilliant discussion of morality and personhood, Read (1955) spoke in similar terms about the Gahuku-Gama of New Guinea. The Gahuku-Gama conception of man "does not allow for any clearly recognized distinction between the individual and the status which he occupies" (255). The Gahuku-Gama do not distinguish an *ethical* category of the person. They fail

... to separate the individual from the social context and, ethically speaking, to grant him an intrinsic moral value apart from that which attaches to him as the occupant of a particular status (257).

The Gahuku-Gama recognize "no common measure of ethical content which would serve as a guide for the moral agent in whatever situation he finds himself" (260). For the Gahuku-Gama, people

are not conceived to be equals in a moral sense: their value does not reside in themselves as individuals or persons; it is dependent on the position they occupy within a system of inter-personal and inter-group relationships (250).

What this means is that for the Gahuku-Gama being human *per se* "does not necessarily establish a moral bond between individuals, nor does it provide an abstract standard against which all action can be judged . . . " (261). Rather, the "specific context", the particular occasion, "determines the moral character of a particular action" (260). For example, the Gahuku-Gama believe it is wrong to kill members of their own tribe

but it is commendable to kill members of opposed tribes, always provided they are not related to him. Thus, a man is expected to avoid his maternal kinsmen in battle though other members of his own clan have no such moral obligation to these individuals (262).

Dumont's (1970:1, 9) observations on India almost sound redundant. He warns us against "inadvertently attributing the presence of the individual to societies in which he is not recognized", and he points to a relational, contextualized "logic" in which justice consists primarily in "ensuring that the proportions between social functions [and social roles] are adapted to the whole [i.e., society as a primary, not derivative, object]".

Geertz, Read, and Dumont contrast Bali, New Guinea, and India with a Western mode of social thought in which the "individual" is abstracted from the social role, and the moral responsibilities of this abstracted, inviolate individual are distinguished from his/her social responsibilities and duties. Read (1955:280) puts it this way: In the West

the moral duties of the person are greater than any of the duties which the individual possesses as a member of society. His moral responsibilities both to himself and others, transcend the given social context, are conceived to be independent of the social ties which link him to his fellows.

In the West, as Trilling (1972:24) so aptly remarks, the person, inviolate in his self-image, supposes that he is

an object of interest to his fellow man [and worthy of respect?] not for the reason that he had achieved something notable or been witness to great events but simply because as an individual he is of consequence.

How are we to interpret this widespread mode of social thought in which the individual is not differentiated from the role, and where the person achieves no abstract, context-independent recognition?

THE PERSON IN CONTEXT: EVOLUTIONARY, UNIVERSALISTIC AND RELATIVISTIC INTERPRETATIONS

The Evolutionary Account

In keeping with their respect for intellectual variety and their desire to rank diverse forms along a scale of progress, evolutionary theorists argue that concrete, occasion-bound thinking (in both the social and non-social domain) is unequally distributed across cultures, and can be explained by reference to one of four types of cognitive "deficits" viz., the absence of (a) cognitive skills; (b) intellectual motivation; (c) pertinent information, or (d) linguistic tools.

1. *Deficit 1: Cognitive skills.* Luria's (1976) work illustrates the evolutionary emphasis on the absence of cognitive skills. He argues that "for some people abstract classification is a wholly alien procedure" (60), and he suggests that illiterate, unschooled peasants in the Uzbekistan and Kirghizan regions of Central Asia lack the *skill* to "isolate (abstract) a common feature" of things "as a basis for comparison" (80–81). Luria credits schools with fostering the ability to abstract, to generalize and to think scientifically (also see Bruner et al. (1966) on schooling effects and Greenfield (1972) and Goody (1977) on literacy effects).

　Kohlberg (1969, 1971) adopts a similar approach. His evolutionary scheme for the ethical category of the person would account for the occasion-bound, socially contextualized person concept of the Balinese, Gahuku-Gama and Hindu by locating it as a stage in the evolution of an adequate moral orientation in which respect for the abstract person transcends social roles. Thus, for example, the Gahuku-Gama view that the moral value of life cannot be separated from the social status of a person, and the cognate view that in a "catastrophe" important people, people of status should be saved first, would be interpreted by Kohlberg as an early childlike form of understanding, an initial step on the ladder ascending to the more mature recognition of universal respect for the value of life *per se*. For Kohlberg, movement through the stages of his evolutionary scheme is ultimately explained by reference to the development of certain cognitive processing skills, e.g., the ability to differentiate, take the perspective of another, and generalize.

2. *Deficit 2: Intellectual motivation*. Levy's (1973:269–270) work illustrates the evolutionary emphasis on intellectual motivation instead of cognitive skill. Levy interprets concrete thinking as an adaptation to life in a "cultural cocoon". Tahitian villagers, he argues, are deeply *"embedded"* in their own mundane daily contexts. They are not *motivated* to reflect upon the alternative cultural practices that surround them (e.g., the Chinese) nor do they have any *need* to conceptually locate their own customs in a more general comparative framework. Consequently, much of Tahitian village behavior "having to do with personal and social description" is marked by an emphasis on "contexts and cases" (262), and is "oriented to richness of detail . . . " (268). Levy speculates that such contextual embeddedness is "not conducive to science [and abstraction] " (269–270).

3. *Deficit 3: Pertinent information*. Horton's (1967) evolutionary interpretation explains concrete thinking by reference to informational limitations. Contextual-embeddedness, he argues, is primarily a cognitive concomitant of living in a "closed intellectual predicament", one too limited in opportunities to become aware of alternative visions of reality. Informational opportunities wax with the development of external trade, literacy and urbanization, and thus these three conditions, Horton argues, are conducive to the development of abstract modes of thought. Also see Super et al. (1977) for a discussion of the informational conditions favoring abstract thought. They conclude that cultures that are "materially simple will rarely require [abstract] categorical organization . . . "

4. *Deficit 4: Linguistic tools*. It is occasionally suggested that concrete thinkers are speakers of impoverished languages, viz. languages lacking *general terms* as a symbolic resource (e.g., Jesperson 1934). Thus, e.g., in Tasmanian each variety of gum-tree and wattle-tree has a name but there is no equivalent for the expression "a tree", while in Bororo (the classic illustration) each parrot has its special name but the general lexical entry "parrot" is absent. Deficient in their symbolic resources, lacking general terms, speakers of such languages are said to be prone to overlook the likenesses between things; hence the failure to abstract.

The Universalist Account

Evolutionary theorists, as we have just seen, argue that some peoples are distinctively concrete in their thinking; this distinctive mode of thought is explained by reference to deficits in cognitive processing skills, intellectual motivation, pertinent information, or requisite tools. Universalists, in contrast, are skeptical of the claim that some peoples are concrete thinkers, others abstract thinkers. From the perspective of the universalist, *attributions* of *differential* concreteness (or abstractness) by one people about another are illusory, and amount to little more than an indication that the category system of the observers fails to align with the category system of the people observed.

There are three claims implicit in the universalist interpretation of concrete and/or abstract thinking. First, it is argued that apparent evidence of concrete and abstract thinking is *equally* present in all cultures (concrete vs. abstract thinking is not a *variable* that can be used to distinguish one culture from another). Secondly, it is argued, the attribution of concreteness or abstractness to other people's thinking is the inevitable result of the confrontation between uncalibrated conceptual systems. More specifically, the universalist argues, we describe other people's thinking as concrete when they overlook likenesses or truths that we emphasize; we describe their thinking as abstract where they emphasize likenesses or truths that we overlook. Finally, it is argued, since no one conceptual system can take note of, or encode, all possible likenesses, or record all possible truths, where conceptual systems clash there will always be areas of *both* apparent concreteness and apparent abstractness. The work of Kroeber (1909) and Frake (1972) illustrates the universalist interpretation.

Frake's (1962) universalist argument is advanced against the evolutionary view of Jesperson (1934) that the mind of the "primitive" is concrete (overlooks likenesses) in its classification of flora and fauna [remember those "parrots"]. Ironically, Kroeber's (1909) universalist argument is advanced against the opposite evolutionary view (Morgan: 1871) that the mind of the "primitive" is excessively abstract (overlooks differences) in its classification of kinsmen (e.g., a "father-in-law" and a "grandfather" are similarly labeled in the Dakota language).

It would be a mistake to conclude from this irony that primitive terminological systems are concrete when it comes to plants and animals yet abstract for kinsmen. Rather the main point of the universalist interpretation is that the contrast between concrete and abstract systems of classification is an *illusion* that:

. . . has its origin in the point of view of investigators, who, on approaching foreign languages, have been impressed with their failure to discriminate certain relationships [e.g., father-in-law and grandfather] between which the languages of civilized Europe distinguish, and who, in the enthusiasm of formulating general [evolutionary] theories from such facts, have forgotten that their own languages are filled with entirely analogous groupings or classifications which custom has made so familiar and natural that they are not felt as such [e.g., overlooking the difference between cousins older and younger than oneself and denoting them both with the same term] (Kroeber 1909:77).

Frake (1962:75) makes a similar point. He remarks that there is "no necessary reason" that other people should heed those particular attributes which, for the English-speaker, make equivalent all the diverse individual organisms he labels "parrots" [see Findley 1979 for an example of the way attribute selection can radically influence which organisms get categorized together]. As Frake notes, any comparison of unaligned category systems will reveal cases where the others' thought seems quite concrete (they overlook likenesses that we emphasize) *as well as* cases where their thought seems quite abstract (they emphasize likenesses that we overlook).

To this point we have described the "logic" of universalist, evolutionary and relativist understandings of other people's understandings, and we have characterized the evolutionary and universalist interpretations of concrete, context-dependent, occasion-bound thinking. We now focus our attention on one specific example of concrete thinking, that is, occasion-bound *social* thinking, more particularly, the concept of the context-dependent person. In presenting the results of a cross-cultural study of person description in India and the United States, we display our reasons for rejecting the evolutionary and universalist interpretations of the Hindu, Balinese, and Gahuku-Gama context-dependent person concept. Finally, we construct an alternative, relativist interpretation which argues that the context-dependent concept of the person is one aspect of a broader sociocentric "organic" (or holistic) conception of the relationship of the individual to society. It is a feature of holistic thinkers that "units" (organs, body parts, groups, individuals, etc.) are believed to be necessarily altered by the *relations* into which they enter (Phillips 1976). We argue that concrete thinking (as a general phenomenon) is a by-product of the commitment to a holistic world view, and we discuss the implications of the sociocentric organic conception of the individual-social relationship for the developing ego's view of its-"self".

CONTEXTS AND CASES: A STUDY OF PERSON DESCRIPTION IN INDIA AND THE UNITED STATES

It is by reference to "contexts and cases" that Oriyas in the old town of Bhubaneswar (Orissa, India) describe the personalities of their friends, neighbors, and workmates. These personal accounts of Oriyas are concrete and relational. They tell you what someone has done; behavioral instances are often mentioned. They tell you where it was done. They tell you to whom or with whom it was done. The descriptive attention of Oriyas is directed towards the behavioral context in which particular behavioral instances occurred, e.g., "whoever becomes his friend, he remembers him forever, and will always help him out of his troubles (Jaha sange thore sango hoichonti, tanku sobudino pain mone rɔkhithanti o tankɔrɔ jɔdi kichi subidha hue, taku dɔbaku cesta kɔrɔnti)", "has no cultivatable land, but likes to cultivate the land of others (Casɔ jɔmi nahi, ɔthɔcɔ pɔrɔ jɔmi casɔ kɔribaku bhɔlɔ paanti)", "when a quarrel arises, cannot resist the temptation of saying a word (GɔndɔgoLɔtae hele pɔde nɔkɔhi rɔhi parɔnti nahi)", "will talk right in the face of even a British Governor (laat saheb hele mɔdhɔyɔ muhe muhe jɔbab diyɔnti)", "comes forward whenever there is an occasion to address a public meeting (Sɔbha sɔmitire kɔhibaku agua)", "behaves properly with guests but feels sorry if money is spent on them (Bɔndhu bandhɔbɔ asile bhɔlɔ byɔbɔharɔ dekhanti, kintu tɔnka pɔisa khɔrcɔ hele dukhɔ korɔnti)."

This concrete-relational way of thinking about other persons differs from the abstract style of our American informants. Americans tell you what is true of a person's behavior (e.g., he's friendly, arrogant, and intelligent) while tending to overlook behavioral context. Below we discuss the results of a comparison of Oriya and American personality descriptions. As we shall see, the striking tendency of Oriyas to be more concrete and relational than Americans does not readily lend itself to evolutionary interpretation in terms of either (a) relative amounts of formal schooling; (b) relative degrees of literacy; (c) relative socio-economic status; (d) the presence or absence of abstract terms in one's language; (e) the absence of skills of abstraction among Oriyas; or (f) relative awareness of alternative behavioral contexts or variations in behavior.

The concrete-relational style of Oriya social thought seems unrelated to variations in cognitive skill, intellectual motivation, available information and linguistic resources. By elimination, we are led to consider the way a culture's world view and master metaphors *per se* influence the relationship between what one thinks about and how one thinks. We consider differences in Indian and American conceptualizations of the relationship of the individual and society with special reference to the sociocentric organic vs. egocentric reductionist view of "man-in-society".

Methodology

1. *Informants*. The 17 informants in the American sample came from three separate groups: (1) counseling psychologists (3 women, 2 men); (2) a college fraternity (6 men), and (3) nursery school teachers (6 women). In each group they had known each other for at least one year. Their ages ranged from 19 to 47, and they all had received or were about to complete a college education. They all lived in or around Chicago, Illinois. Socio-economically they were predominantly middle-class.

The 70 Indian informants resided in the old town of Bhubaneswar, Orissa. They were selected on the basis of caste criteria as part of a general enquiry into household composition and caste interaction patterns. Thus, the full range of the local caste hierarchy was represented. With two exceptions the Oriyas were all males and spanned a wider age range than the Americans (18–70).

Educational variability among them was also greater, ranging from no formal education to the attainment of the M.A. degree. Seventeen informants had no education at all. Eighteen informants were illiterate.

Caste, formal schooling and literacy are not orthogonal in the Indian sample. Informants from the lower castes tend to be less educated and illiterate although there are a number of informants from the upper castes who are literate but relatively unschooled. The confounding of caste, literacy and schooling in the sample is less worrisome than it might at first appear. The cultural differences in concrete-relational thinking, to be reported below, are stable across the entire Indian sample and do not vary by caste, education or literacy. Unschooled, illiterate untouchables and highly educated, literate Brahmans differ from Americans in the same way and do not significantly differ from each other.

2. *The task*. Informants in both populations responded to the task of describing a close acquaintance. However, in the Indian group each informant described up to three friends, neighbors, or workmates, whereas in the American group each described the other four of five members of his/her group. There were also slight differences in the instructions and format of the descriptive task between the two cultures, an inevitable consequence of the fact that they had originally been associated with independent studies. Indian informants were presented with the instructions: Tankɔrɔ cɔritrɔ, prɔkruti, o byɔbɔharɔ bisɔyɔre mɔte bhalɔbhabɔre kuhɔntu, (Tell me in depth about so-and-so's character, nature [personality] and behavior), whereas Americans were asked: "How would you characterize so-and-so's personality?" Indians could respond in as many or few ways as they chose (they averaged between seven and eight descriptive phrases) whereas Americans were asked to provide 20 descriptive sentences or phrases. Finally, Indians responded orally while Americans wrote out their description.

Because these procedural differences could have interacted with the cultural difference observed on the various dependent variables (see results section), the following "ex-post facto" study was done with a sample of 10 Americans. Informants were divided into two groups and given one or the other of the two instructions mentioned above. In each of these groups some informants were permitted to make as many responses as they wished, the others told to give 20 responses. All responses were given orally. While the different instructions had a slight, statistically nonsignificant effect on the tendency of informants to give concrete or abstract descriptions, this effect was nominal in comparison with that associated with cultural differences, as reported in the results section.

3. *The coding of descriptions*. To facilitate coding, all descriptions were broken down into constituent sentences. Where a sentence was compound or complex, it was further broken down into units each of which contained no more than one subject-predicate-object sequence. These units were subsequently referred to as "descriptive phrases". Each descriptive phrase was typed onto a 3 x 5

card. In this fashion a total of 3,451 descriptive phrases for both cultures was obtained.

A coding system was developed to enable judges to decide on the presence or absence of a number of features related to concrete thinking, in particular (a) descriptive reference to abstract traits; (b) descriptive reference to concrete action; (c) descriptive incorporation of contextual qualifications.

An abstract trait reference (abbreviated "*T*") was operationally defined as any attribute that answered the question, "What kind of person *is* the ratee?" The judgment was made independently of the presence or absence of contextual qualifications in the descriptive phrase. Thus "she is stubborn" and "she is stubborn about family matters" would both be coded "*T*" although the final coding for the two phrases would differ in the specification of additional contextual qualifiers.

An action reference ("*A*") answered the question, "Is this something the ratee does?" This judgment also was made independently of the presence or absence of contextual qualifiers. Thus, "she uses dirty language" and "she uses dirty language when her friends give her advice about family matters" would both be coded "*A*" though they differ in the specification of additional contextual qualifiers.

Pure emotive-evaluative terms ("*TE*") such as "he is a good man" were not considered traits ("*T*") in our final analysis. One reason for drawing the distinction was the reference to (moral) "character" ("coritro") in the Oriya instructions. This tended to elicit a ritualized initial response from most informants. They would first say "he is a good man" or "he is not a good man" and then go on with their description. "*TE*" phrases in both the American and Oriya descriptions were dropped from the analysis discussed below. The total number of descriptive phrases actually analyzed numbered 3,209 (1,524 Oriya, 1,685 American).

Contextual qualifications were coded under the following categories:

Personal Reference: (a) reference to a specific individual, often denoted by a proper or common noun (e.g., "he gets angry with his father") coded "*P1*", (b) reference to a specific group of others (e.g., "he makes fun of his family") coded "*P2*", (c) reference to people or others in general (e.g., "he is honest with others") coded "*P3*", (d) reference to the person described himself (e.g., "he gets angry with himself") coded "*SR*", (e) reference to the rater (e.g., "he gets angry with me") coded "*RR*".

Qualification: (a) temporal: statement of when or how frequently the attribute occurs (e.g., "last year he did favors frequently") coded "time", (b) locale: statement of where or in what location the attribute occurs (e.g., "At school she puts on a front") coded "place", (c) general qualification: any statement of the conditions under which an attribute occurs or obtains (e.g., "He gets irritable if provoked") coded "qual", (d) inferential qualification: statement of the conditions under which the *rater* makes the attribution (e.g., "judging from what others say, he is reserved") coded "inf", (e) any phrase which states an action, trait, etc. *without* qualification is coded "No qualification" (Noqual).

A coding category called *Miscellaneous Types* allowed us to make more refined judgments about the presence or absence of references to traits of actions:

Miscellaneous Types: (a) a reference to what the ratee *likes* (*L* or *LA*), (b) *wants, seeks*, or *desires* (*D* or *DA*), (c) *experiences* (*E* or *EA*), (d) *feels* (*F* or *FA*), (e) is *interested* in (*I* or *IA*), (f) is *capable* of or *able* to do (*C* or *CA*), (g) *values* (*V* or *VA*), (h) a reference to what *type* of person the ratee is (e.g., "he's a joker, a friend," etc.) (*R*), (i) a reference to the *social role* the ratee fills (e.g., "he's a leader," "he's a teacher," etc.) (*R* social), or (j) a reference to the *physical characteristics* of the ratee (*Phys*).

The coding system provided explicit criteria, with positive examples, for the identification of all the preceding categories. Phrases which were refractory to any of the categories were coded "questionable" (?). Two illustrations of a descriptive "phrase" and its coding according to the above system follow:

(a) "He jokes with his friends" (Coding: *A, P*2).
(b) "She is stubborn" (Coding: *T*, Noqual).

Several composite categories consisting of combinations of those listed above were also defined. These categories can be arranged along two dimensions of abstractness – concreteness, which, following Levy (1973), we shall label "Cases" and "Contexts". They are defined as follows:

Cases: The contrast between trait-type references ("*T*" or "*R*" or "*R*Social") (e.g., "he is a leader"), on the one hand, and action references ("*A*" or "*LA*" or "*DA*") (e.g., "he lends people money"), on the other hand.

Contexts: The contrast between context-free references ("Noqual") e.g., ("he is verbally abusive"), on the one hand, and context-dependent references ("P_1" or "P_2" or "P_3" or "time" or "place") e.g., ("he is verbally abusive to his father-in-law whenever they meet at his home"), on the other hand.

4. *Reliability and the determination of consensual codings*. Four judges, all graduate students, were trained to use the coding system. At least two judges independently coded all 3,451 phrases comprising the basic data. In a majority of cases three or all four of the judges coded the phrase.

Judges were originally asked to provide their first, second, third, etc. alternative codings of a phrase in cases where there was some ambiguity about the correct coding. Only the first coding of each judge was used in our study. If anything, this reduced intercoder agreement (reliability) from what it would have been if the "closest" codings of a phrase among all of the two, three, or four judges' several alternatives had been used.

For the final data analysis it was necessary to arrive at a single, common coding for each phrase. Two alternative procedures suggested themselves at this point: (1) judges might have discussed the discrepancies among their independent codings for each phrase and achieved a consensus or (2) a mechanical procedure could be used to derive a "consensual coding" from among the two to four alternatives for each phrase. The latter procedure was chosen for two reasons.

First, time considerations advised against the laborious process of having judges reconcile their differences for each of the 3,451 phrases. Secondly, a mechanical procedure ensured that exactly the same impartial procedure would be applied to each set of alternative codings for a phrase. Otherwise consensual codings would have been based upon the subjective decisions of different combinations of judges.

A computer program was devised to consider the alternative codings for a particular phrase and include in the final, consensual coding, any category (i.e., trait, action, personal reference, etc.) which occurred in 2 out of 2 independent codings, 2 out of 3, 3 out of 3, 3 out of 4, 4 out of 4 (thus, e.g., excluding cases where the category occurred in only 2 out of 4 codings). To illustrate, suppose four judges' codings of a particular item were as follows: (1) T, $P3$, time, qual; (2) T, $P1$, qual; (3) R, $P3$, qual; and (4) T, qual. The consensual coding here, on the basis of the above criterion, would be "T, qual".

Out of a total of 3,451 phrases, this procedure achieved a consensual coding for 3,290 phrases or 95% of the corpus. This in itself suggests a relatively high level of interjudge agreement. Interjudge reliability was operationalized more precisely, however, by determining the percentage out of the total number of instances of all categories among the alternative codings of a phrase which were represented in the consensual coding. To illustrate, in the above example the two categories comprising the consensual coding — "T" and "qual" — occur seven times among the various alternative codings. Since the total number of instances of all categories among the alternatives is 12, it follows that 7/12, or approximately 58% of the alternative codings, are represented in the consensual coding. In brief, this particular reliability index estimated the proportion of variance among the alternative codings which was "common" or consensual.

Averaging over the interjudge reliability estimates for the total of 3,290 phrases for which consensual codings were obtained, the mean estimate was found to be 77%. This level of agreement seems both satisfactory and surprising, given the difficulty the judges reported in applying the coding system.

5. *Data analysis.* With the consensual codings of phrases available, it was possible to compare the frequency and proportion of occurrence of any category between the two cultures or among caste, literacy, or educational groups within India. This constituted the first step of the data analysis.

Chi square tests were performed to test the significance of the difference in frequencies observed for each comparison from the expected frequency. The major results are reported in the following section.

The second step of the data analysis examined the relationship between the two composite categories representing the "cases" and "contexts" dimensions of abstraction discussed above. Each dimension was dichotomized. The "cases" dimension was scored 1 or 0 depending upon whether a particular phrase contained a trait, type, or social role attribution (T, R, Rsocial) or any of the action attributions included under the composite category (A, LA, DA) (see the section on the coding system above). The "contexts" dimension was scored 1 if the phrase contained any instance of the category P_1, P_2, P_3, time, place, and 0 if it contained no qualification (i.e., was coded NoQual).

Results

1. *Contexts*. Oriyas are more likely to say "she brings cakes to my family on festival days". Americans are more likely to say "she is friendly". Contextual qualifications having to do with personal reference ("P_1", "P_2", "P_3"), "time" and "place" each occur significantly more often in Oriya descriptions of personality ($p = < .001$ for all five variables). American descriptions are noteworthy for the frequency of descriptions that are entirely unqualified by context ("Noqual") ($p = < .001$). There are two exceptions. Americans use more self-referential qualifiers ("SR") (e.g., "she is beginning to accept herself"; "he is hard on himself") than Oriyas ($p = < .001$). Americans also use more inferential qualifiers ("inf") (e.g., "judging from what others say, he is very reserved") ($p = < .001$). Earlier we discussed a composite variable entitled "Contexts" (P_1, P_2, P_3, time, place vs. Noqual). The ratio of context-free to context-dependent phrases is 3 to 1 in the American descriptions and 1 to 1 in the Oriya descriptions.

2. *Cases*. Oriyas tell you what someone has done, e.g., he shouts curses at his neighbors. The emphasis is upon behavioral occurrences or "cases". Americans tell you what is true of what someone has done, e.g., he is aggressive and hostile. Americans describe personality by means of trait ("T") (e.g., "friendly") and type ("R") (e.g., "a friend") concepts ($p = < .001$). Oriyas describe personality by reference to actions ("A", "LA", "DA") ($p = < .01$ for all three variables). The only time Americans are more likely than Oriyas to mention what someone does is when they describe a person's capabilities ("CA"; $p = < .05$) or interests ("LA"; $p = < .01$).

Earlier we discussed a composite variable entitled "Cases" (A, LA, DA, vs. T, R, RSocial). The ratio of abstractions to actions is 3 to 1 in the American descriptions but only 1 to 1.8 in the Oriya descriptions.

3. *Contexts and cases*. Case reference and context reference are not entirely independent descriptive acts although their associational relationship, while statistically significant ($p = < .001$) is only weak to modest (Phi = .30 for the Oriyas and .18 for the Americans). The relationship can be summarized as follows: There is a greater tendency to contextualize descriptions that make reference to a behavioral case. One is more likely to contextualize "he curses" [his mother-in-law] than "he is aggressive" [to his mother-in-law]. "He is aggressive" is more likely to stand alone. We emphasize again that the positive association between cases and contexts is weak to modest.

Discussion

Oriyas are more concrete than Americans in their descriptions of personality.

80% of Oriya descriptions are either contextually qualified (P_1, P_2, P_3, time, place) or make reference to a behavioral instance (A, LA, DA) (in contrast to 56% for the Americans). 46% of American descriptions are *both* context-free (Noqual) and abstract (T, R, R Social) (in contrast to 20% for the Oriyas). This result compares favorably with the findings of Fiske and Cox (n.d.). When American informants were asked to describe someone "so that someone else would know what it's like to be around this person" 40% of the items were abstract traits. Trait attributions were twice as frequent as references to behavioral patterns.

How is this cross-cultural difference in the thinking of Americans and Oriyas to be explained? We believe that each of the following plausible evolutionary hypotheses is *not* supported by the evidence.

1. *Hypothesis 1*: The Oriyas have less formal schooling than the Americans. Therefore, they are more concrete.

Formal schooling is often viewed by evolutionary theorists as a condition for the development of skills of abstraction (e.g., Bruner et al. 1966; Luria 1976). Considered as an aggregate the Oriyas are less educated than the Americans. 24% of the Oriya descriptive phrases came from informants who had never been to school. 65% came from informants with less than three years of schooling. Nevertheless, the relative concreteness of the Oriya personality descriptions is not related to this difference in education. Table I shows that the descriptive phrases elicited from Oriyas with an educational level comparable to the Americans (beyond high school) are more concrete than the American descriptive phrases. In the Oriyan sample concreteness does not significantly vary across educational levels for either "cases" (p = n.s.) or "contexts" (p = n.s.). Concrete thinking in the personality domain transcends variations in formal schooling experience. See Table II.

2. *Hypothesis 2*: The literacy level of the Oriyas is less than the Americans. Therefore, they are more concrete.

Literacy is often cited by evolutionary theorists as a condition for the development of skills of abstraction (e.g., Greenfield 1972; Luria 1976; Goody 1977). The overall literacy level of the Oriyas is certainly less than the Americans. 25% of the Oriya descriptive phrases were elicited from entirely illiterate informants. Nevertheless, this relative difference in literacy levels does not explain the relative concreteness of Oriya descriptions of personality. Literate and illiterate Oriyas do not significantly differ in the relative concreteness of their personality descriptions for either "cases" (p = n.s.) or "contexts" (p = n.s.). Concrete thinking in the personality domain transcends variations in literacy in Orissa. Moreover, if the illiterate Oriya informants are eliminated from the sample, the difference in concrete thinking between Americans and literate Oriyas continues to be significant. See Table I.

TABLE I

Comparison of the relative emphasis on contexts and cases in the descriptive phrases of all Americans, all Oriyas, and various sub-groups of Oriyas

	All Americans	Oriyas						
		All Oriyas	Beyond high school	No school	Literate	Illiterate	Brahmans	Bauris
Context-dependent (P_1, P_2, P_3, time, place)	28.3%	49.6%	48.3%	51.8%	48.4%	53.2%	50.6%	50.4%
Context-free (Noqual)	71.7%	50.4%	51.7%	48.2%	51.4%	46.8%	49.4%	49.6%
$n =$	1685	1505	215	357	1135	370	494	244
Actions (A, DA, LA)	25.4%	64.8%	58.8%	66.7%	64.6%	65.5%	66.1%	70.1%
Abstractions (T, R, RSocial)	74.6%	35.2%	41.2%	33.3%	35.4%	34.5%	33.9%	29.9%
$n =$	1333	1194	117	282	901	293	392	201

TABLE II

Comparison of the relative emphasis on contexts and cases across educational levels within the Oriya sample

	Formal schooling				
	None	1–3 years	4–7 years	8–11 years	Beyond high school
Contexts					
Context-dependent (P_1, P_2, P_3, time, place)	51.8%	50.0%	48.2%	49.6%	48.4%
Context-free (Noqual)	48.2%	50.0%	51.8%	50.4%	51.6%
$n =$	357	328	455	125	215
Cases					
Actions (A, LA, DA)	66.7%	62.5%	68.2%	64.4%	58.8%
Abstractions (T, R, RSocial)	33.3%	37.5%	31.8%	35.6%	41.2%
$n =$	282	259	349	104	177

3. *Hypothesis 3*: The Oriyas are of lower socio-economic status than the Americans. Therefore, they are more concrete.

Social and economic impoverishment is sometimes cited by evolutionary theorists as a condition retarding the development of skills of abstraction (e.g., Luria 1976). Considered as an aggregate, the Oriya sample is probably of lower socio-economic status than the American. We say "probably" because the notion of relative socio-economic status is difficult to apply in a comparison of India and the United States. A high status Brahman can be relatively impoverished without serious threat to his/her caste position. Wealthy and powerful informants can come from middle-level or even relatively low-status castes. However, since 16% of the descriptive phrases came from Bauris, an untouchable or so-called "scheduled" caste, and since these informants were uniformly impoverished, it seems safe to conclude that by most standards the Oriyas, as an aggregate, are not as high status as the Americans.

Socio-economic status, an elusive cross-cultural yeardstick, does not seem to explain the relative difference in concrete thinking in the personality domain between the two cultures. Within Orissa, concrete thinking does not vary by caste status for either "cases" (p = n.s.) or "contexts" (p = n.s.). A comparison of Brahman informants to American informants continues to reveal a cultural difference in concrete thinking. Brahman informants differ little from the overall Oriyan sample (see Table I). In fact, the truly remarkable feature of Tables I and II is the stability of the evidence of concrete thinking across all the Oriyan sub-samples. In Orissa the concrete style of personality description transcends variations in education, literacy and caste.

4. *Hypothesis 4*: Concrete-Abstract thinking is a global cognitive process variable that distinguishes Oriyas from Americans. Oriyas lack the skill to abstract or generalize across cases.

5. *Hypothesis 5*: The Oriya language lacks general terms with which to refer to individual differences in behavior. Therefore Oriyas are deficient in linguistic resources for generating abstract descriptions of personality.

An investigation carried out by Shweder (1972: see Chapters 2 and 4 for a detailed discussion) makes it apparent that hypotheses 4 and 5 are not very helpful. The study concerned the influence of pre-existing conceptual schemes and taxonomic structures on judgment. A sub-set of the descriptive phrases elicited from our Oriya informants played a part in the study. The study revealed the ability of our Oriya informants to generate and intellectually manipulate abstract behavioral descriptions, and to recognize and utilize conceptual likenesses among them.

Ninety-nine representative descriptive phrases were written on cards and presented to 43 Brahman informants from the community whose concrete style of personality description we have been discussing. Most of these 99 phrases were concrete, i.e., they were either case specific or contextually qualified or both. A full list appears in Shweder (1972:56–60).

Each of the 43 informants was asked to sort the descriptive phrases into piles, placing together in the same pile items that might "go together" in the same person. Each informant was then asked to name or label the piles he had created. Informants were free to make as many piles as they liked and to place as many descriptive phrases in each pile as they wished. After making an initial sorting and labeling their piles, informants were asked to collapse their piles into fewer, more general piles. They were asked to name or label these new piles. This process of collapsing their groupings of phrases and naming their new groupings went on as long as the informant was willing to produce fewer and fewer piles, with more and more descriptive phrases in each.

The crucial point for our present discussion is that the sorting task success-fully generated abstract and general terms (trait and type concepts) for describ-ing personality from every one of the 43 informants. Using 43 informants, 420 different abstract trait and type terms were generated by means of the sorting task. English translations of 81 of these terms are shown in Figure 2 (see Shweder 1972:65–66) for the original Oriya terms). (A casual perusal of G. C. Praharaj's seven-volume lexicon of the Oriya language, 1931–1940, should dissuade anyone who believes our Oriya informants speak a language that is lacking in abstract personality trait and type concepts.)

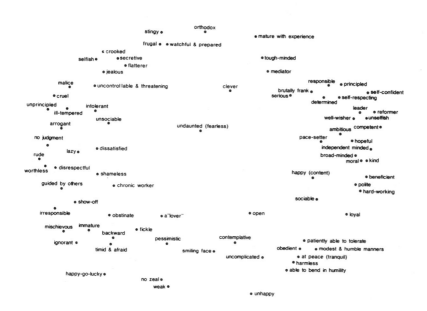

Fig. 2. Two-dimensional scaling of 81 Oriya personality terms (for original Oriya terms, see Shweder 1972:65–66).

Oriya informants have no difficulty recognizing and arranging things in terms of overarching conceptual likenesses. This was most clearly revealed by a second sorting task study. 81 personality trait and type concepts (see Figure 2) were selected to represent the 420 terms that had been generated in the first sorting task. They were written on cards and presented to 25 Brahman informants from the community whose concrete style of person description we have been discussing. Except for one additional feature, the sorting task was identical to the one previously discussed. Informants were asked to place items together that "went together" in people. They were asked to label (or describe) the piles. They were *also* asked to indicate which items in each pile were exemplary instances of the concept suggested by the pile. After an initial sorting they were asked to construct abstract hierarchies or taxonomies by collapsing the initial piles into a small number of general categories. Again they were asked to label (or describe) the categories, etc. The hierarchies of all 25 informants can be found in Shweder (1972:Appendix 1).

A measure of association between all possible pairs of 81 terms was calculated on the basis of the sorting task data. The particular measure has been described by Burton (1968:81–84). It is a normal variate score which is sensitive to three indices of "proximity" between a pair of terms. The primary index of "proximity" is the number of times two terms are placed together in the same pile over a sample of informants. This simple frequency count is adjusted to the number of terms in the pile in question (the larger the pile, the less proximate the two terms) and the total number of piles made by the particular informant (the fewer the piles, the less proximate the two terms). The final measure of association is a Z score. It was calculated using each level in the hierarchy of each informant as if it were the sorting task of a different informant. The measure was thus based on 73 partitionings of the 81 terms into piles. Subsequent analysis revealed that a simple frequency count of the number of times two items appear together in a pile over each of the hierarchical levels of each of the informants correlates .98 (person r) with the Z score used in our analysis.

The matrix of association among all possible pairs of 81 terms generated from the second sorting task was scaled in two-dimensional space using the multidimensional scaling program (MDSCALE) devised by Donald C. Olivier. A two-dimensional spatial representation of the associational relationships among the 81 terms is shown in Figure 2.

The most relevant feature of the scaling solution for our present discussion is that it demonstrates that our Oriya informants have consistently classified the terms on the basis of two independent underlying conceptual likenesses that they have abstracted from the 81 terms. The vertical axis in Figure 2 is interpretable as a "dominance vs. submission" (or "power") dimension. The horizontal axis is interpretable as a "social desirability" dimension. In its abstractness, generality and dimensional content the Oriya scaling solution in Figure 2 is comparable to the conceptual organization of the personality domain discovered in America (see, e.g., Leary and Coffey 1955; Lorr and McNair 1963, 1965; also see White (1980) on the possible universality of the scaling solution in Figure 2). Figure 2 suggests that the concreteness displayed by our Oriya informants when they freely describe personality or answer a request for information about someone's character, personality (nature) and behavior is *not* an indication of a deficit in the cognitive skills of abstraction and generalization. Hypothesis 4 and Hypothesis 5 must be rejected.

6. *Hypothesis 6*: Oriyas live in a "closed" intellectual environment in which they never have to confront alternative customs, behavioral styles, or viewpoints. However, abstract thinking (the search for likenesses between diverse phenomena) presupposes that one has access to information about variant phenomenon and different perspectives. Oriyas, lacking such information, are disinclined to abstract or generalize across cases.

Hypothesis 6 can be construed at a global level or at a level that is specific to the way Oriyas freely describe personality. At a global level it might be argued that Oriyas are so culturally insulated that they ought to display concrete thinking in all domains. We have already discussed the evidence that has led us to reject the notion that Oriyas lack the ability to abstract (see Hypothesis 4). There are also a number of features of life in the old town of Bhubaneswar and India in general that make it difficult to even seriously entertain the hypothesis that Oriyas live in a "closed" informational environment.

There are 24 Oriya castes (including five major Brahman sub-castes) represented in the residential wards and quarters of the old town of Bhubaneswar. There is considerable consensus concerning the relative status position of these castes, a judgment that takes into account the relative "purity" of the customs and behavior of a caste community. The concept of a caste hierarchy itself pre-supposes (a) an awareness of the diverse life styles of interdependent communities (e.g., do they eat meat, do they let their widows remarry, do they cut their own hair, wash their own clothes, etc.); (b) the ability to evaluate and rank caste communities in terms of the common yeardstick of "purity" (see, e.g., Dumont 1970). India is a land where diversity has always been accommodated by means of the sophisticated device of explicit hierarchical interdependence. Oriyas, evolutionists to the core, encourage diversity and rank it.

Caste disputes over relative status are a frequent occurrence in Orissa. Whenever they occur, one has the opportunity to observe social cognition in action over matters of importance to the participants. What one sees is a keen sensitivity to behavioral variations and to the way those behavioral variations will be judged from a third person perspective, e.g., in the eyes of a particular outside community or in the eyes of the general community.

A characteristic pattern of Oriyan social thought surfaces in disputes over the relative status of caste communities. Consider a typical instance. Three untouchable castes are involved in a dispute over the relative status of the two lowest. The issue at stake is simply, "who is the lowest of the low?" In order of relative "purity" the cast of castes includes community A (they are washerman), community B (they are agricultural laborers), and community C (they are scavengers, basketmakers, and drummers). A's wash other people's dirty linen. The "unclean" nature of this work guarantees their untouchable status. Nevertheless, A's are unquestionably higher in rank than either of the other two communities; their relative superiority is asserted and in part constituted by their refusal to wash B or C clothing. B's and C's are too impure even for the A's. The A's are the highest of the untouchable castes. Their superiority is never assailed in the dispute that arose between the B's and C's. In fact, the competitive status claims of the B's and C's could only be resolved because both communities accepted unquestionably the A's persepctive on matters of "purity". At the time the dispute surfaced, the C's were generally thought to be the most "polluted" of all the castes. Their caste position was asserted and in part constituted by their traditional activity of cleaning the latrines (and thus handling excrement) in the wards of other castes. But then events got underway.

(a) The status ploy by the C's. They refuse to clean the latrines in the B ward, thus, symbolically asserting their superiority. The move is effective. The B's have a serious dilemma. Either the B's must let their ward latrines accumulate excrement, etc., thereby polluting their neighborhoods, associating themselves with filth, confirming their untouchable status, and aggravating an already unpleasant living condition, or else they must clean their own latrines, thereby sacrificing the one taboo or restraint they have to their credit that distinguishes them from the C's in the eyes of outside communities. What to do?

(b) B—A status negotiations. B representatives approach representatives of the A community. They seek a trump card to use against the C's. In fact, they seek no less than to convince the A's to wash their clothes. "Impossible", assert the A's. "Your linen would pollute us and disgrace our community." The B's persist. They remind the A's that without the B's, A weddings could not take place. B's blow the conch shell at A weddings; they threaten to withdraw. The ploy is effective. Either the A's must cease marrying their children (that's no option) or else they must blow the conch shell themselves or find someone else to do it (Would it really be a wedding?).

(c) B—A Compromise. A compromise is struck. The A's will wash B clothing. Not all B clothing. Not even most B clothing. They will wash the ritual clothing that B performers wear in one particular religious ceremony on one particular day. It is reasoned that ritual cloth is not polluted even if worn by a B. The B's are pleased. At least the A's wash their clothing on some occasion. They never wash the C's clothes (as the C's are soon to be informed, and redundantly reminded). The A's are pleased. They can continue marrying their daughters at no cost to their community's status. And the C's? They go back to cleaning the latrines in the B ward. The absence of diversity and the non-recognition of alternative perspectives is just not an Indian problem.

However, hypothesis 6 might be construed narrowly. It might be argued that Americans are more likely to experience their intimates in diverse behavioral settings, and thus are more likely to abstract out a common feature of their behavior for personality diagnosis. We can only suggest that the situation with our Oriya and American informants may be the reverse of that supposed by hypothesis 6. Ethnographic observation suggests that our Oriya informants experience their intimates in a relatively small and standard set of contexts, e.g., at work, in family affairs, in ritual contexts, at public meetings, etc. They also have much second-hand knowledge via gossip and rumor. However, the number of settings in which teachers in a nursery school, college students in a fraternity and psychologists in a counseling center experience one another may be even less. Hypothesis 6 does not seem relevant to the cultural differences we have discovered in the concrete vs. abstract way Oriyas vs. Americans describe individual differences.

We seem to be left in an explanatory void. In their free descriptions of personality Oriyas are more concrete than Americans. They describe their intimates by reference to behavioral instances (cases) and they qualify their descriptions by reference to contexts. These differences hold up even when one is comparing Americans to literate Oriyas, educated Oriyas, and high caste Oriyas. Within the Oriya community, the concrete style of describing individual differences is stable across castes and across educational and literacy levels. The difference cannot be explained in terms of the "intellectual predicament" of the Oriyas. They are aware of alternative behavioral styles. It is not a reflection of a deficiency in skills of abstraction. In sorting tasks, Oriyas display a facile ability to think abstractly. The difference has little to do with education, literacy, socio-economic status or language. It seems to be a cultural phenomenon, and it is perhaps as a cultural phenomenon that we should try to understand it.

A RELATIVIST THEORY OF THE CONTEXT-DEPENDENT SELF: HOLISM AND ITS COGNITIVE CONSEQUENCES

As we have seen, Oriyas are less prone than Americans to describe people they know in abstract, context-free terms. Instead of saying so-and-so is "principled" they tend to say "he does not disclose secrets". Instead of saying so-and-so is "selfish" they tend to say "he is hesitant to give away money to his family". While this difference in person perception is only a "tendency" (e.g., 46% abstract, context-free descriptions from Americans, 20% from Oriyas), it is a pervasive tendency, stable across Oriya sub-samples, a tendency significant enough to reject a universalist interpretation of context-dependent thinking.

Our results also lend little support to an evolutionary interpretation. As noted earlier, Oriya informants do not lack skills of generalization and abstraction. They are aware that the behavior of someone who "does not become partial while imparting justice" and "does not disclose secrets" can be described as "principled" (nitibadi); they recognize that there are likenesses that link together such very different behavioral occurrences as imparting justice and keeping secrets. If asked to select from a corpus of concrete behaviors those that generally "go together" in people, Oriyas, like Americans, will utilize conceptual likenesses to assist them in the task ("all those are principled behaviors"; see hypothesis 5 above; also Shweder 1972, 1975, 1977a, b, 1980a, b; D'Andrade 1965, 1973, 1974; Shweder and D'Andrade 1979, 1980). Similarly, our results suggest that the concrete mode of person perception of our Oriya informants cannot be explained by reference to deficient information, motivation, or linguistic resources (see hypothesis 1–6 above). Why then are Oriyas more prone than Americans to describe their intimates by reference to "cases and contexts".

How to Construct a Relativist Interpretation of Concrete Thinking

Relativists acknowledge that concrete, contextualized, occasion-bound thinking is unequally distributed across human cultures. However, it is the position of the relativist that the prevalence of context-dependent thinking in some cultures tells us little about underlying deficits in cognitive processing skills, intellectual motivation, available information or linguistic tools. The trick for the relativist is to acknowledge diversity while shunning the evolutionary notion of "cultural deficits". How can this be done?

1. *Distinguish ideational products from intellectual processes*. Why are Oriyas more prone than Americans to describe their intimates by reference to "cases and contexts?" Relativists answer this question by drawing a sharp distinction between intellectual *process* and ideational *product*. The relativist hypothesizes that cultures differ less in their *basic* cognitive skills (e.g., generalization, abstraction, reversibility) than in the metaphors by which they live (Lakoff and Johnson 1980), the world hypotheses (Pepper 1972) to which they subscribe, and the ideas underlying their social action. Thus, according to a relativist account, the Oriyas, Balinese and Gahuku-Gama are perfectly competent information processors, not unskilled at differentiating, generalizing and taking the perspective of others, etc. What really distinguishes them from us is that they place so little *value* on differentiating (e.g., person from role), generalizing (e.g., "treat outsiders like insiders") or abstracting (e.g., the concept of "humanity"); and, the relativist is quick to point out, they show so little interest in such intellectual moves because Oriyas, Balinese, and other such folk live by a metaphor and subscribe to a world-premise that directs their attention and passions to particular systems, relationally conceived, and contextually appraised. Indeed, a central tenet of a relativist interpretation of context-dependent person perception is that *the metaphors by which people live and the world views to which they subscribe mediate the relationship between what one thinks about and how one thinks.*

2. *Holism: A mediating world premise*. Holism is a mode of thought elaborating the implications of the "part-whole" relationship: viz., (a) what's true of, or

right for, the whole is not necessarily true of, or right for, any or all of the parts of the whole [e.g., "an arm can throw a football", and "an elbow is part of the arm" does not imply that "an elbow can throw a football"]; (b) diverse parts of the whole are not necessarily alike in any crucial respects [e.g., while different "kinds of" canines, say terriers and spaniels, are alike in some characteristic ways, different "parts of" a body, say finger nails and red blood cells, or different "parts of" an automobile, say the axle and the fan belt, need not commune in any way whatsoever]; (c) each part is defined by the particular relationships into which it enters within the specific whole of which it is a part [e.g., try defining a "tongue" or "brake" without functional, relational, or contextual references]. For a holist, "unit" parts are necessarily altered by the relations into which they enter (Phillips 1976).

From a holistic perspective unit-parts (e.g., an elbow) change their essential properties when isolated from the unit-wholes (e.g., an arm) of which they are a part. Thus, the holist concludes, it is not possible to understand or appraise an entity in isolation, in the abstract. The holist is prone to seek contextual clarification before making a judgment; the holist is disinclined to examine or judge things in vacuo.

3. *The body: "A metaphor people live by"*. All societies are confronted by the same small set of existential questions, and some societies even try to answer them. A minimal set includes: (a) the problem of "haves" vs. "have nots". It is a fact of life that the things all people want are unequally distributed within any society. Have nots must be told in convincing terms why they have not. "Haves" must have confidence that their privileges are justifiable and legitimate; (b) the problem of *our* way of life vs. *their* way of life. Diversity of custom, value, belief and practice is also a fact of life. Why should I live this way and not some other way? "There but for fortune goes you or goes I" is not a satisfying answer; (c) the problem of the relationship of nature to culture. Are we merely "naked apes", or better yet "rational featherless bipeds", or still yet better "the children of god"; (d) the problem of the relationship of the individual to the group, to society, to the collectivity. There seem to be relatively few "solutions" to this last problem; the "sociocentric" solution subordinates individual interests to the good of the collectivity while in the "egocentric" solution society becomes the servant of the individual, i.e., society is imagined to have been created to serve the interests of some idealized autonomous, abstract individual existing free of society yet living in society.

Holistic cultures seem to embrace a sociocentric conception of the relationship of individual to society, a sociocentric conception with an organic twist. Some Indologists (see Dumont 1960, 1970:184–186; Marriott 1976), for example, have noted that the concept of an autonomous, bounded, abstract individual existing free of society yet living in society is uncharacteristic of Indian social thought. "Man-in-society", for Indians, is not an "autonomous, indivisible, bounded unit" (see Marriott 1976). Like most peoples, Indians do have a concept of "man-in-society" but "man-in-society" is not an autonomous individual. He is regulated by strict rules of interdependence that are context-specific and particularistic, rules governing exchanges of services, rules governing behavior to kinsmen, rules governing marriage, etc. (See our earlier discussion of negotiations over caste status; hypothesis 6 above.)

The idea that man-in-society is not an autonomous individual is not unique to India. Selby's (1974, 1975) discussion of Zapotec culture in Oaxaca, Mexico makes this apparent. Selby (1974:62—66, 1975) argues that the "folk explanatory model that puts responsibility for morality and cure on the individual" is "deeply rooted in Western thought". It is "as old as Thucydides, who wrote 2,400 years ago and was rediscovered and glorified in the Renaissance and Reformation". [Indeed, in the West, the fact that good works (e.g., scientific discoveries) are often the products of base motives (e.g., envy) is treated as a disturbing anathema, a glaring insult to our faith in the individual as the ultimate measure of all things.] It is otherwise among the Zapotecs. Selby explicates the Zapotec expression "we see the face, but do not know what is in the heart" as follows: It is

not an expression of despair. They [Zapotecs] do not have to know what is in the heart, because it isn't defined as being very interesting and it shouldn't have anything to do with human relations.

With regard to perceptions of deviant behavior, Selby notes

[Zapotecs] do not, therefore, have to overcome their own prejudices about the *character* of people who go wrong. They know their own society and how it works, and they are aware of the sociological nature of deviance. They have no need to peer into people's hearts and minds . . . [my emphasis].

Selby presents case material indicating that even blatantly deviant acts (e.g., murder) do not elicit characterological attributions.

Oriyan culture is not Zapotec. Indians do peer into one another's hearts and minds; Indians unlike the Zapotecs do have a concept of "autonomous individualism". But, and this is the main point, for an Indian to be an autonomous individual one must leave society. The autonomous individual is the holy man, the renouncer, the sadhu, the "drop out: (Dumont 1960, 1970). Yet even here his goal is not to find one's distinctive identity but rather to merge one's soul with the soul of others. When Indians peer into one another's hearts and minds they are more likely than most peoples to look for the ultimate universal, the ground of all things, God.

What makes Western culture special, then, is the concept "autonomous distinctive individual living-in-society". What makes Indian culture special is the concept "autonomous non-distinctive individual living-outside-society". When it comes to "man-in-society" Indian views are not unique (indeed, their views are prototypical and lucid expressions of a widespread mode of social thought), but they do diverge considerably from the "natural man" tradition of Western social thought. In America, men-in-society conceive of themselves free of the relationships of hierarchy and exchange that govern all social ties and are so central to theories of the self in Orissa.

The sociocentric conception of the individual-social relationship lends itself to an organic metaphor. Indeed in holistic sociocentric cultures like India the human body, conceived as an interdependent system, is frequently taken as a metaphor for society (and society, conceived as an organic whole, is sometimes taken as a metaphor for nature).

The human body is a pregnant metaphor. It has its ruler (the brain), its servants (the limbs), etc. Political affairs, interpersonal dyads, family organiza- tion are all easily conceived after a model of differentiated parts arranged in a hierarchy of functions in the service of the whole.

What we think follows from a holistic world view and sociocentric organic solution to the problem of the individual-social relationship are some of the features of the context-dependent, occasion-bound concept of the person: (a) no attempt to distinguish the individual from the status s(he) occupies; (b) the view that obligations and rights are differentially apportioned by role, group etc.; (c) a disinclination to ascribe intrinsic moral worth to persons merely because they are persons. [To ask of a holist: "Is killing wrong" is like asking a morphologist or physiologist to assess the value of a body part or organ without knowledge of, or reference to, its function in the interdependent organic structure of this or that particular species.] Indeed, with their explicit cultural recognition and even deification of obligatory, particularistic interdependence, Oriyas would seem to be culturally primed to see context and social relationships as a necessary condition for behavior.

By contrast, in the West, as Dumont (1970) notes, each person is conceived of as "a particular incarnation of abstract humanity", a monadic replica of general humanity. A kind of sacred personalized self is developed and the individ- ual qua individual is seen as inviolate, a supreme value in and of itself. The "self" becomes an object of interest *per se*. Free to undertake projects of personal expression, personal narratives, autobiographies, diaries, mirrors, separate rooms, early separation from bed, body and breast of mother, personal space – the autonomous individual imagines the incredible, that he lives within an inviolate protected region (the extended boundaries of the self) where he is "free to choose" (see Friedman and Friedman (1980) for the purest articulation of this incredible belief), where what he does "is his own business".

More than that, the inviolate self views social relationships as a derivative matter, arising out of consent and contract between autonomous individuals. Society is viewed as mere "association" (see Dumont 1970). It, thus, hardly seems surprising that despite much evidence to the contrary (Hartshorne and May 1928; Newcomb 1929; Mischel 1968; D'Andrade 1974; Shweder 1975, 1979a; Nisbett 1980), our culture continues to promote the fiction that within the person one can find a stable core "character". Nor is it surprising that this abstract individual, "man-as-voluntary-agent", is protected by deeply enshrined moral and legal principles prescribing privacy and proscribing unwanted invasions of person, property and other extensions of the self. Americans are culturally primed to search for abstract summaries of the autonomous individual behind the social role and social appearance.

4. *From concrete thinking in particular to concrete thinking in general.* We have argued that concrete, "cases and contexts" person perception is an expression of a holistic world premise and sociocentric organic conception of the relationship of the individual to society. But, what of concrete thinking in other domains? For example, what about the evidence on "functional complexes", i.e., the tendency for informants in some cultures to respond to requests about how things are alike by linking the things together in an action sequence or activity structure? Consider one of Luria's (1976:56) informants. The informant is presented with four objects (hammer-saw-log-hatchet). He is asked: "which of these things could you call by one word". He is told: " . . . one fellow picked three things – the hammer, saw, and hatchet – and said they were alike". The informant responds: "a saw, a hammer, and a hatchet all have to work together. But the log has to be there too . . . if you have to split something you need a hatchet".

To interpret this type of finding within a relativist framework one might speculate that from the point of view of a holistic thinker it makes no sense to ignore the functional interdependencies among objects and events. Indeed, Luria's illiterate, unschooled peasants repeatedly try, in vain, to explain to him that it is "stupid" to ignore the way objects and events fit together in action sequences (e.g., 1976:54, 77). One is reminded of Glick's (1968) Kpelle informant who insisted on grouping objects into functional complexes while commenting "a wiseman can do no other". Only when asked, "How would a fool group the objects" did he give the Westerner what he wanted, a linguistically-defined equivalence structure!

Is it far-fetched to imagine that holism, the sociocentric conception of the individual-social relationship, and the organic metaphor have a generalized influence on cognition. Perhaps! But, one should not overlook the following fact about the cultural organization of knowledge. Although in our culture it is the "natural" sciences that have an elevated position, in many non-Western cultures (see Fortes 1959; Smith 1961; Durkheim and Mauss 1963; Horton 1968) much of the intellectual action is in the arena of *social* thought. For us it is the organization of knowledge in physics and chemistry that is adopted wholesale as the ideal for social understanding. More than a few social scientists are busy at work searching for a "periodic table" of social elements. Many more have been enamored of physical metaphors (forces, energy, mechanisms, etc.). In the West, the physical world has become the model of the social world. Why should not a reverse extension take place in other cultures, the social order as the model of nature. Metaphors, deliberately selected to guide our thinking, often have generalized effects on how we think.

Privacy and the Socialization of the Inviolate Self

We have sketched the outline of a relativist interpretation of both "cases and contexts" person perception, in particular, and concrete thinking in general. The concept of the context-dependent person, we have argued, is one expression of a broader sociocentric organic view of the relationship of the individual to society which in turn is an aspect of the holistic world view adopted by many cultures. The holistic model, the sociocentric premise and the organic metaphor focus one's attention on the context-dependent relationship of part to part and part to whole; the holist, convinced that objects and events are necessarily altered by the relations into which they enter is theoretically primed to con-textualize objects and events, and theoretically disinclined to appraise things in vacuo, in the abstract.

To the question "Does the Concept of the Person Vary Cross-Culturally?" our answer is obviously "yes"; we have tried to identify two major alternative conceptualizations of the individual-social relationship, viz., the "egocentric contractual" and the "sociocentric organic". It is crucial to recognize that neither of these conceptualizations of the relationship of the individual to society has the epistemological status of a scientific category. They are not inductive generalizations. They are not the discoveries of individual perception. Quite the contrary, the egocentric and sociocentric views of man are creations of the collective imagination. They are ideas, *premises* by which people guide their lives, and only to the extent a people lives by them do they have force. How do people live by their world views? It is instructive to reflect, for example, on the socialization of autonomy in the West.

We find it tempting to argue that Western individualism has its origins in the institution of privacy — that privacy promotes a passion or need for autonomy, which for the sake of our sense of personal integrity, requires privacy (see Trilling 1972:24). Socialization is terroristic. The young are subject to all sorts of invasions, intrusions and manipulations of their personhood, autonomy and privacy. Where they go, when they sleep, what they eat, how they look, all the intimacies of the self are managed for them, typically without consent. Heteronomy is the universal starting point for socialization; it may or may not be the end point.

It is sobering to acknowledge that our sense of personal inviolatability is a violatable social gift, the product of what *others* are willing to respect and protect us from, the product of the way we are handled and reacted to, the product of the rights and privileges we are granted by others in numerous "territories of the self" (Goffman 1971) (e.g., *viz-à-viz* eating, grooming, hair length, clothing style, when and where we sleep, who we associate with, personal possessions, etc.). Simmel (1968:482) notes that "the right to privacy asserts the sacredness of the person". And, where are these "assertions" redundantly (even if tacitly) reiterated? Well, the assertion is there in the respect shown by a parent for a child's "security blanket". It's there as well when an adult asks of a three-year-old "What do you want to eat for dinner?" and again in the knock on the door before entering the child's personal space, his private bedroom, another replica of the assertion.

The ego's view of its-"self" is the product of the collective imagination. In the West, the messages implicit in many of our child handling *practices* may well socialize deep *intuitions* about the "indecency" of outside (external) intrusions, regulations or invasions of our imagined inviolatable self. Practices cultivate intuitions, intuitions about what's decent, which then support such Western notions as "free to choose" (Friedman and Friedman 1980), "autonomy in decision-making", "sanctuary" and "my own business" (see the literature on privacy law, e.g., Bostwick (1976); Gerety (1977)).

Of course not all cultures socialize autonomy or redundantly confirm the right of the individual to projects of personal expression, to a body, mind, and room of his own. To members of sociocentric organic cultures the concept of the autonomous individual, free to choose and mind his own business, must feel alien, a bizarre idea cutting the self off from the interdependent whole, dooming it to a life of isolation and loneliness (Kakar 1978:86). Linked to each other in an interdependent system, members of organic cultures take an active interest in one another's affairs, and feel at ease regulating and being regulated. Indeed, others are the means to one's functioning and vice versa.

It is also sobering to reflect on the psychic costs, the existential penalties of our egocentrism, our autonomous individualism. There are costs to having no larger framework within which to locate the self. Many in our culture lack a meaningful orientation to the past. We come from nowhere, the product of a random genetic accident. Many lack a meaningful orientation to the future. We are going nowhere — at best we view ourselves as "machines" that will one day run down. The social order we view as the product of our making — an "association" based on contract and individual consent. In our view, society is dependent on us. And what are our gods? Personal success and wealth; "the tangible evidences of financial success have come to symbolize . . . the whole expectancy of ego satisfaction" (Smith 1952:398). Cut adrift from any larger whole the self has become the measure of all things, clutching to a faith that some "invisible hand" will by slight of hand right things in the end.

Of course what we've just said about egocentrism and autonomy in the West could easily be rewritten in terms of psychic benefits and one should not forget that sociocentrism has severe costs as well. Perhaps the real point is that the costs and benefits of egocentrism and sociocentrism are not the same (*pace* universalism), nor are the benefits mostly on one side and the costs mostly on the other (*pace* evolutionism).

CONCLUSION

In 1929 Edward Sapir remarked that "the worlds in which different societies live are distinct worlds, not merely the same world with different labels attached".

In this essay we have tried to show that different peoples not only adopt distinct world views, but that these world views have a decisive influence on cognitive functioning.

People around the world do not all think alike. Nor are the differences in thought that do exist necessarily to be explained by reference to differences or "deficits" in cognitive processing skills, intellectual motivation, available information, or linguistic resources. It is well known in cognitive science that what one thinks about can be decisive for how one thinks (e.g., Wason and Johnson-Laird 1972). What's not yet fully appreciated is that the relationship between what one thinks about (e.g., other people) and how one thinks (e.g., "contexts and cases") may be *mediated* by the world premise to which one is committed (e.g., holism) and by the metaphors by which one lives (Lakoff and Johnson 1980).

REFERENCES

Austin, J. L.
  1962 How To Do Things With Words. Oxford: Clarendon Press.
Benedict, R.
  1946 The Chrysanthemum and the Sword. New York: New American Library.
Berlin, B. and P. Kay
  1969 Basic Color Terms: Their Universality and Evolution. Berkeley: University of California Press.
Bostwick, G. L.
  1976 A Taxonomy of Privacy: Repose, Sanctuary, and Intimate Decision. California Law Review 64:1447–1483.
Bruner, J. S., R. R. Olver, and P. M. Greenfield
  1966 Studies in Cognitive Growth. New York: John Wiley and Sons.
Burton, M. L.
  1968 Multidimensional Scaling of Role Terms. Unpublished Ph.D. dissertation. Stanford University.
Collingwood, R. G.
  1972 An Essay on Metaphysics. Chicago: Henry Ragnery Co.
Conklin, H.
  1955 Hanunoo Color Categories. Southwestern Journal of Anthropology 11:339–344.
D'Andrade, R. G.
  1965 Trait Psychology and Componential Analysis. American Anthropologist 67:215–228.
  1973 Cultural Constructions of Reality. *In* Cultural Illness and Health. L. Nader and T. W. Maretzki (eds.). Washington: American Anthropological Association.
  1974 Memory and the Assessment of Behavior. *In* Measurement in the Social Sciences. T. Blalock (ed.). Chicago: Aldine-Atherton.
Durkheim, E. and M. Mauss
  1963 Primitive Classification. Chicago: University of Chicago Press.
Dumont, L.
  1960 World Renunciation in Indian Religions. Contributions to Indian Sociology 4:3–62.
  1970 Homo Hierarchicus. Chicago: University of Chicago Press.

Evans-Pritchard, E. E.
    1937 Witchcraft, Oracles and Magic Among the Azande. Oxford: Clarendon.
Feyerabend, P.
    1975 Against Method. Atlantic Highlands. NJ: Humanities Press.
Findley, J. D.
    1979 Comparisons of Frogs, Humans and Chimpanzees. Science 204:434–435.
Fiske, S. T. and M. G. Cox
    n.d. Describing Others: There's More to Person Perception Than Trait Lists. Unpub-
          lished manuscript, Department of Psychology and Social Relations, Harvard
          University.
Fortes, M.
    1959 Oedipus and Job in West African Religion. Cambridge: Cambridge University
          Press.
Frake, C. O.
    1962 The Ethnographic Study of Cognitive Systems. In Anthropology and Human
          Behavior. T. Gladwin and W. C. Sturtevant (eds.). Washington: Anthropological
          Society of Washington.
Friedman, M. and R. Friedman
    1980 Free To Choose. New York: Harcourt, Brace and Jovanovich.
Geertz, C.
    1973 Interpretation of Cultures. New York: Basic Books.
    1975 On the Nature of Anthropological Understanding. American Scientist 63:47–
          53.
Gerety, T.
    1977 Redefining Privacy. Harvard Civil Rights-Civil Liberties Law Review 12:233–
          296.
Glick, J.
    1968 Cognitive Style Among the Kpelle. Symposium on Cross-Cultural Cognitive
          Studies. Unpublished manuscript, American Education Research Association,
          Chicago.
Goffman, E.
    1971 Relations in Public. New York: Harper and Row.
Goodman, N.
    1968 Languages of Art. New York: Bobbs-Merrill.
    1972 Seven Strictures on Similarity. In Problems and Projects. N. Goodman (ed.).
          New York: Bobbs-Merrill.
Goody, J.
    1977 The Domestication of the Savage Mind. New York: Cambridge University Press.
Greenfield, P. M.
    1972 Oral or Written Language: The Consequence for Cognitive Development in Africa,
          the United States, and England. Language and Speech 15:169–178.
Hart, H. L. A.
    1961 The Concept of Law. London: Oxford University Press.
Hartshorne, H. and M. A. May
    1928 Studies in the Nature of Character, Volume 1. Studies in Deceit. New York:
          Macmillan.
Hempel, C. G.
    1965 Science and Human Values. In Aspects of Scientific Explanation. C. G. Hempel
          (ed.). New York: Free Press.
Horton, R.
    1967 African Traditional Thought and Western Science, Part 2. Africa 37:159–187.
    1968 Neo-Tylorianism: Sound Sense or Sinister Prejudice? Man 3:625–634.
Jespersen, O.
    1934 Language: Its Nature, Development, and Origin. London: Allen and Unwin.

Kakar, S.
  1978 The Inner World: A Psychoanalytic Study of Childhood and Society in India. Oxford: Oxford University Press.
Kohlberg, L.
  1969 Stage and Sequence: The Cognitive-Developmental Approach to Socialization. *In* Handbook of Socialization Theory and Research. D. A. Goslin (ed.). New York: Rand McNally.
  1971 From Is To Ought: How To Commit The Naturalistic Fallacy And Get Away With It In The Study of Moral Development. *In* Cognitive Development and Epistemology. T. Mischel (ed.). New York: Academic Press.
Kroeber, A. L.
  1909 Classificatory Systems of Relationship. Journal of the Royal Anthropological Institute 39:77–84.
Kruskal, J. B. and R. Ling
  1967 How To Use The Yale Version of MDSCALE, A Multidimensional Scaling Program. Unpublished manuscript.
Lakoff, G. and M. Johnson
  1980 Metaphors We Live By. Chicago: University of Chicago Press.
Leary, T. and H. S. Coffey
  1955 Interpersonal Diagnosis: Some Problems of Methodology and Validation. Journal of Abnormal and Social Psychology 50:110–124.
LeVine, R. A.
  1976 Patterns of Personality in Africa. *In* Responses to Change. G. A. DeVos (ed.). New York: Van Nostrand-Reinhold.
Levi-Strauss, C.
  1963 Structural Anthropology. New York: Doubleday.
  1966 The Savage Mind. Chicago: University of Chicago Press.
  1969a The Elementary Structures of Kinship. Boston: Beacon Press.
  1969b The Raw and the Cooked. New York: Harper and Row.
Levy, R. I.
  1973 Tahitians: Mind and Experience in the Society Islands. Chicago: University of Chicago Press.
Lorr, M. and D. M. McNair
  1963 An Interpersonal Behavior Circle. Journal of Abnormal and Social Psychology 2:823–830.
  1965 Expansion of the Interpersonal Behavior Circle. Journal of Personality and Social Psychology 2:823–880.
Luria, A.
  1976 Cognitive Development: Its Cultural and Social Foundations. Cambridge, Mass.: Harvard University Press.
Marriott, M.
  1976 Hindu Transactions: Diversity Without Dualism. *In* Transactions and Meaning. B. Kapferer (ed.) Philadelphia: Institute for the Study of Human Issues.
Mischel, W.
  1968 Personality and Assessment. Stanford: Stanford University Press.
Morgan, L. H.
  1871 Systems of Consanguinity and Affinity of the Human Family. Smithsonian Contributions to Knowledge, No. 218. Washington, D.C.: Smithsonian Institution.
Nerlove, S. and A. K. Romney
  1967 Sibling Terminology and Cross-Sex Behavior. American Anthropologist 69:179–187.
Newcomb, T. M.
  1929 The Consistency of Certain Extrovert-Introvert Behavior Patterns in 51 Problem Boys. Contributions to Education 382. Teachers College, Columbia University.

Nisbett, R. E.
    1980 The Trait Concept in Lay and Professional Psychology. *In* Forty Years of Social
          Psychology. L. Festinger (ed.). New York: Oxford University Press.
Osgood, C. E.
    1964 Semantic Differential Technique in the Comparative Study of Cultures. American
          Anthropologist 66:171–200.
Pareto, V.
    1935 The Mind and Society. New York: Harcourt Brace.
Pepper, S. C.
    1972 World Hypotheses: A Study in Evidence. Berkeley: University of California Press.
Perelman, C.
    1963 Idea of Justice and the Problem of Argument. Atlantic Highlands, Humanities
          Press.
Phillips, D. C.
    1976 Holistic Thought in Social Science. Stanford, California: Stanford University
          Press.
Piaget, J.
    1966 Need and Significance of Cross-Cultural Studies in Genetic Psychology. Interna-
          tional Journal of Psychology 1:3–13.
Praharaj, G. C.
    1931– Purnnachandra Ordia Bhashokosha (A Lexicon of the Orya Language), Vol.
    1940 1–7. Cuttack: Utkal Sahitya Press.
Price-Williams, D. R.
    1975 Explorations in Cross-Cultural Psychology. San Francisco: Chandler and Sharp.
Read, K. E.
    1955 Morality and the Concept of the Person Among the Gahuku-Gama. Oceania 25:
          233–282.
Rorty, R.
    1979 Philosophy and the Mirror of Nature. Princeton, N.J.: Princeton University Press.
Sapir, E.
    1929 The Status of Linguistics as a Science. Language 5: 207–214.
Searle, J. R.
    1979 A Taxonomy of Illocutionary Acts. *In* Expression and Meaning. J. R. Searle
          (ed.). New York: Cambridge University Press.
Selby, H. A.
    1974 Zapotec Deviance. Austin: University of Texas Press.
    1975 Semantics and Causality in the Study of Deviance. *In* Sociocultural Dimensions
          of Language Use. M. Sanches and B. G. Blount (eds.). New York: Academic
          Press.
Shepard, R.
    1962a The Analysis of Proximities: Multidimensional Scaling with an Unknown Distance
          Function I. Psychometrics 27:125–140.
    1962b The Analysis of Proximities: Multidimensional Scaling with an Unknown Distance
          Function II. Psychometrics 27:219–246.
    1963 Analysis of Proximities as a Technique for the Study of Information Processing
          in Man. Human Factors 5:33–48.
Shweder, R. A.
    1972 Semantic Structures and Personality Assessment. Unpublished Ph.D. dissertation.
          Cambridge: Harvard University. University Microfilms, Ann Arbor, Michigan,
          Order #72–79, 584.
    1975 How Relevant is an Individual Difference Theory of Personality? Journal of
          Personality 43:455–484.
    1977a Likeness and Likelihood in Everyday Thought: Magical Thinking in Judgments

About Personality. Current Anthropology 18:637–658. Reprinted in Thinking: Readings in Cognitive Science. P. N. Johnson-Laird and P. C. Wason (eds.). Cambridge: Cambridge University Press. (1978).

1977b Illusory Correlation and the MMPI Controversy. Journal of Consulting and Clinical Psychology 45:917–924.

1979a Rethinking Culture and Personality Theory Part I: A Critical Examination of Two Classical Postulates. Ethos 7:255–278.

1979b Rethinking Culture and Personality Theory Part II: A Critical Examination of Two More Classical Postulates. Ethos 7:279–311.

1980a Factors and Fictions in Person Perception: A Reply To Lamiell, Foss and Cavenee. Journal of Personality 48:74–81.

1980b Rethinking Culture and Personality Theory Part III: From Genesis and Typology to Hermeneutics and Dynamics. Ethos 8:60–94.

Shweder, R. A. and R. G. D'Andrade

1979 Accurate Reflection or Systematic Distortion? A Reply to Block, Weiss and Thorne. Journal of Personality and Social Psychology 37:1075–1084.

1980 The Systematic Distortion Hypothesis. In Fallible Judgment in Behavioral Research: New Directions for Methodology of Social and Behavioral Science, No. 4. R. A. Shweder (ed.). San Francisco: Jossey-Bass, Inc.

Simmel, A.

1968 Privacy. International Encyclopedia of the Social Sciences 12:480–487.

Smith, H.

1961 Accents of the World's philosophies. Publications in the Humanities No. 50. Department of Humanities, Massachusetts Institute of Technology. Cambridge, Massachusetts.

Smith, M. W.

1952 Different Cultural Concepts of Past, Present and Future. Psychiatry 15:395–400.

Super, C. M., S. Harkness, and L. M. Baldwin

1977 Category Behavior in Natural Ecologies and in Cognitive Tests. The Quarterly Newsletter of the Institute for Comparative Human Development 1(4). Rockefeller University.

Trilling, L.

1972 Sincerity and Authenticity. Cambridge, Mass.: Harvard University Press.

Wason, P. C. and P. W. Johnson-Laird

1972 The Psychology of Reasoning. London: Batsford.

Werner, H. and B. Kaplan

1956 The Developmental Approach to Cognition: Its Relevance to the Psychological Interpretation of Anthropological and Ethnolinguistic Data. American Anthropologist 58:866–880.

White, G. M.

1980 Conceptual Universals in Interpersonal Language. American Anthropologist 82:759–781.

Wittgenstein, L.

1968 Philosophical Investigations. New York: Macmillan.

SECTION II

CULTURAL CONCEPTIONS OF MENTAL DISORDER

BYRON J. GOOD AND MARY-JO DELVECCHIO GOOD

5. TOWARD A MEANING-CENTERED ANALYSIS OF POPULAR ILLNESS CATEGORIES: "FRIGHT ILLNESS" AND "HEART DISTRESS" IN IRAN

INTRODUCTION

In recent publications, Marsella outlined an approach to cross-cultural psychiatric epidemiologies. He suggests that such studies begin with an "emic determination of disorder categories", utilizing ethnoscience techniques "to evolve categories of disorder and their experiential components which are meaningful to the cultures under study" (Marsella 1978:351; cf. Marsella 1979:246; 1980:49). These illness categories should then be submitted to epidemiological research, establishing baseline data and using multivariate analysis to determine objective patterns of disorder for particular societies. Such culture-specific studies should precede cross-cultural comparison. This approach will be welcomed by many anthropologists as having significant advantages over traditional psychiatric epidemiologies, of the sort Kleinman has called "the old transcultural psychiatry" (Kleinman 1977). Anthropologists experienced in studying illness across cultures will recognize also that the most fundamental aspect of such research — the emic determination of categories of disorder — is fraught with important methodological and theoretical difficulties.

This paper will examine the relationship between mental disorders and culture-specific or "emic" categories. At issue are the following kinds of questions. How are we to discover culture-specific illness syndromes? Can we rely on ethnoscience techniques to identify such categories? Can we expect folk categories to be used as labels for particular syndromes of symptoms? Can we expect popular or folk illness categories to map onto Western psychiatric diagnostic entities? Are epidemiologies of such folk categories feasible? These questions lead directly to more general issues concerning the relationship of psychiatric disorders and the system of shared meanings in terms of which suffering is experienced and communicated in a society. How are we to study the meanings associated with illness and healing across cultures? What is the status of cultural "explanations" of psychiatric disorders? What does the anthropologist, engaged in detailed cultural analysis and case studies, have to offer the psychiatric epidemiologist?

In this paper we argue that any approach to studying illness cross-culturally is embedded in a particular theory of language and meaning. We first demonstrate that traditional epidemiologies and some anthropological theories share an "empiricist theory of language". This paradigm is criticized and a "meaning-centered approach" that incorporates semantic and hermeneutic analyses proposed. We then contrast the Iranian categories "illness by fright" and "heart distress" to raise questions about the nature of emic categories of disorder. We

A. J. Marsella and G. M. White (eds.), Cultural Conceptions of Mental Health and Therapy, 141–166.

conclude with a discussion of the implications of cultural analysis for psychiatric epidemiology.

FOLK ILLNESSES, EPIDEMIOLOGY AND THE EMPIRICIST THEORY OF MEDICAL LANGUAGE

Cross-cultural theories of illness and healing are grounded, explicitly or implicitly, in a particular epistemology and theory of language. Assumptions are made about the nature of disease and its relationship to the empirical or phenomenological data observed by the clinician or researcher; about the status of various forms of medical discourse (e.g., the complaint of a sick person, the clinician's diagnostic or therapeutic discourse, the scientist's theory); and about how the meaning of discourse is constituted. One of the most significant changes in the human sciences in the past two decades has been the recognition of the centrality of discourse and the importance of discourse analysis for understanding social, political and personal realities. Examples of this change include the emergence of linguistic philosophy and a renewed interest in Wittgenstein, the growth of interest in Foucault's discursive analysis among historians of medicine, the development of socio-linguistics and interpretive theories in anthropology, and a reconceptualization of the role of language in psychoanalysis. Despite these changes, many anthropological theories of medicine, along with psychiatric epidemiology and biomedical theory, remain grounded in a positivist understanding of discourse we may call "the empiricist theory of language". If efforts to carry out epidemiology in terms of categories of illness meaningful to the society under study are to be successful, the empiricist paradigm must be subjected to critical analysis and new techniques developed that are grounded in emerging symbolic and discursive paradigms.

The empiricist tradition of anthropological studies of folk illnesses and cross-cultural psychiatric research have shared the following basic assumptions. Diseases, it is assumed, are grounded in biological or psycho-physiological processes and therefore are universal. Their phenomenological appearance, however, is shaped by culture. Culture systematically selects some symptoms associated with a disease and suppresses others. Given the same set of body sensations, members of different cultural groups will selectively attend to, complain about, and seek professional help for some symptoms and not others. In cases of thought disorders, the content of the symptoms will be culturally variable as well. Folk medical systems provide a classificatory scheme that maps symptoms onto discrete folk illness categories, which may or may not be equivalent to "real" (biomedical) disease categories.

This paradigm suggests a clear logic and strategy for research. First, anthropologists should study how folk theories lead members of a society to attend to particular experiences and complain about them as symptoms, while other experiences remain unlabeled and untroubling. The most valuable result of such a study for clinicians and epidemiologists would be a culture-specific code describing the correct mapping of verbal expression onto underlying physiological processes. Second, the anthropologist should study the mapping of culturally meaningful symptom expressions onto the categories of folk nosology. Third, the results of these studies should allow the clinician or epidemiologist to map folk illness categories or sets of symptoms onto the diagnostic entities of scientific medicine and psychiatry. Such a strategy would allow the researcher to move beyond the phenomenal expression of suffering to the underlying disease entity.

The anthropological and cross-cultural literature is replete with studies assuming this logic. Cross-cultural psychiatrists have often sought to establish that the culture-bound disorders are known psychiatric diseases in cultural garb. For example, anthropologists and psychiatrists have debated whether *susto* should be considered an anxiety reaction associated with acute psychic stress or a depressive disorder (e.g., Gillin 1948; Kiev 1972). Epidemiologists have sought increasingly rigorous methods for identifying diagnostic entities in a culture-free manner. This research has often failed to produce results that are both culturally meaningful and epidemiologically significant.

Counter to this universalist position, cultural relativists have argued that each society constructs its own psychiatric disorders by distinguishing normal and deviant forms of experience and behavior. Some studies argue explicitly that the fact that societies differentially respond to particular behaviors and that different syndromes of deviance exist across cultures provides evidence that there *are* no psychiatric diseases, that psychiatric entities are produced by keepers of order in a society, and that such production is therefore essentially political. Dispute over this contention has led to unproductive debate over the ontological status of mental diseases and over the specificity with which culture-bound illnesses are linked to biologically real diseases. Such debate often obscures important cross-cultural findings and theoretical advances. As recently as 1976 in *Science*, Murphy implicitly identified social response theory with the position that psychiatric diseases do not exist and sought to discredit such theory by showing that all societies really do have mental illness.

Both the universalist position and the logic of the debate with the social labeling theories are grounded in an empiricist theory of medical language. A number of authors have criticized the methodology and philosophical assumptions of the universalist position (Kleinman 1977; Marsella 1978; Fabrega 1972). We will briefly focus on the theory of discourse in which this position is embedded to provide the basis for a positive critique and an alternative approach. Biomedicine, cross-cultural epidemiologies, and a number of recent approaches to medical anthropology share many of the assumptions of what Harrison calls "the empiricist theory of language" (1972). The meaning of discourse, according to this paradigm, is constituted by its relationship to empirical reality. Meaning attaches to basic utterances in language through a conventional association between a "language element" and a particular "world element" (Harrison 1972: 33; cf. Good 1977:52). In Foucault's terms, this paradigm holds that the "order of words" has meaning through an ostensive relationship to the "order of things"

(Foucault 1970; cf. White 1973). The validity of a configuration of the symbolic or discursive order is thus judged by the accuracy with which it reflects the empirical order.

The history of empiricist theories of language and medicine are deeply entwined. Givner (1962) argues that Locke modeled this theory of language on the medical experiments of his friend Sydenham. The two primary functions of language, Locke believed, are *designation* and *classification*. Similarly, the foremost task of clinical research, according to Sydenham, is the accurate identification of naturally-occurring disease entities, the discovery of their distinctive clinical features, and the establishment of nosologies that reflect their natural interrelationships.

The dominant medical model employed in contemporary medical research and clinical practice is grounded in an empiricist theory of language. Diseases are conceived as universal biological or psychophysiological entities, resulting from somatic lesions or dysfunctions. Somatic or biochemical disorders produce experiences of distress and suffering that are communicated as complaints, and physiological and behavioral abnormalities that may be measured by clinical, laboratory or psychometric procedures. The patient's discourse is thus interpreted as a "manifestation" of an "underlying abnormality" and is "ultimately ascribed to a particular diagnostic entity" (Feinstein 1973:220). The primary tasks of clinical medicine are diagnosis — the interpretation of patients' symptoms by relating them to underlying disease entities — and "rational treatment" (Kety 1974) aimed at intervention in the biological sequence of causes of disorder. Whatever the cultural form or rhetorical function a patient's discourse may have, and however untrustworthy a patient's discourse may be, the primary interpretive strategy of clinical medicine is to link complaints to underlying processes and ultimately to disease entities. The semantic elements of medical discourse have as their referents elements in the physiological order.

Many cross-cultural medical and psychiatric studies not only assume an empiricist theory of medical language, but are modeled specifically on biomedical theory and clinical practice. This has been particularly important for the study of folk illness categories. Ethnoscience and ethnosemantic studies of folk nosologies, prominent in the 1960s, serve as examples. Ethnoscience provided a procedure for eliciting and analyzing elements in native classificatory schemata in terms of the distinctive features that mark the boundaries of the categories. This approach was modeled on biomedical theory in several ways. First, it assumed the disease world (both in empirical reality and in folk knowledge) to be made up of discrete and mutually exclusive disease entities, each having a name of its own. For example, Frake described Subanun disease classification as follows:

Conceptually the disease world, like the plant world, exhaustively divides into a set of mutually exclusive categories. Ideally every illness either fits into one category or is describable as a conjunction of several categories (Frake 1961:131).

Second, it assumed the distinctive features used to discriminate among disease entities to be symptoms (e.g., Kay 1979; Fabrega and Silver 1973:ch. 7). Third, diagnosis was understood to be the linking of a patient's condition to a disease category through the interpretation of symptoms as distinctive features (e.g., Frake 1961). Thus, along with Locke and Sydenham, the ethnosemanticists held designation and classification to be the primary functions of medical discourse. The logical conclusion of such an approach was to map folk categories onto biomedical categories (see Fabrega and Silver 1973), thus providing a basis for evaluation of the validity of folk categories and a procedure for epidemiologists who want to work within culturally relevant categories.

The empiricist theory of medical language and its application to cross-cultural research may be criticized on a number of grounds. First, assumptions made about the nature of illness categories and diagnosis have not been borne out by empirical research. For example, illness categories in a number of societies have not been found to be defined as a distinctive set of symptoms or clinical signs as the ethnoscientists expected. Gilbert Lewis found that "the Gnau do not depend on observation of the physical signs or symptoms of illness to discriminate between them ... " (Lewis 1976:75). Fabrega's detailed analysis of Zinacanteco illness categories showed that "most illness terms seemed to be linked with a number of general symptoms" (Fabrega 1970:305) and that several illness terms share the same distinctive features (Fabrega and Silver 1973: 116). This raises the question, as Fabrega recognizes, of whether symptoms are the distinctive features of many illness categories, or whether "the critical features of folk illnesses may refer to the social and moral characteristics of the person who is ill" (Fabrega 1970:312).

In other societies, as our experience in Iran suggests, some illness categories are defined in clinical/symptomatic terms while others are not. Second, traditional forms of diagnosis have often been assumed to be a process of linking symptom clusters to illness categories. Again, the literature on healers demonstrates that explicit elicitation of symptoms is often not part of the diagnostic process. For example, prayer writers in Iran may gather astrological information about a client, sometimes in the absence of the client, and determine the illness category (fright, jinns, evil eye, etc.) without inquiring in any detail about symptomatology. Finally, it is often assumed by cross-cultural studies grounded in the empiricist paradigm, that folk illness categories are disease-specific or at least specific to culturally patterned illness syndromes. Our research, which will be described below, questions even this assumption. Thus, research findings raise serious questions about using emic categories determined through ethnoscience techniques as the basis for epidemiological research.

The empiricist theory of medical language can also be challenged on more fundamental theoretical grounds. First, empiricist theories assume folk taxonomies to more or less accurately reflect empirical reality. Since biomedical categories reflect actual diseases with increasing accuracy, the validity of folk nosologies can be determined by comparing them with biomedical categories. This reasoning produces what Kleinman calls the "category fallacy":

Having dispensed with indigenous illness categories because they are culture-specific, studies of this kind go on to superimpose their own cultural categories on some sample of deviant behavior in other cultures, as if their own illness categories were culture-free (Kleinman 1977:4).

Second, the conception of cultural categories as conjunctions of discrete features which divide reality into discrete, mutually exclusive units has come under criticism. Eleanor Rosch (1975) argues that "the prevailing 'digital' model of categories in terms of logical conjunctions of discrete criterial attributes is inadequate and misleading when applied to most natural categories" (Rosch 1975:178). She proposes an alternative "analog" model, "which represented natural categories as characterized by 'internal structure'; that is, as composed of a 'core meaning' (the prototype, the clearest cases, the best examples) of the cateogory, 'surrounded' by other members of decreasing similarity and decreasing 'degree of membership'" (179). This view raises fundamental questions about characterizing illness categories, as they are used either in folk practice or by clinicians, as discrete and mutually exclusive. Rosch's work suggests findings corresponding with this view of illness categories may be an artifact of the research methodology employed (e.g., ethnoscience elicitation procedures). Third, recent work in cognitive psychology suggests that in practice, categories join traits that have semantic similarity rather than those that correspond in actual behavior. In a careful analysis of how observers rate behaviors of individuals in experimental settings, D'Andrade found that:

... traits the observer considers similar will be recalled as applying to the same person, even when this is not the case. As a result of this effect, the correlations found between traits prove to be due more to the observer's conception of "what is like what" than to covariation in the behavior of the subject (D'Andrade 1974:161).

These findings challenge the view that "language elements" and "world elements" are isomorphic and suggest further research is needed to discover how semantic structures influence diagnostic judgments. Finally, the empiricist paradigm conceives meaning as a relationship between language and a reality that lies outside of language, and therefore as essentially independent of social and cultural context. Such a view fails to call into question precisely those variables most important in cross-cultural psychiatric studies.

We argue that *the meaning of medical discourse is constituted in relationship to socially constructed illness realities*, which are developed in interaction with physiological and psychophysiological processes but are not simple reflections of them. From this perspective, analysis of the nonreferential and theoretical functions of medical discourse takes on new importance. Medical discourse is conceived as a constructive process embedded in social, institutional, and cultural contexts. The semantic structure of illness discourse and the interpretive use of medical models to construct illness realities become central foci of research.

A MEANING-CENTERED APPROACH TO THE STUDY OF
FOLK ILLNESS CATEGORIES

A variety of recent studies in the social sciences focusing on meaning, discourse, interpretation theory, and reality construction provides the theoretical framework and methodology for what we have called a "meaning-centered approach to medical anthropology" (Good and Good 1980, 1981). This approach provides an alternative to the "disease-centered" empiricist paradigm outlined above. We will briefly outline several aspects of this approach, then turn to an analysis of two categories of illness in Iran.

A meaning-centered approach to medical anthropology begins with two underlying assumptions. First, it assumes that meaning in discourse is not constituted primarily by an ostensive relationship between a symbol (signifier) and an objective reality in the physical universe (signified). Meaning is rather constituted as coherent networks of symbols through which experienced realities are constructed. Meaning is constituted in the interpretive experience, through which subjects make sense of some part of their lived-in world. Second, a meaning-centered medical anthropology assumes that medical idiomata provide interpretive frameworks used in the construction of personal and social realities. The concept "illness reality" may be used to bridge biological and sociocultural aspects of disease (Good and Good 1981). Following Berger and Luckmann, we define "reality" as "a quality appertaining to phenomena that we recognize as having being independent of our own volition (we cannot 'wish them away')" (Berger and Luckmann 1966:1). Illness is a paramount reality in human experience. It appears as a natural phenomenon in all societies, beyond control, invading life as ultimately threatening. At the same time, the reality revealed by sickness varies by society and according to the social and meaningful form of the illness experience. Sickness reveals the reality of spirits in one society, bioamine deficiences in another. Illness realities are thus biologically constrained and culturally constructed. Medical language provides the medium through which illness realities are constructed, constituted as skilled performances, interpreted and re-interpreted retrospectively, used to achieve conscious and unconscious results, and responded to by a variety of actors in the social field of the sufferer (cf. Fischer 1977). On the other hand, individuals and societies are narrowly constrained in this process: constrained by psycho-physiological processes and ecological relationships, constrained by the structure of medical discourse, constrainted by medical institutions that define the objects of therapeutic enterprise. The social construction of illness realities exploits universal human potentials and responds to universal limits in a culturally unique fashion.

A meaning-centered approach to medical anthropology provides a framework for the study of illness categories that is alternative to both biomedical approaches and cultural relativist analyses. This approach avoids debates over whether psychiatric illnesses are ontologically real. It makes the central issue of study the comparison of alternative constructions of illness realities — alternative forms of medical language and knowledge, alternative modes of use of medical idiomata in clinical praxis, alternative foci of clinical activity, alternative structures of relevance that determine what phenomenal realities are attended to as relevant.

A variety of methods for studying systems of discourse and meaning have been developed in the past decade, each of which may make a contribution to analyzing the semantic structure of illness realities. We outline two forms of analysis useful for studying illness categories: semantic network analysis and investigation of the social construction of illness realities. *Semantic network analysis* is based on an understanding of meaning as configurations or semantic fields, which link key public symbols both to primary social values and to powerful personal affects. The medical culture of a society and particular illness categories may be analyzed in these terms. Each illness in a culture condenses a specific semantic network. An illness reality, from this perspective, is "a 'syndrome' of typical experiences, a set of words, experiences, and feelings which typically 'run together' for the members of a society", a "set of experiences associated through networks of meaning and social interaction" (Good 1977:27).

Freud understood that a psychiatric symptom or dream symbol condenses a network of conscious and unconscious meanings, and that the most powerful symbols are those that are the most dense or "polysemic" and are linked to the most powerful affects. Similarly, an illness or a symptom condenses a network of meanings for the sufferer: personal trauma, life stresses, fears and expectations about the illness, social reactions of friends and authorities, and therapeutic experiences. The meaning of illness for an individual is grounded in – though not reduceable to – the network of meanings an illness has in a particular culture: the metaphors associated with a disease, the ethnomedical theories, the basic values and conceptual forms, and the care patterns that shape the experience of the illness and the social reactions to the sufferer in a given society (Good 1977; Sontag 1977). In any episode of major illness, personal meanings are grounded in networks of signification and linked to basic values of a society or subculture. Such networks shape the experience of individual sufferers; they are developed, sustained and changed as individuals use medical language to articulate their suffering. Semantic illness networks thus link conscious and unconscious personal experience to cultural configurations of a society.

A semantic network analysis of an illness category should identify the central images or core symbols in the medical discourse that are related to the illness. The culturally-marked experiences or units of meaning associated with the illness category may be explored by observing how key themes are used in specified medical contexts, by investigating the stressful experiences linked to the illness, and by eliciting the explanatory models and affect-laden images associated with the category. These units of meaning will be linked to the illness category and to each other through various "semiotic connectives" or associational relationships, including metaphoric, syntagmatic (indicating proximity in space or experience), causal and symbolic relationships. The resulting configuration provides insight into the integration of elements of the medical lexicon into typical syndromes of experience in a society and thus into the unique meaning an illness category — biomedical or folk — has in a particular society. This approach is modeled on symbolic studies of ritual (Turner 1967) and ritual texts (Fox 1975). Published semantic network analyses of illness categories include our studies of heart distress in Iran (Good 1977; Good 1980), Amarasingham's (1980) analysis of a case of madness in Sri Lanka, Kleinman's (1980) analysis of medical culture in Taiwan, and Blumhagen's (1980) study of hypertension in America.

Illness categories, in addition to condensing a semantic network, provide interpretive frameworks used in the construction of personal and socially validated illness realities. While the "clinical construction of illness realities" (Kleinman et al. 1978) has been analyzed to some extent in American psychiatric and medical settings (Gaines 1979; Scheff 1968; Emerson 1970; Atkinson 1977; cf. Frank 1979), surprisingly few cross-cultural accounts detail the construction of illness realities in either popular or clinical contexts. (Kleinman, (1980) is the notable exception; cf. Kleinman and Mendelsohn (1978).) Medical culture provides frames for interpreting sickness and determining the nature of the illness involved. Clinicians, whether physicians or folk specialists, have a repertoire of clinical models that are used explicitly to elicit a client's complaint, identify certain data as relevant, abstract that data from the complex totality of the sufferer, interpret the data, and construct a clinical reality that becomes the object of therapy. (See Good and Good (1980) for a detailed analysis of the interpretive dimension of clinical practice; cf. Good and Good, (1981).) Popular illness models are employed by individuals and members of their primary networks in a similar manner to construct illness realities. In either case, the illness models have a fundamental "hermeneutic" dimension: they are used to interpret subjective and symbolic data "to bring to light an underlying coherence or sense" (Taylor 1979:25) by determining the nature of the pathological condition and revealing the illness reality.[1]

In a recent analysis of an African folk nosology, Louis Mallart Guimera (1978) distinguished "descriptive" and "etiological" illness categories. The Evuzok medical system, he found, has two autonomous and complementary taxonomies: one classifying illness in purely descriptive terms, one classifying illnesses in terms of religious, magical and social causes. While many illness categories include both descriptive and etiological elements, it may be useful to make this distinction among illness categories both in terms of their primary interpretive function and their primary means of relating to clinical syndromes. Such a distinction may be particularly critical if epidemiological research is to be carried out in terms of folk categories. Etiological categories are applied to the sufferer in order to name the cause of the experienced disorder. They may be associated with diverse clinical syndromes rather than a particular behavioral entity. They may be used primarily to diagnose aspects of the social and behavioral environment of the individual rather than a symptom cluster. Descriptive categories, on the other hand, are associated with a particular set of clinical phenomena that are essential to the identification of particular illness realities. There may indeed be other forms of illness categories, such as treatment categories (illness best treated by x). Investigation of the interpretive use of illness models is required if we are to understand the relationship between popular illness categories and behavioral syndromes in a society. After providing data from Iran, we will return to this issue in the Conclusion.

What we have called a meaning-centered analysis of popular illness categories is likely to produce quite a different picture of the relationship of some folk illnesses to culture-bound syndromes than that resulting from enthosemantic or other empiricist theories. Data from Iran will illustrate.

FRIGHT ILLNESS AND HEART DISTRESS IN IRAN

The Context of the Research

Data presented in this paper were collected from 1972 to 1974 as a part of a study of social hierarchy, medical change and medical discourse in Maragheh, a provincial town in Azerbaijan in northwest Iran. The town is a subprovincial capital and major agricultural and commercial center. It has a population of over 63,000, the vast majority of whom speak Azerbaijani Turkish. The research methodologies included participant observation, numerous lengthy interviews and a stratified random sample survey on health, illness and fertility of 771 individuals in Maragheh and three nearby villages.

There are three salient medical traditions practiced in contemporary Maragheh: Galenic-Islamic medicine, which is based on Greek humoral theory; sacred medicine, which uses astrological techniques and curative prayers; and cosmopolitan-professional medicine. Each tradition continues to be practiced by specialists, from folk healers who do cupping or bone setting or who recommend and sell herbal remedies, to prayer writers and diviners, to biomedical health professionals. There are also popular home-based practices for each tradition.

Distress (Narahati) in Maragheh

Iranians who experience what we would call emotional upset often complain of being *narahat* — distressed, upset, or uncomfortable. Such distress may be associated with general malaise (*daruxlux*), weak nerves, quickness to anger or edginess (*asabanilix*), heart distress (*narahatiye qalb*), and in extreme cases with madness. According to popular explanatory frameworks, *narahati* may be caused by fright, evil eye or jinns and treated by sacred-religious cures, or caused by problems of blood, nerves, or humoral imbalance and treated with herbal or modern medicines. Individuals may be made susceptible to *narahati* by general social and personal pressures or by a specific configuration of stress (such as sudden fright) that is associated with a particular illness. While each of these forms of *narahati* has a distinctive configuration of meaning, they are not sharply bounded categories. Rather they represent a network of terms and illness syndromes that occupy overlapping semantic space.

We will briefly discuss two categories of illness in Iran – illness caused by fright, and heart distress – to illustrate some of the problems of carrying out research in terms of categories of disorder. Some of our discussion will be speculative and raise questions for further research. The two categories pose an interesting contrast. While fright illness is clearly a category and a framework for constructing illness realities in Iran, it does not seem to be associated with a particular syndrome of symptoms or a particular psychiatric disease. In contrast, heart distress seems to be associated with a typical behavioral or symptomatic syndrome.

Illness Caused by Fright

When we first began our research in Maragheh, we discovered that people frequently spoke of illness as caused by "fright". It appeared that sudden fright (shock, trauma) was an important element in Iranian medical culture. We began to speculate whether we had encountered an Iranian culture-bound disorder, and whether any specific psychiatric disorder, such as conversion symptoms, hysteria, and anxiety reactions, or night terrors in children, was associated with fright illness. However, when we saw several cases of fright and analyzed our health survey data, the existence of a particular clinical syndrome associated with the category fright illness was called into question.

Although many Iranians believe that if a person receives a start or sudden fright it may cause illness,[2] the reported symptoms of the resulting illness vary widely. There is general agreement that the sufferer turns pale or yellow. It is said colloquially that fright may "hurt ones gall bladder" or "cause ones spleen to explode", causing yellowness of the skin. Other symptoms may include turning pale, fever, excessive nervousness, weak nerves, becoming "jumpy" or easily startled (*tez tez disjinir* – he is frequently or easily startled), and shaking or quivering. Sudden shock may also cause heart palpitations and eventuate in chronic "heart distress" (*narahatiye qalb*). Less common results of "fright" may include deformity or twisting of one's mouth or eyes, development of paralysis, or even madness.

A wide variety of therapeutics is used to treat illness caused by fright. More modern people in Maragheh believe it is most appropriate to go to a doctor for such illnesses. Others recommend herbal medicines (used often as pharmaceutic "simples" to treat stomach problems, colds, or "weak nerves"). The standard traditional prescription for treating illness due to fright is one of several forms of religious cures. The most common is to have a prayer (*du'a*) written by a religious practitioner (*du'a nevis*), who divines the cause of illness through religious or astrological techniques and who treats illness primarily by writing special Arabic prayers or verses from the Qur'an.

TABLE I

Reported symptoms of fright by social group

Symptoms of fright	Professionals, civil servants	Bazaaris	Workers	Villagers	Total
Respondents (n)	156	191	146	233	726
Turns pale or yellow	44%	42%	50%	26%	40%
Has nervous problems	21%	14%	19%	20%	19%
Fever	17%	20%	14%	30%	21%
Heart palpitations	12%	14%	10%	15%	13%
Mouth or eye problems (becomes twisted, tics, squints, etc.)	1%	4%	3%	5%	3%
Becomes crazy	5%	5%	3%	4%	4%
Total responses	210	259	189	222	880

* This table analyzes answers to the question: "What are the symptoms of fright illness?" Up to two responses were recorded per respondent. Percentages refer to the percentage of respondents who gave a particular response. The sum of the percentages may thus reach a maximum of 200% for any social group.

TABLE II

Fright cures by social group

Fright cures	Professionals, civil servants	Bazaaris	Workers	Villagers	Total
Respondents (n)	156	191	146	233	726
Go to doctor	68%	41%	19%	51%	31%
Use herbs or cupping	14%	16%	18%	8%	9%
Religious cures (write prayers, use *zar*, ingest pollution, divination, shock)	49%	83%	100%	100%	59%
It cures itself	5%	2%	1%	-0-	1%
Total responses	211	270	204	373	1,058

* This table analyzes answers to the question: "What should you do if you are sick from fright?" Up to two responses were recorded per respondent. Percentages refer to the percentage of respondents who gave a particular response. The sum of the percentages may thus reach a maximum of 200% for any social group.

Another set of cures are aimed at "driving the fright out of the sufferer". Some of these simple rites have an almost mechanical logic. A hot wire or piece of burning thread will be touched to the patient, causing him to start and causing the fright to be "frightened" out of the body. Another set of rites involves the ingestion of pollution by the sufferer. Tea made from bones found in the graveyard, sugar cubes dipped in urine, *kebab* made from the feces of a white dog, smoke from burning wood tables used for washing corpses – any of these may be forced upon the patient. These cures are often justified by saying the individual is shocked by the polluted matter, causing fright to leave; but clearly underlying these cures is the symbolic logic of driving out disease by pollution. Another set of cures involves divining the cause of the fright and then dispelling this cause by casting the collected image out of the household. For example, an oily rock (*zar*) from Mecca is put in a copper bowl of water, held over the patient, and the picture that forms is interpreted as the cause of the fright. The water is then thrown over the courtyard wall in the direction of Mecca. Another rite involves creating a small dummy replicating the patient, wrapping the dummy in a shroud, then carrying the dummy to the graveyard and burying it, reciting (three times), "I place death, I take life; ... " The prevalent Iranian theory of fright is symbolically parallel to the theory of invasion or possession by jinns. While full possession cults exist in only a few limited parts of Iran (along the Persian Gulf), the model of illness invading the body and the logic of cure through dispelling an invading substance are common in Persian folk medicine.

Epidemiological data on the incidence and social distribution of illness caused by "fright" were gathered by asking respondents to our survey if anyone in their household had been ill because of fright since the New Year (eight months) and in the past two weeks. If respondents answered yes, the age and sex of the person with the illness were noted. The data indicate that women report more cases of fright illness in the household than do men, and that both women and men from more traditional social groups report more episodes than do respondents from the professional and civil servant social group.

The age and sex distribution of the illness is noteworthy, with 45% of all reported cases occuring in infants and children four years or younger. For this group, the mother's concern about a child who awakes terrified or who is unusually cranky plays an important role in the labeling process.

Two cases, one from our study in Iran and one of an Iranian student in the U.S., illustrate the social construction of fright illness.

Case I: Dr B., a general practitioner and public health physician in Maragheh, left his 13-year-old daughter in the care of his elderly, traditional mother while he and his wife went to Mecca on the pilgrimage. During their absence, which lasted over a month, his daughter became ill. He recounted his daughter's case to us.

A strange thing happened to my daughter while my wife and I were in Mecca. My daughter

TABLE III

Prevalence of "fright" and "heart distress" by social class and sex

	Professionals and high civil servants[1]	Bazaaris[1]	Workers	Villagers
Female Respondents (n)	51	87	64	64
Fright (No. cases/ household/8 mos.)	0.29	0.37	0.33	0.43
Heart Distress (No. cases/ household/8 mos.)	0.35	0.55	0.62	0.56
Male Respondents (n)	61	60	74	82
Fright (No. cases/ household/8 mos.)	0.08	0.13	0.19	0.18
Heart Distress (No. cases/ household/8 mos.)	0.20	0.43	0.25	0.34

* Respondents were asked to report for their total household; e.g., "How many people in your household have had fright illness since New Year's?" (eight months before the interview).

[1] The low civil servants and high bazaaris classes are omitted for the sake of clarity.

TABLE IV

Age distribution of reported cases of fright and heart distress

Age	Fright	Heart distress
0–1	12%	–0–
1–4	34%	1%
5–14	23%	2%
15–44 Female	23%	55%
15–44 Male	6%	16%
45+ Female	1%	18%
45+ Male	1%	7%

lost her voice and had terrible fevers every night. The doctors here who looked at her thought her illness was a complication of influenza. But my mother was certain that my daughter was ill with something else — with "fright". My mother noticed that one day when she came home from school, my daughter had lost her voice and that evening she began to have these fevers. Even after we returned from Mecca my daughter continued to have laryngitis and night fevers. I took her to an ENT specialist in Tehran. He could find nothing wrong with her and told me her larynx was physically fine. He felt it was something else which caused her to lose her voice, perhaps a form of hysteria. A psychiatrist was visiting with our friends in Tehran where we were also staying. We told him of my daughter's illness. He called her into a separate room and talked to her for no more than 15 minutes. She came out cured. He called me in to see that she was cured and could speak again. In 15, perhaps 10 minutes she was cured. We were all impressed by the psychiatrist. Our host said that he had not believed in psychiatry until that moment when he saw the results. My daughter has not had a relapse since that time.

My mother was correct when she said that the problem my daughter was suffering from was something other than influenza. My daughter had had a dream in which she saw us in a car accident in Mecca. The next day she claimed she was nearly hit by a car when she was crossing the street on the way home from school. She felt that her near-miss accident confirmed her dream. And it was from that moment that she lost her voice, and that evening, her fevers started.

Dr B. attributed his daughter's hysteric symptoms to "fright", which in his view, resulted from her being separated from her parents for an extended period, her fears for their safety in a foreign country, and the startling effects of the dream and the near-miss accident. To us, it appeared that Dr B.'s daughter suffered from conversion aphonia.

Case II: We were invited to give consultation to the psychiatrists in care of a 23-year-old Iranian male student, "Ali", who had suffered two episodes of acute manic psychosis. The hospital staff was upset by the constant presence on the ward of the student's distraught mother, Mrs A., who they believed was disruptive and over-involved in her son's care. Our relationship to patient and mother included lengthy interviews held weekly for two months. Ali had spent the past four years enrolled at various American colleges and had recently moved to California. During these four years, he suffered from severe back pains and was told by physicians that his pain was a result of nervous tension. Two weeks prior to his first psychotic episode, he was diagnosed as having a congenital defect of both kidneys with severe impairment of kidney function. He reported that the physician abruptly told him he had a life threatening illness, but that it would be corrected by two surgical operations if done immediately. Ali was stunned and terrified. In desperation, he called his mother in Iran and asked her to join him. She arrived after the first surgery was successfully completed. Three days after being discharged to his mother's care, he was admitted to the psychiatric ward because of increasingly bizarre behavior. He became grandiose, agitated, insomniac, verbally abusive to his mother and friends. He became obsessed with sexual fantasies and with the fear that his mother would be sexually assaulted. He was diagnosed as having an acute psychotic episode, responded well to treatment, and was released after one week. His second kidney operation was also successful, but several days after discharge he was readmitted to the psychiatric ward in graver condition than on first admission. He was hospitalized for two weeks, again responded well to anti-psychotic drugs, and was discharged with a diagnosis of acute manic episode. He spent two months in out-patient therapy and was maintained on Lithium. During this period his physical and mental health steadily improved.

Mrs A. attributed the onset of her son's psychiatric episodes to the "fright" he had suffered when abruptly told he had a life-threatening illness that would require immediate surgery. In her view, Ali was particularly susceptible to a "fright" disorder because he was in a new environment, living alone and socially isolated from close family and friends. Thus he had to bear the news of the illness himself. In addition, Mrs A. felt that Ali's frequent episodes of severe back pain over the past four years, his unfruitful visits to numerous physicians who could give no clear diagnosis, and especially his unwillingness to share his concerns about his health with his parents, added to his vulnerability. The final stressor was the kidney ailment and major surgery, which physically weakened her son. Mrs A. also acknowledged that her son's personality may have contributed to his vulnerability. She recalled that he was a "sensitive" and "nervous" boy, a difficult child who was quick to anger. She attributed Ali's seemingly slow recovery from his physical and mental disorders to his body's weakness.

Mrs A's attempts to understand the source of the sexual content of Ali's manic thoughts and behavior were also expressed in terms of fright or "shock" induced illness. She noted that two years earlier her son had become extremely agitated by his roommate's sexual promiscuity and that he was disturbed by American sexual mores in general. She saw her son, a conservative Muslim boy living in America, as suffering from culture "shock", which heightened his vulnerability to mental illness accompanied by inappropriate sexual behavior.

Ali's mother gave meaning to his psychotic episodes by interpeting them as a manifestation of a fright disorder. The problems she believed were associated with his illness — social isolation, a "sensitive" personality, and a frightening event — are all part of the typical semantic network of fright illness in Iran. While Ali reacted in a culturally patterned way to the news that he needed surgery, the illness reality was constructed retrospectively as his mother sought to make sense of the illness. Her interpetation was in sharp contrast to that of the psychiatrists, who used a psychophysiological model of manic depressive psychosis as well as a psychodynamic model to interpret the nature of the pathology. A bipolar affective disorder was indicated both by symptoms and course of the sickness and by a history of depressive illness in the mother's family. The coincidence of the onset of symptoms with Ali's being in an unusually intimate situation with his mother (helpless, cared for by her, sleeping with her in a one-room apartment) were interpreted psychodynamically as arousing unresolved Oedipal issues. Until we became involved as consultants, the discrepancies in interpretation and illness realities led to an impasse in communication between the staff and Ali and his mother. Difficulties were resolved to a great extent when the physicians came to understand the meaning of the illness to the family.[3]

These two cases of fright clearly raise the question of the nature of popular illness categories. Fright, it seems, is not distinguished primarily by physical symptoms or particular behaviors, although certain symptoms are commonly associated with the illness in people's minds. Fright illness does not seem to be associated with a single psychiatric syndrome or culture-specific disorder. In addition, in the two cases reported, fright language did not provide a "repertoire of behavior" (Carr 1978:289) that patterned symptoms and experience into a unique illness syndrome. Rather, the diagnosis of fright was used primarily by patients and their families retrospectively and interpretively, to make sense of otherwise baffling symptoms and to construct an illness reality appropriate to Iranian culture. This interpretation had significant implications for social response to the sufferer and expectations about prognosis.

These two cases also demonstrate some of the more important aspects of the semantic network. The coincidence of sudden danger or sudden loss, of "sensitivity", and of social isolation are believed by Iranians to pose a very grave threat to one's health. Persons away from home will often not be told of bad news, the excuse being given that "they will be startled or shocked". For example, families may reassure a member studying abroad that all is well for several years after there has been a death in the family. As a result, good news may be mistrusted. When bad news is broken, it will be broken indirectly, with extreme care, and ideally in the presence of strong social support. Some persons are believed to be particularly sensitive, and that sensitivity will be heightened if they are away from their family and home.

The view of the person as seriously threatened by emotional trauma is embedded in the Iranian view of the nature of the self and of patterns of social interaction. The ideal person is one who keeps a pure and calm interior self (safa-yi batin), negotiating outward relationships in such a way as to protect the inner self from either disclosure or exposure to anger or shame (Bateson et al. 1976; Bateson 1979). Iranians engage in a highly ritualized form of social interaction that prevents either intimacy or open conflict in public arenas (Beeman 1976).

The illness reality in the two cases reported condensed important parts of the semantic network of fright. In both cases, the themes of social isolation, sensitivity, and a sudden threatening event were present. Both Dr B. and Ali's mother felt their children were susceptible to fright because they were separated from their parents. In Ali's case, his social isolation was more severe because he was living in a foreign country and had recently enrolled in a new college. Both parents also considered their children to be particularly "sensitive". Ali's mother associated her son's sensitivity with his quickness to anger and excessive nervousness. In addition, she related his weakened physical condition to his susceptibility to illness from fright. Both parents also focused on one or two startling events as they reconstructed what they believed the course of the illness to have been.

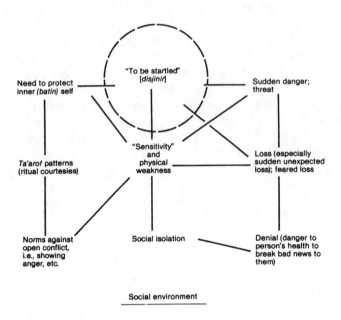

Fig. 1. Semantic network of 'fright'.

A full analysis of fright illness would need to give additional attention to cases reported among infants. In these cases, the diagnosis of fright is usually not based on a self-report of a frightening event. Aspects of the social context, rather than a psychological trauma or a peculiar set of symptoms, lead to a diagnosis of fright illness among infants. Our attention is thus shifted from an individual's experience to the cues in the broader social setting that determine when a person will be labeled ill because of fright.

Given the interpretation we have been developing here, it is clear that "illness due to fright" is not a simple, discrete disease category. Fright-caused illness occupies some of the same semantic space occupied by madness and illness due to jinns, nerves, and heart distress. It has some of the same symptoms as these disorders; it shares some of the same typical stresses in Iranian culture associated with those disorders; and its connotative meanings overlap with these other disorders. At the same time, "fright" can be understood as a symbol that condenses a *unique* configuration of meanings for Iranians. It does not seem to be used to label a unique configuration of symptoms or a particular psychiatric disease. Certain aspects of the social and cultural context, rather than the symptoms, are evaluated in the diagnostic process, and fright as an etiological model is used to make sense of an illness and condense a set of meanings. The category fright thus provides an interpretive framework used to construct and socially validate an illness reality.

Heart Distress

Heart distress is a category of illness that provides an important contrast with illness caused by fright. While we have analyzed this syndrome in great detail elsewhere (Good 1977; Good 1980), a brief description will allow us to draw the implications of this contrast for our understanding of popular illness categories.

When we arrived in Maragheh, we discovered that people commonly complained about problems of the heart. They complained of a physical sensation of their hearts pounding, quivering, or feeling squeezed or pressed. When asked the cause of their heart distress, they told us of several clusters of stresses and problems of living they believed caused the illness: those associated with the problematics of female sexuality, the status of women, and the religious pollution attributed to child birth, menstruation and bleeding; those associated with grief, loss and old age; and the experiences of family conflict, anxiety and worry. For example, women complained that the contraceptive pill caused heart distress, or individuals told how a particular conflict or loss had led to the sickness of heart distress.

While they experienced heart distress as a physiological sensation, the people of Maragheh were also aware that it was closely associated with affective life, in particular with feelings of sadness, anxiety, and feelings of being trapped. Their explanatory model of the heart was based in Galenic-Islamic medicine, where the heart was considered an organ of affect rather than a means of circulation of blood. Many of the people in Maragheh still hold to this understanding of the heart. The idiom of the heart is used to articulate affective experience associated with clusters of stresses that are particular to Iran. Heart distress thus condenses a configuration of meanings and culturally marked experiences for Iranians.

The social distribution of heart distress is quite different from that of illness caused by fright (see Tables III and IV). Unlike fright, the incidence of heart distress is highest among adult women. Of all reported cases 75% were among women 15 years of age or older. It is also highest among the lowest social classes, again especially as reported by women.

Heart distress is often associated with several other complaints: feelings of weakness, weak nerves, general malaise, anxiety, lack of patience and physical symptoms. Persons we saw who suffered from heart distress were mildly depressed, sometimes with anxiety or symptoms akin to neurasthenia. We did not see enough cases of severe depression to determine whether heart distress was a major complaint. In Afghanistan, however, Waziri (1973:215) notes that many depressed patients "described their feeling 'as if a strong hand were squeezing' their 'hearts' . . . This was the most stressed symptom from which the patient wanted relief".

It is our belief that unlike illness caused by fright, heart distress is an illness category associated with a culturally-specific illness syndrome. This syndrome

appears to be a depressive illness; it is not clear to us, however, the exact relationship between clinical depression and heart distress. We do not know, for
example, whether heart distress is associated with all depressive illness or only
some particular forms of depression. This analysis suggests hypotheses for
further research.

CONCLUSION

We began this paper asking about the relationship between popular illness categories and psychiatric disorders. We argued that empiricist theories, especially
ethnoscience, may not enable the researcher "to evolve categories of disorder
and their experiential components which are meaningful to cultures under
study" (Marsella 1978a:351). We have suggested that a meaning-centered theory
of medical language offers an alternative to empiricist theories, and used this
approach to examine our Iranian data. We will use our research findings as the
basis for making several observations.

First, it cannot be assumed that popular illness categories are associated
with particular clinical syndromes. We would expect some clinical syndromes,
which may have distinctive cultural forms, not to have their own label and unique
explanatory model in the popular medical culture of a society. On the other
hand, some illness categories may not be associated with particular syndromes.
The distinction between "descriptive" and "etiological" categories may be
useful for contrasting those associated with particular behavioral syndromes
(descriptive categories) and those that identify causation but are not specific
to particular clinical syndromes (etiological categories). While the explanatory
models of both heart distress and fright include both etiological and descriptive
explanations, heart distress seems to function as a descriptive category and
fright as an etiological category. We hypothesize that the category fright is used
to construct an illness reality that condenses a culture-specific configuration
of life stresses, but that it is not associated typically with any one clinical
syndrome. On the other hand, we hypothesize that heart distress is constructed
in the presence of dysphoric affect and specific syndromes of experience, and
is therefore associated with specific clinical or behavioral phenomena.

Other "folk illnesses" need to be submitted to such analysis. For example,
it is interesting that after many years of research we still do not know whether
susto is primarily descriptive or etiological. However, whereas earlier reports
assumed *susto* to be a descriptive category, recent data suggests this is probably
not true. O'Nell (1975) reported that "fright" is used as a framework to interpret the cause of a condition retrospectively, much as our data indicates for
Iran. In some cases, the illness was identified as due to fright and then a frightening event was searched for in the client's history. O'Nell and Rubel (1976)
found that *susto* is not associated with level or type of psychiatric impairment, but that it is associated with high levels of stress around the issue of
role performance. Our theory predicts that a semantic network anaysis would

lead to hypotheses about distinctive configurations of stress associated with *susto*.

Second, we need further investigations of the relationship between popular illness categories and particular physiological and psychological processes. Two recent studies indicate a fascinating interaction between universal psychophysiological processes and culturally patterned illness behavior. Simons' (1980) research on *latah* suggests that in all societies a part of the population is hypersensitive to being startled, but that only in some societies are hyperstartlers identified and their susceptibility exploited to construct a culture-specific syndrome. Simons claims that he, rather than the cultural theorists (e.g., Geertz 1968; Kenny 1978) can "explain" the phenomenon. What is suggested is that *latah* as a meaning syndrome has cultural roots, but the illness was developed as a framework for interpreting and exploiting a particular physiological process. Interdisciplinary research can lead to understanding of the subtle interactions between particular psychophysiological processes and the use of popular illness frameworks to interpret and react to such processes. Ness's (1978) analysis of the "old hag phenomenon" as a culturally-patterned interpretation of sleep paralysis is a second example of a similar phenomenon. It should not be expected that all culture-bound syndromes will be susceptible to such clear analysis: most disorders are far more pathoplastic than the startle reflex or sleep paralysis. For most psychiatric disorders more subtle interactions between physiological, psychological and interpretive processes must be identified and analyzed.

Third, we need many more detailed analyses of how illness models are used to construct illness realities. Analysis of clinical practice (professional and folk) may provide a framework for such research. Clinicians have a repertoire of clinical models that they use to abstract data from a patient's complaints and total condition, focusing on some data and interpreting it as resulting from a particular pathological entity (see Good and Good (1980) for a detailed analysis). Each clinical model thus has several characteristics. First, it posits a pathological entity that becomes the object of therapeutic attention (a fright, a biological lesion, a spirit, etc.). Second, it has a "structure of relevance" (Schutz 1970): it makes relevant certain data that will be considered in the diagnosis. While symptoms may be made relevant by some clinical models, aspects of the social context, family structure, or astrological conditions may be more important for others. Third, each model has certain elicitation procedures (divination, laboratory tests, consultation with spirits). Fourth, a clinical model employs a particular "interpretive strategy" for constituting the meaning of the data elicited and interpreting the client's discourse. And finally, each model has a therapeutic goal and a means of treating pathology. For many popular illness models, we have little idea about what data is made relevant in the labeling of a case. We might expect that in practice, both explicit and implicit structures of relevance are used. Spiritualist healers explicitly acknowledge only what they "see" or what their spirit guides convey to them. We believe that very subtle cues of body language and verbal responses to their statements are included in the "implicit structure of relevance", much as social class and race can influence diagnosis.

Finally, a meaning-centered medical anthropology makes a variety of symbolic and linguistic models relevant to the study of popular illness categories. Medical discourse has distinct rhetorical and performative functions in a variety of culturally-specific contexts. Sociolinguistic analysis may help us understand the processes of the construction of illness realities, the nature of the "persuasion" of healers, the functions of diverse medical rituals such as hospital admissions or healing rites, and the nature and use of sources of authority (statistics, proofs, oracles) in medical discourse.

Semantic network analysis provides an important opportunity for investigating the phenomenological structure of particular illness categories and the relationship between medical meanings and medical discourse. It is surprising how little we know about the symbolic structure of illnesses that have great symbolic potency in our own society — obesity, cancer, mental illness — and how changes in medical culture are altering the meaning of these disorders for those who suffer and for social response to these disorders. For example, "personal responsibility", a central value in Western society, but one heretofore not part of a medical sick role though explicitly part of a psychiatric one, is increasingly being associated with cancer. The social origins of such changes and their implications for the meaning of cancer have not been researched. Semantic network analysis provides an important method for analysis of changes in medical culture.

The call to base cross-cultural psychiatric research on "detailed local phenomenological descriptions" (Kleinman 1977:4) and on the "emic determination of disorder categories" (Marsella 1978:351) provides both challenge and opportunity to medical and psychiatric anthropologists. It is our belief that anthropologists need to develop their own "meaning-centered" theoretical approaches to meet this challenge, rather than relying on empiricist theories that are derivative of biomedicine. Only from this perspective can they make a fundamental contribution to medicine, psychiatry, and anthropology.

ACKNOWLEDGMENTS

Support for the research in Iran upon which this paper is based was provided by a Foreign Area Training Fellowship from the Social Science Research Council for Mary-Jo Good, a U.S. Public Health Service Traineeship for Byron Good, and a grant from the Pathfinder Fund. The writing was supported in part by N.I.M.H.-Psychiatry Education Branch, Grant No. MH 14022. Special thanks to Geoffrey White for his critical reading of the paper.

NOTES

1. The "hermeneutic" or "interpretation theory" approach to studying social reality has been made accessible through publication of Ricoeur (1976) and the introductory collection edited by Rabinow and Sullivan (1979).

We use the term "hermeneutics" in this paper to refer to the process of translating across diverse sets of meanings, which is inherent in all clinical transactions. This process, as Ricoeur (1976) argues, is analogous in important ways to textual interpretation, the subject of classical hermeneutics. As Taylor (in Rabinow and Sullivan 1979:25) indicates, both seek to make a coherent interpretation from incomplete or confusing texts or statements:

> Interpretation, in the sense relevant to hermeneutics, is an attempt to make clear, to make sense of . . . a text, or a text analogue, which in some ways in confused, incomplete, cloudy, seemingly contradictory – in one way or another unclear. The interpretation aims to bring to light an underlying coherence of sense.
> This means that any science which can be called "hermeneutical", even in an extended sense, must be dealing with one or another of the confusingly interrelated forms of meaning. And both construct interpretations by moving dialectically from the meaning of the text to the text's larger context, and back to the text itself, with ever increasingly rich interpretations.

2. In our survey, 91% of the women and 96% of the men reported that fright causes illness.
3. For a more detailed analysis of some aspects of this case, including the psychiatrist's interpretations, see Good and Good (1981).

REFERENCES

Amarasingham, L. B.
  1980 Movement Among Healers in Sri Lanka: A Case Study of a Sinhalese Patient. Culture, Medicine and Psychiatry 4:71–92.
Atkinson, P.
  1977 The Reproduction of Medical Knowledge. *In* Health Care and Health Knowledge. R. Dingwall, C. Health, M. Reid, M. Stacey (eds.). London: Croom Helm.
Bateson, M. C.
  1979 "This Figure of Tinsel": A Study of Themes of Hypocrisy and Pessimism in Iranian Culture. Daedulus, pp. 125–134 (Summer).
Bateson, M. C. et al.
  1976 Safa-yi Batin: A Study of the Interrelations of a Set of Iranian Ideal Character Types. *In* Psychological Dimensions of Near Eastern Studies. L. Carl Brown and Norman Itzkowitz (eds.), pp. 257–274. Princeton: The Darwin Press.
Beeman, W. O.
  1976 The Meaning of Stylistic Variation in Iranian Verbal Interaction. Ph.D. dissertation. University of Chicago: Department of Anthropology.
Berger, P. L. and T. Luckman
  1966 The Social Construction of Reality. New York: Doubleday & Co., Inc.
Blumhagen, D.
  1980 Hypertension: A Folk Illness With a Medical Name. Culture, Medicine and Psychiatry 4:197–228.
Carr, J. E.
  1978 Ethno-Behaviorism and the Culture-Bound Syndromes: The Case of Amok. Culture, Medicine and Psychiatry 2:269–293.
D'Andrade, R. G.
  1974 Memory and the Assessment of Behavior. *In* Measurement in the Social Sciences. H. B. Blalock (ed.), pp. 159–186. Chicago: Aldine Publishing Company.
Emerson, J.
  1970 Behavior in Private Places: Sustaining Definitions of Reality in Gynecological Examinations. *In* Recent Sociology No. 2. P. Dreitzel (ed.), pp. 73–100. London: The Macmilan Company.

Fabrega, H.
   1970 On the Specificity of Folk Illnesses. Southwest Journal of Anthropology 26: 305–314.
   1972 The Study of Disease in Relation to Culture. Behavioral Sciences 17:183.
Fabrega, H. and D. B. Silver
   1973 Illness and Shamanistic Curing in Zinacantan. Stanford: Stanford University Press.
Feinstein, A. R.
   1973 An Analysis of Diagnostic Reasoning, Parts I and II. Yale Journal of Biology and Medicine 46:212–232, 264–283.
Fischer, M. M. J.
   1977 Interpretive Anthropology. Reviews in Anthropology 4:391–403.
Foucault, M.
   1970 The Order of Things: An Archaelogy of the Human Sciences. New York: Vintage Books.
Fox, J. J.
   1975 On Binary Categories and Primary Symbols: Some Rotinese Perspectives. In Interpretation of Symbolism. Roy Willis (ed.), pp. 99–132. New York: Halsted.
Frake, C. O.
   1961 The Diagnosis of Disease Among the Subanun of Mindanao. American Anthropologist 63:112–132.
Frank, A. W.
   1979 Reality Construction in Interaction. Annual Review of Sociology 5:167–191.
Gaines, A.
   1979 Definitions and Diagnoses: Cultural Implications of Psychiatric Help-Seeking and Psychiatrists' Definitions of the Situation in Psychiatric Emergencies. Culture, Medicine and Psychiatry 3:381–418.
Geertz, H.
   1968 Latah in Java: A Theoretical Paradox. Indonesia 3:93–104.
Gillin, J. P.
   1948 Magical Fright. Psychiatry 11:387–400.
Givner, D. A.
   1962 Scientific Preconceptions in Locke's Philosophy of Language. Journal of History of Ideas 23:340–354.
Good, B.
   1977 The Heart of What's the Matter: The Semantics of Illness in Iran. Culture, Medicine and Psychiatry 1:25–58.
Good, B. J. and M. J. D. Good
   1980 The Meaning of Symptoms: A Cultural Hermeneutic Model for Clinical Practice. In The Relevance of Social Science for Medicine. L. Eisenberg and Arthur Kleinman (eds.), pp. 165–196. Dordrecht, Holland: D. Reidel Publishing Co.
   1981 The Semantics of Medical Discourse. In Sciences and Cultures: Sociology of the Sciences Vol. 5. E. Mendelsohn and Y. Elkana (eds.), pp. 177–212. Dordrecht, Holland: D. Reidel Publishing Co.
Good, M. J. D.
   1980 Of Blood and Babies: The Relationship of Popular Islamic Physiology to Fertility. Social Science and Medicine 14B: 147–156.
Guimera, L. M.
   1978 Witchcraft Illness in the Evuzok Nosological System. Culture, Medicine and Psychiatry 2:373–396.
Harrison, B.
   1972 Meaning and Structure: An Essay in the Philosophy of Language. New York: Harper and Row.

Kay, M.
  1979 Lexemic Change and Semantic Shift in Disease Names, Culture, Medicine and Psychiatry 3:73−94.
Kenny, M. G.
  1978 Latah: The Symbolism of a Putative Mental Disorder. Culture, Medicine and Psychiatry 2:209−231.
Kety, S.
  1974 From Rationalization to Reason. American Journal of Psychiatry 131:957−963.
Kiev, A.
  1972 Transcultural Psychiatry. New York: Free Press.
Kleinman, A.
  1977 Depression, Somatization and the "New Cross-Cultural Psychiatry". Social Science and Medicine 11:3−10.
  1978 Clinical Relevance of Anthropological and Cross-Cultural Research: Concepts and Strategies. American Journal of Psychiatry 135:427−431.
  1980 Patients and Healers in the Context of Culture. Berkeley: University of California Press.
Kleinman, A., L. Eisenberg, and B. Good
  1978 Culture, Illness and Care: Clinical Lessons from Anthropologic and Cross-Cultural Research. Annals of Internal Medicine 88:251−258.
Kleinman, A. and E. Mendelsohn
  1978 Systems of Medical Knowledge: A Comparative Approach. Journal of Medicine and Philosophy 3:314−330.
Lewis, G.
  1976 A View of Sickness in New Guinea. In Social Anthropology and Medicine. J. B. Loudon (ed.). pp. 49−103. New York: Academic Press.
Marsella, A. J.
  1978 Thoughts on Cross-Cultural Studies on the Epidemiology of Depression. Culture, Medicine and Psychiatry 2:343−357.
  1979 Cross-Cultural Studies of Mental Disorders. In Perspectives in Cross-Cultural Psychology. A. J. Marsella, R. Tharp, and T. Ciborowski (eds.), pp. 233−262. New York: Academic Press.
  1980 Depressive Experience and Disorder Across Cultures. In Handbook of Cross-Cultural Psychology, Volume 5: Culture and Psychopathology. H. Triandis and J. Draguns (eds.). Boston: Allyn and Bacon.
Murphy, J.
  1976 Psychiatric Labeling in Cross-Cultural Perspective. Science 191(4231):1019− 1028.
Ness, R. C.
  1978 The Old Hag Phenomenon as Sleep Paralysis: A Biocultural Interpretation. Culture, Medicine and Psychiatry 2:15−40.
O'Nell, C. W.
  1975 An Investigation of Reported "Fright" as a Factor in the Etiology of Susto, "Magical Fright". Ethos 3:268−283.
O'Nell, C. W. and A. J. Rubel
  1976 The Meaning of Susto (Magical Fright). Actas del XLI Congreso Internacional de Americanistas (1974) 3:342−349.
Rabinow, P. and W. M. Sullivan, eds.
  1979 Interpretive Social Science. Berkeley: University of California Press.
Ricoeur, P.
  1976 Interpretation Theory: Discourse and the Surplus of Meaning. Fort Worth: Texas Christian University Press.

Rosch, E.
   1975 Universals and Culture Specifics in Human Categorization. *In* Cross-Cultural
         Perspectives on Learning. R. W. Brislin, S. Bochner, and W. Lonner (eds.), pp.
         177–206. New York: John Wiley and Sons, Sage Publications.
Scheff, T.
   1968 Negotiating Reality: Notes on Power in the Assessment of Responsibility. Social
         Problems 16:3–17.
Schutz, A.
   1970 Reflections on the Problem of Relevance. R. M. Zaner, (ed.). New Haven: Yale
         University Press.
Simons, R. C.
   1980 The Resolution of the Latah Paradox. Journal of Nervous and Mental Disease
         168:195–206.
Sontag, S.
   1977 Illness as Metaphor. New York: Farrar, Straus and Giroux.
Taylor, C.
   1979 Interpretation and the Sciences of Man. *In* Interpretive Social Science: A Reader.
         P. Rabinow and W. M. Sullivan, (eds.), pp. 25–71. Berkeley: University of Cali-
         fornia Press.
Turner, V.
   1967 The Forest of Symbols: Aspects of Ndembu Ritual. Ithaca: Cornell University
         Press.
Waziri, Rafiq
   1973 Symptomatology of Depressive Illness in Afghanistan. American Journal of
         Psychiatry 130:213–217.
White, H.
   1973 Foucault Decoded: Notes from Underground. History and Theory 12(1):23–54.

ATWOOD D. GAINES

6. CULTURAL DEFINITIONS, BEHAVIOR AND THE PERSON IN AMERICAN PSYCHIATRY

INTRODUCTION

This paper extends work presented earlier (Gaines 1979b) on the relation of psychiatric actors' definitions of mental illness, seen as folk theories, to professional behavior. A summary of earlier work sees American psychiatry as ethnopsychiatry and examines the role of cultural assumptions in psychiatric theory and emergency room practice. The paper then shows how actors' definitions affect not only cognitive behaviors such as diagnosis, but also the temporal dimension of interaction with patients themselves. It is shown that differences in etiological definitions affect the length of time a resident spends with a patient before making a disposition. The next section of this paper does two things: First, it suggests that it is useful and possible to distinguish two major "Great" cultural traditions in the West. For each tradition, aspects of world view are sketched. Second, two conceptions of person which correspond to the cultural traditions distinguished, the indexical and referential, are delineated. Lastly, some implications of these differing conceptualizations for psychiatric practice are presented with reference to case material considered in the second section of the paper.

The Culture of Psychiatry

In any culture, there exist notions of dysfunction which Westerners have tried to categorize as either mental or biological. These categorizations reflect our own conception of human beings and of the domains in which problems may occur. Researchers have tended to describe and explain indigenous systems and popular psychiatric health systems in terms of Western beliefs and practices. These attempts usually compare an indigenous system to the Western (Kiev 1968) or, more frequently, force illness experiences of others into Western psychiatric nosological systems (Yap 1969) or dynamic configurations (Murphy 1976). However, little research has focused attention on the standard of comparison, Western psychiatry *qua* ethnopsychiatry. The conceptual bases of Western psychiatric theory and practice are often assumed *a priori* to be culturally neutral scientific and therefore applicable cross-culturally.

This lack of attention to American psychiatry, conceived as a cultural system on a par with other such systems, allows for the perpetuation in researchers' minds of a dichotomy between modern and traditional medicine (Kleinman 1977a), between modern/scientific psychiatry and traditional/non-scientific ethnopsychiatry. The dichotomy is also one of rationality vs. irrationality, and

167

A. J. Marsella and G. M. White (eds.), *Cultural Conceptions of Mental Health and Theory*, 167–192.

of instrumental vs. expressive forms of practice and knowledge. Hence, while *we* have psychiatry, *they* have ethnopsychiatry. However, it can be argued (Gaines 1979a, b) that both "we" and "they" have kinds of ethnopsychiatric systems, one no less culturally constructed, informed and communicated than another. I do not suggest, as per the harmful reverse ethnocentrism in medical and cross-cultural psychiatric research remarked upon by Kleinman (1980a), that because we too have an ethnopsychiatric system, other systems are better or just as efficacious. For, "while it is often stated that these (indigenous) treatment systems are effective, few studies have been mounted to investigate the outcome of indigenous and primary care for mental health problems" (Kleinman 1980a:9). As cultural systems, they all have equal status ontologically and are equally valid ways of perceiving and dealing with a world so perceived. Whether one is more efficacious than another remains to be seen.

Folk Knowledge and Theory

This paper is concerned with two levels of culture as they relate to ethnopsychiatry. One level is what may be termed folk knowledge or theory. Cognitive anthropologists have increasingly concerned themselves with "how people construct knowledge, (in) the kinds of units in which knowledge is packaged and stored in memory, and (in) the ways in which these knowledge structures are interconnected" (Quinn 1979:2). They are less concerned with taxonomies and other logical schemata criticized by Geertz (1973a) as an overly rational and logical view of human thought.

My interest in folk theories of mental illness lies in actors' use of cultural knowledge and assumptions to generate ideas and theories about certain things — things such as mental illness. This knowledge may be called a folk theory, and as such "is more culture-specific, since the knowledge it contains does not permit interpretation of different events enacted in diverse institutions and even in widely different societies" (Quinn n.d.:1). My concern here will be the relationship of folk theories of mental illness held by psychiatric residents and their behavior in the emergency room.

Ideology

The second level of culture with which I will deal is unconscious. That is, I will be looking at sets of assumptions which are not articulated and which are unconscious. They cannot be thought of as knowledge which actors can marshall to explain particular domains such as marriage (Quinn 1979) or mental illness. Rather, assumptions about the world and people in it form the bedrock of understanding which allows actors to make sense of experience and of one another. Elsewhere I have referred to such sets of assumptions as ideology (Gaines 1979a). Again, this level is unconscious and should be seen as underlying ethnopsychological or ethnopsychiatric descriptions given by ethnographic researchers. It refers to ideas abstracted from ethnographic data which provide insight into the nature of the assumptions which structure knowledge about personality (White 1978), morality (Boehm 1980), psychology (Strauss 1977; Valentine 1963) or psychopathology (Townsend 1975; 1978). These assumptions organize knowledge units to provide a cultural hermeneutic, or meaningful interpretation of experience.

This paper focuses on but one aspect of this assumptive ideology of culture (Geertz 1973b), the concept of person. The concept of person is little more than a vague outline waiting to be filled in by cultural specifics and has no meaning outside of a cultural context. The self is part and parcel of the same level of cultural assumptions. Other persons are conceiveable only in terms of the self, for the self is the key and central point of reference which makes it possible for other selves, called persons, to be characterized, described, and perceptually apprehended.

The last section of this paper will delineate two conceptions of person found in Western society, which may be expressions of two distinct Western cultural traditions, as I have suggested elsewhere (Gaines 1979a, b, c). The discussion below enlarges upon these ideas as central to ethnopsychiatric and cultural psychiatric research. This discussion views American psychiatry *qua* ethnopsychiatry, and describes the cultural "webs of significance" in which American psychiatry is suspended.

SOME PREVIOUS RESEARCH

In earlier works, a number of issues were addressed which related to Western psychiatry as an ethnopsychiatric system or, in other words, as a cultural system (Gaines 1979a, b). Before considering the influence of cultural definitions and conceptions of the person on actions in the emergency room, it is necessary first to recall some of the findings of the earlier work.

Research on psychiatric residents taking part in a residency program in a public non-profit hospital in a West Coast urban area in 1977 examined the relationship of residents' ideas about mental illness to their functioning as professionals. Initially, I had supposed that the residents' definitions of the psychiatric emergency [including their views of patients, their own role in that context (their 'job'), and the disturbances which confronted them] formed their behavior in emergency psychiatric contexts.

Interviews with residents and readings of at least one quarter of all their records of emergency room consultations, including diagnoses, showed that there was variation among the residents in their definitions and consequent actions. Diagnostic styles were shown to be grounded in and to follow logically from psychiatric residents' definitions of the psychiatric situation. It was shown that psychiatrists' definitions of the situations, especially their notions of etiology of mental disorders, play a prominent, but generally unnoted, role in the development of diagnostic variability. Pre-existing definitions led actors to emphasize or de-emphasize various aspects of the clinical picture. There was consistency, however, in each resident's diagnostic style over time. From a resident's very first consultation to his last, he showed a consistent diagnostic style.

Consistent diagnostic styles seen in my research, taken together with Light's (1976) comments about the unchanging nature of residents' work styles in an Eastern psychiatric residency training program, suggest that the definitions which serve as the foundation for residents' interpretations of medical discourses and clinical presentation are cultural, i.e., folk definitions. As such, they may be seen as cultural ideas which precede professional socialization/training and which influence scientific judgments. Such ideas need not be homogenous. There did not seem to be a single medical, or biomedical model of mental diseases among the residents observed. Rather there were a number of biological/medical models as well as others which co-existed in a single psychiatric setting. These models may be seen as variations of a particular somatic/physical or empiricist theme in Western medicine, psychiatry and culture.

In the earlier research (Gaines 1979b), models of mental illness were elicited from each of four residents who represented one half of the residents in the training program. These models again reflected residents' definitions and their diagnostic styles.

In terms of diagnostic styles, the biologically oriented residents diagnosed patients in psychiatric terms only, and no other problems were noted. One of the biologically-oriented residents saw patients as having genetically-based biological deficits while the other saw his patients as exhibiting neurological dysfunctions expressed in mental disorders. Each attributed an empirical disease to their patients on the basis of clinical presentations and medical discourse (previous records were not available to these residents).

Another resident saw the problems besetting individuals as being the result of situational problems to which they were *reacting*. In other words, patients were seen as reacting to external events and social problems not as *having* particular psychiatric diseases or conditions, a view or theory I termed 'psychosocial'.

I pointed up that diagnostic styles appeared related to etiological assumptions. That is, those with etiological assumptions which were biological (of which there were two varieties as noted above) used a uni-axial diagnostic style, while the two residents who viewed etiology in terms that were not exclusively biological were also the two who employed a multi-axial style (Gaines 1979b:407). Uni-axial diagnostic styles are as variable as multi-axial styles, two versions of each being represented in my small sample.

The earlier study did not involve actual observations being made, but used only patients' charts (read to me by each resident). Later research (1978–1979) in a larger psychiatric department with teaching and clinical functions allowed me to see and, in some instances, participate in the diagnosis of patients in emergency room contexts. In this next section I will show the influence of actors' definitions on their handling of patients seen in the emergency room of a large hospital set in an extremely ethnically diverse urban area. This section focuses on a temporal dimension of psychiatric practice, e.g., the time residents spend with their patients in emergency contexts. I hope to show that the length of time a resident spent with a patient in the emergency room was dependent upon his definition of the etiology of mental illness. These etiological definitions involve unconscious assumptions about the cause of mental illness.

TIME AND THE DEFINITION OF MENTAL ILLNESS

The following discussion focuses on the interaction of two psychiatric residents with their patients in the emergency room of a large metropolitan hospital. The hospital and the city are to be found in the western United States some distance from the city of Morningside and Madera General reported on earlier (Gaines 1979a, b) and summarized above. A total of 17 hours was spent in the emergency room with these two residents handling an equal number of patients. With Dr Bonner, the first of the residents, I spent a total of 11 hours in the emergency room while with the second resident, Dr Lauren, I spent more than six hours on two different shifts of about 3.25 hours each. This work gave me the opportunity to make additional points about the relationship of definitions to psychiatric practices that I could not have made earlier without observation of the actual interactions involved.

The aspect of diagnostic activities that I want to show is influenced by residents' definitions is, simply, the amount of time a psychiatrist will spend with a patient. That is, the definition of mental illness held by a psychiatrist will influence the amount of time which he/she will spend in direct contact and interaction with the patient, from which a diagnostic label is generated.

The two residents which I will discuss here are both male and shared a level three status (third year of a four year residency) during the time of the ethnographic present (1979). The hospital is a large, 600-bed general hospital near the downtown area of a large multi-ethnic urban center. The residency program in this hospital was approximately one-third larger than the first program reported on. Residents were required to rotate as the resident-on-call to the emergency room and had to be physically present in the hospital when on duty. The two residents I will discuss hold divergent views on the character of mental illness.

Dr Bonner adhered to a biological view of the etiology of mental illness and emphasized the genetic component of mental disorders as did Dr Smith in my earlier study. Dr Lauren, however, felt that mental disorders could be caused by biogenic, macro- or micro-sociogenic or psychogenic factors. This view is not a kind of holistic view as that held by Dr Sohm in my first study. Rather, Dr Lauren was asserting that any and/or all of these sorts of factors could be causal agents. Basically, he was asserting an open position, rather than a holistic view. Dr Lauren did not 'know' which was the most significant etiological element, and therefore could not assert that all made a contribution in varying degrees, as in the holistic viewpoint of Dr Sohm. Now let us look at the cases.

The Cases:

Dr Bonner. To characterize the way in which each resident went about work, I will provide cases from each. The first case is that of a 27-year-old white male, a Ph.D. candidate in chemistry at the local university. The patient was brought to the emergency room by his wife of three (or four) years. The patient, she thought was depressed. When asked by Dr Bonner "How do you feel?", the patient himself said, "I'm depressed, I guess". Dr Bonner asked the patient if he had been depressed before, and the patient answered that he had been some years ago. His wife noted that he periodically went on "work binges".

During the period in which Dr Bonner posed questions, the patient sat upright on a guerney in a medical examination room. As was standard practice, patients were first seen by medical staff and all vital signs checked. The patient was casually dressed and looked slightly disheveled, hair uncombed, and had a pained look on his face (though I'm unsure whether or not the patient was aware of his facial expression). He seemed slightly ill-at-ease and did not quite know why he had been brought to the hospital. The patient responded to the few questions put to him by Dr Bonner, although his responses evidenced some psychomotor retardation.

The patient's wife, after hearing what seemed to be unexceptional questions, addressed Dr Bonner and informed him that her husband had been writing letters to various people, including President Carter, Fidel Castro, Leonid Breznev and other world leaders. The patient's wife said that she had been keeping the letters for her husband who was concerned that they might get lost or otherwise go undelivered. She said the patient believed that he had very important information concerning world peace which he felt should be communicated to important world political leaders.

Dr Bonner asked the patient about the letters, but the patient simply shrugged his shoulders as if to say there was not really anything to discuss. He did ask his wife if she was keeping them safely. The patient's wife then asked to speak to Dr Bonner and me outside of the examination room. Upon leaving the room, the patient's wife extracted some papers from her purse. These papers were at least some of the letters of which she had spoken. She asked if we would like to see them. She seemed anxious and concerned that we should see the letters in order to know how ill her husband was. Dr Bonner replied, "No (I don't need to see them), I think I know what is going on". With that he turned and left, heading for the emergency room office to begin the paper work which is an inevitable accompaniment of patient dispositions.

Aside from the questions mentioned above, the other questions posed by Dr Bonner were more or less routine queries about the patient's vegetative symptoms or about occupation and residence. We were with the patient for about 4 or 5 minutes. He did not use standard interrogative devices of the formal mental status examination such as serial sevens and proverbs. The diagnosis of the patient was "manic-depressive, depressed". Dr Bonner said that he would be starting the patient on lithium but wanted to run a series of tests to ascertain whether or not the patient might have any problem metabolizing the drug.

In this brief time which I have outlined, Dr Bonner provided the patient with the services of the emergency room related to psychiatric emergencies with a minimum of delay. Other patients whom Dr Bonner saw rarely required more time, though some less. One patient was seen for about 10 seconds, a schizophrenic who was acting out and under restraint, guarded by several policemen. (The patient was a prisoner and had been brought in to obtain something to calm him.)

Dr Bonner saw some patients for a few minutes more than others, but he generally spent less than 10 minutes with each patient. It is, however, important to remember that the psychiatrist's involvement with a patient may entail large sums of time outside of the actual contact time. The disposition of a patient may involve calling a patient's regular psychiatrist, relatives, friends, medical consults, the hospital psychiatric ward or the state hospital. The latter two possibilities may take up much time if arrangements must be made to accommodate the patient at one of those psychiatric facilities. As well, one has to wait for the records of the patient before a disposition can be made. All of these contacts can add up to an hour or more for each patient.

Dr Lauren. Now Dr Lauren presents a striking contrast to the methods of Dr Bonner. In one case, Dr Lauren spent two and a half hours talking with a patient for whom it was clearly ascertainable early on that nothing could be done, due to the fact that the patient was a tourist from New Zealand who resisted hospitalization for the problem for which she had been brought in by her tour guide. The problem was not, properly speaking, psychiatric. Hospitalization would have been a means of separating combatants in a domestic war.

The patient was a woman in her fifties, the wife of a physician and a resident of New Zealand. She and her husband were on tour in the area with a group. The tour director had brought the woman in because he was at his wits' end about what to do with the doctor and his wife. It seems the couple spent most of their time in their hotel rooms drinking and fighting. They rarely took part in the tour group's activities, preferring to keep one another company with drink and fist. The patient, as she appeared in the emergency room, bore several bruises on her face and scalp; her hair was a mess. She was interviewed in one of the psychiatric interview rooms by Dr Lauren and myself. The tour guide remained throughout.

By turns in the interview, the woman refused to come into the hospital, to separate temporarily or permanently from her husband, to cease drinking, to cease fighting with her husband or to change in any other way. She maintained that her husband was, "basically, a good man and provided very well" for her. As her husband and her provider, she felt she could not criticize him for beating her. In fact, she said it was her "duty to God" to be beaten, "it was her lot in life" and she should beat it. She was a charismatic Catholic, as I ascertained during the interview.

So, for several hours, knowing that there was nothing which could be done for the woman, we talked with her, trying to reason with her. We suggested in several ways that perhaps the tour should end of for them, or at least one of them. No, she did not want to "spoil" their vacation by going home early. The tour guide felt that one or the other of them would be killed at some point in the tour. He did not want that responsibility. He hoped that the psychiatrist on duty would be able to relieve him of the burden which the couple represented to him. The woman, for her part, was in fact quite proud of her suffering. She felt she was a good and decent woman for bearing it. She felt separation or divorce were completely out of the question. Only a 'bad' woman would even think of such a thing (As she said, "what kind of woman would even . . . ").

Even confronted with this rather inflexible individual, Dr Lauren sought to provide some advice and to gain some understanding of the patient, her problems and her motivations. (Until I pointed it out, he did not recognize the relationship of the religious beliefs to her intractability.) It is, however, true that none of his knowledge or understanding could contribute to the improvement of services which he, as the psychiatrist on duty, could provide. All of the patients whom I saw with Dr Lauren were handled in this lengthy, non-directive manner. The patient mentioned above was given the diagnosis of "reactive depression caused by a family situational problem".

Another patient, a young, attractive 20 year-old woman, was brought in by her husband. The young woman evidenced extreme emotional lability moving from smiles and laughter to tears and back again in moments. Her thoughts were markedly tangential and she talked of her 'pregnancy' (she wasn't) and pap smears (which were all bound up in her notion of pregnancy). Dr Lauren and I spent over an hour with this patient. Before we began the interview, Dr Lauren had heard that there were no beds for females in either of the hospital's two wards (closed and open).

At the end of the hour, which included a fairly full psychiatric evaluation interspersed with the patient's tangential ramblings and emotional outbursts, she was sent home with her husband. Both were born-again Christians and had earlier sought advice from their minister. He had recommended vitamins in large doses for the "schizophrenia" he diagnosed in the patient. The husband was advised by Dr Lauren not to seek further advice about his wife's illness from the minister but instead was told to make sure he took his wife to the mental clinic in their own neighborhood. Dr Lauren would call to inform them she would be there in the morning.

The patient was diagnosed as having a "schizophrenic episode". One of the physicians on the emergency room staff had seen the patient a year earlier. This episode had been described by the husband. The physician said that the patient was perhaps a little worse during the previous visit. Dr Lauren thought that the young woman was schizophrenic and was beginning to decompensate as she got older – a pattern most residents in the program identified as common.

It is now possible to summarize briefly this component of the relationship of ideology to practice. Dr Bonner sought to provide quick and efficient service to his patients. As he articulated, service provision is not enhanced by spending large amounts of time with patients, learning of their lives, motivations, etc. "Besides", he said, "I've seen hundreds of schizophrenics. I don't need to spend hours with them to help them in the emergency room". He does not need to understand a patient in order to help him or her. Before a patient is seen, Dr Bonner has established the range of possibilities, the range of options he has. As in the example given above, Dr Bonner needs only to know what condition his patient has. Relatively little time is required for him to ascertain that condition. Knowing the condition, Dr Bonner can set about doing something for the patient.

In the case of the prisoner, Dr Bonner needed only to ascertain that the patient was indeed psychotic and acting out in order to provide assistance – an order for a psychopharmacologic treatment. He needed only to walk into the police room and see this shirtless, aggressive, shouting (delusional) man in handcuffs to confirm the need for a soporific antipsychotic. He did not need to get to know the patient to provide the basic services of the facility for that particular psychiatric emergency.

Dr Lauren, on the other hand, regularly spent a great deal of time with each patient. He tried to get to know each of the patients and to obtain from them enough information to formulate an opinion about the precipitating causes of the episode, the dynamics of the individual and, ultimately, some understanding of the person's crisis. Dr Lauren's non-directive manner meant that some time had to be spent with each patient in order to obtain enough information to 'explain' what was going on with the patient. Thus, it is possible to see that the goal of the intervention for each resident is different.

One seeks to provide quick, efficient service and feels that he best handles the problems presented in the emergency room by seeing them quickly and making for dispositions with dispatch. His handling of emergency patients is consistent with his biological definition of mental illnesses. Given that illnesses are seen in biological terms, understanding has little place in the interactional equation. His view resembles 'the empiricist theory of language' (Harrison 1972), wherein a label is thought to have an empirical referent (cf., Good, this volume). Dr Lauren, on the other hand, uses a sort of interpretive scheme which requires much information for him to assess the plight of the patient. He is concerned, too, that the patient get a chance to air his/her views. He too, however, seeks to apply a label to a "real" phenomenon. Thus, both residents, while they differ in their definitions of the character and etiology of mental illness, adhere to empiricist medical thinking. However, while acting in the emergency context in terms consonant with their definitions, each fulfills certain cultural premises or values which make sensible each set of actions even though they may differ.

Dr Bonner, acting on his biological model, produces uni-axial diagnoses, as did the residents I studied earlier who held biological models. He also provides a model of objective and distant demeaner with his patients as I suggested would occur with psychiatrists holding such views (Gaines 1979b:406–407). Abram and Meador (1976) make a similar point with regard to primary care physicians.

One might ask how it is that two completely different approaches could be appropriate in the single context of the emergency room. It may be suggested here that each, though different, fulfills cultural commandments which are meaningful and understandable at the folk level. That is, Dr Bonner works in the emergency room providing services which satisfy personal and cultural notions (the two may be seen as nearly isomorphic) of efficiency and economy (or elegance) of time and effort. Dr Lauren works in terms of personal interest in and cultural understanding of the Other, in this case, the patient. More importantly, Dr Lauren's position reflects a second personal and cultural set of meanings, those related to the notion of insight.

Because efficiency, economy and insight are all valued and meaningful cultural constructs, the acts of the residents here and in my earlier study are meaningful to them individually and collectively as psychiatric residents, as well as to other medical personnel working in tandem with them. Thus, each view, with its associated behaviors, "makes sense" in cultural terms to self and others in the context of psychiatric practice even though actual practice differs. This latter point is worth emphasizing before moving on to consider another cultural construct, the person.

While recent research rightly has been guiding us in the direction of a consideration of the meanings of illness experience (as distinct from disease), part of the healing nexus may be omitted by researchers. That is, the meaningfulness of the acts of the healers may be overlooked. I mean to suggest, simply, that not only is the illness experience meaningful to the patient (Kleinman 1980b; Good 1977; Good and Good 1980), but also that the illness and disease experiences presented to the ethnopsychiatrist (or ethnophysician) are also meaningful to these practitioners in *both* professional and lay terms.

The model of research suggested by Kleinman (1977b) and subsequently elaborated (Kleinman et al. 1978; Kleinman 1980b) seems appropriate for understanding cultural constructs in the healing context. In Kleinman's formulation, Explanatory Models (EMs) of patient, family and popular culture as well as that of the healer, must be explicated and understood. Each is an equally important ingredient of the cultural construction of illness and of clinical realities. I want to add that the meaningfulness of professional healers' actions in psychiatry and medicine, as well as the healing traditions of other areas, may not derive from 'professional' evaluations of conduct, but from cultural criteria which are used to make sense of and evaluate their behavior, such as those of elegance and insight mentioned above.

This paper now turns to a brief consideration of conceptions of self and of person – the central cultural construct which informs experiences of illness and diseases, communication about such states, and their interpretation by members of the popular, folk and professional health care sectors.[1] The reflection of cultural conceptions of person may be glimpsed, if not met head on, in virtually all of the 10 categories of phenomena which comprise the autonomous subject matter of cultural psychiatry and ethnopsychiatry, as these were outlined by Kleinman (1980a).

PRACTICE AND THE SELF

It is axiomatic that patients' beliefs inform and construct illness experience and behaviors, such as help-seeking, associated with illness episodes. "Such beliefs are central to the psychosocial experience of illness and the communicative context of health care" (Kleinman 1977b:103). And just as "illness and affects are socially (i.e., culturally) constructed through the effect of cultural categories and interpersonal transactions" (Kleinman 1980b:147), so too is the culturally specific construct of the person and the person as self.

On logical grounds, it is possible to show that all human thought has at its base the distinction of self and other (including other things). As Hallowell (1955) has argued, the concept of self is basic to human social life as self awareness is a generic human trait.

One of the distinguishing features of human adjustment, as compared with that of animals lower in the evolutionary scale, rests upon the fact that the human adult, in the course of ontogenetic development, has learned to discriminate himself as an object in a world of objects other than himself. Self awareness is a psychological constant, one basic facet of human nature and of human personality (Hallowell 1955:75).

If an object exists in isolation from all others, it may be said not to exist. That is, for that object to be characterized, described, even experienced and perceptually apprehended as an object it must be compared, implicitly or explicitly with another object; description is comparison.

The concept of self, then, is a prerequisite for the experience of other objects. While we can assume that some concept of person, that of the self, is a universal, a particular conception or set of conceptions need not exist cross-culturally. The cultural criteria of distinction, the elements of the behavioral environment, are surely not universal, and so could not serve to create a universal construct. The concept of person, as it is found in a particular culture, may be considered a key or core conception crucial to the distinctive organization of a given culture, and would seem to be logically prior to other cultural elements, such as themes (Cohen 1948; Opler 1945), values (Vogt 1951), integrative concepts (DuBois 1936), value profiles (DuBois 1955; Kluckhohn 1950) or ethoses (Bateson 1976).

The concept of the self needs to be seen not just as a social construct as in social interactionism, but also as a cultural construct as Hallowell (1955) defines it. Furthermore, we should see person conceptions not in ethnopsychological terms, as knowledge of psychology which members of a society may articulate, but as an implicit cultural construct which serves as a hermeneutic device in the interpretation and comprehension of experience, including illness experiences. Normal and abnormal, defined relative to some notion of person and of self, are states which are experienced not just by persons, but by particular kinds of persons. As such, the person construct may be seen as an essential and major ideological component in the clinical (Kleinman et al. 1978), popular (Good 1977; Townsend 1978), and professional (Gaines 1979b) construction of illness realities.

Earlier writers who considered conceptions of self and provided a basis for the study of the person and the self cross-culturally were generally interested in issues other than medical praxis (Lee 1959; Hallowell 1955). However, more recent research in medical anthropology and cross-cultural psychiatry has pointed to the centrality of the concept of self in therapeutic contexts (Lebra 1976; Kapferer 1979; Bourguignon 1965; Marsella et al. 1973; Tanaka-Matsumi and Marsella 1976; Marsella 1979). Researchers have come to recognize that healing, religious or secular, often entails a transformation of self, a redefinition of one's notion of self to achieve desired ends (Kapferer 1979; Wallace 1978). It is possible to suggest that there is, in fact, a certain amount of 'deconstruction' of self conceptions sought in religious and secular healing traditions, including Western medicine, as one suddenly takes on the role of patient (see T. Lebra, this volume).

I would like to argue that there are two conceptions of self in the West. While this presentation may not advance the study of the person in any material way, the elucidation of two conceptions of person and self in the West may provide a corrective to ethnopsychiatric and ethnomedical research which have been based on unitary models of Western culture. The discussion below will briefly sketch these major cultural traditions in the West and show their distinct conceptions and modes of presentation of the self.

Two Traditions

Elsewhere I have argued that Christianity should not be seen as a single cultural ethic (Gaines 1979b, c, n.d.). Comparative researchers often contrast "the West" to the "East" or some other area of the world, or contrast "Western" ideas with local or parochial ideological systems or components (Fabrega 1974; Kleinman 1980b). My research in Western Europe and a reading of the now-growing anthropological literature on Western society suggest that the West is not constituted by one major cultural tradition. Rather, it may be suggested that there are two distinct major cultural traditions in the West. Below, I will briefly sketch these two cultural traditions and characterize aspects of world view for each. I will then argue that these two major traditions have distinct conceptions of person implicit in them and that these differing conceptions of person have consequences for clinical interactions.

What are these two Great Traditions in the West? Basically, we can distinguish the Northern European Culture Area from the Mediterranean Culture Area. While in each area there are a plethora of ethnic groups, one should be aware that ethnic distinctions are not necessarily cultural distinctions. Many distinct ethnic groups bear the same cultural heritage, representing mere variations of a cultural core. Much like language, a cultural tradition is the total of its variations rather than any one of them and is known through its representatives, as with a musical theme we come to know only through its variations.

For each tradition, the fundamental distinguishing feature is not economy, for both groups have developed economies based upon agriculture or herding of hooved animals (Arensberg 1963) without developing similar ideologies.[2] Rather, the basic differences can be traced to religion and its impact upon social organization (cf. Boissevain 1980). Northern Europe is home to the world view which Weber (1964) referred to as "disenchanted" and is heir to the Magisterial Protestant Reform which symbolized a practical, empiricist, non-magical approach to the social and natural world. Goals of this world are to be achieved by action in this world, not by the intercession of preternatural forces and beings into this life. Action in this world is caused by physical factors, not by fate, immaterial saints, genies (as in Islamic lands), devils or miracles (which are the touch of divinity itself).

The disenchanted world view deriving from the Protestant Reformation in Europe is found in Northern Europe, referred to here as Protestant Europe as it includes Switzerland. But Anglicanism does not differ significantly in doctrine from Catholicism and so must be considered not as part of Protestant Europe, but as part of Mediterranean Europe. Latin Europe, a species of Mediterranean tradition, is that of the enchanted world view (Erickson 1976) and evidences the dualistic cosmology (the City of God is contrasted with and opposed to the City of Man) which contrasts with the monistic cosmology of Protestant Reformers (e.g., God's world is this world, all work is God's work, God is omnipresent) (Ebeling 1970; Gaines 1979c, n.d.).

In research in Alsace on ethnicity and religious affiliation (Gaines 1979c, 1980, 1982, n.d.) I found striking differences in aesthetics, social organization and magical beliefs and practices between Catholic and Protestant (Calvinist and Lutheran) Alsatians. These differences could not be accounted for by socioeconomic measures or length of urban residence. Rather, such differences were associated with religious affiliation. Alsace may be seen as a microcosm of Europe mirroring the cultural contrasts between Protestant and Latin Europe. These European traditions led to a fundamental division within American society as well.

Thus, in Alsace certain Protestant groups are also seen as similar to Catholics (e.g., Evangelicals). Clearly, the same should be said for America. Evangelical, Pentecostal, Southern Baptist and other forms of fundamentalist religiosity termed "Protestant" in America may be seen as returns to traditional Mediterranean ideology, one form of which is Roman Catholicism. The Bible, the major

source of inspiration for these groups, serves as a vehicle for the transportation
of ideology to an ostensibly other culture, time and place. Since these groups
use literalist interpretations of Scripture, the sacred text becomes, in essence,
a sacred ethnography. Exegesis of the sacred ethnography serves as a model of
and for social behavior and morality. In this way role relations (patriarchy,
patripotestality, matrifocality, familial and personal honor) become highly
similar in fundamentalist and Catholic Christian societies.

There are, of course, distinctions among the ethnic groups, such as mariology
among Mediterranean Latin groups, but there are numerous ideological and
social organizational elements which *are* shared. These include patripotestality,
matrifocality (Stack 1974; Wolf 1969), familism, bilateral kinship (Wolf 1969),
embedded social networks (where one's neighbors, friends, work-mates and
relatives tend to be the same people) (cf. Bott 1971), masculine honor, familial
honor, female sexual shame (Peristiany 1974; Campbell 1964), extreme concern
for and attempted control of women's sexuality (Rogers 1975; Friedl 1967;
Peristiany 1974), sharply defined sexual roles and spacio-temporal domains
(external public domain for males, internal domestic domain for women) (Rogers
1975; Boissevain 1980; Friedl 1967), gossip as a basic social activity and means
of social control (Bailey 1971; Stack 1974), and authoritarianism (Wolf 1969).
These and other similarities make understandable fundamentalist and Catholic
alliances on issues such as abortion and the Equal Rights Amendment in America.

Fundamentalist and Catholic groups share in the belief in a magical, enchanted world wherein threads of this world and those of the world beyond
are woven together into a single fabric of perception and experience as in the
medieval (e.g., Latin) world view (cf., Erickson 1976). Thus the enchanted
world view of the Mediterranean area and its daughter cultures in the Old and
the New World conceives of illnesses as having either natural or supernatural
etiologies. So we see that in Mexican-American groups illness, either physical
or psychological, has a supernatural or preternatural (e.g., evil eye) origin (Clark
1959; Kiev 1968; Rubel 1971). Foster (1953) has shown that the essentials
of Mexican and Mexican-American medical beliefs are derived from Spanish
folk medicine, itself a variant of older pan-Mediterranean beliefs and practices
(e.g., humoral pathology). Strikingly similar beliefs are found among widely
separate but culturally close ethnic groups, such as Puerto Ricans (Harwood
1977), Haitians (Weidman 1979), Italians (Foulkes et al. 1977) and others.

The belief in the evil eye is found throughout the Mediterranean area and
in all daughter cultures in Central or South America and the Caribbean. "*Susto*"
and other phenomena such as malevolent witches are likewise found throughout
Latin groups though names for specific disorders may vary from place to place
(Fabrega 1974). "Falling out" is another case in point. It is a folk illness which
appears in both Black and White (southern) fundamentalist groups as well as
in Latin Caribbean groups, although several different terms for the disorder
are in use among the different ethnic groups (Weidman 1979; Lefley 1979).
Researchers have also pointed out that hexing and rootwork (malign magic

involving herbs and spells) are not confined to southern Blacks (Hall and Bourne 1973; Snow 1977) but are also found among southern Whites (Hillard 1978). These forms, along with *susto* and notions of soul loss and possession, recall Homeric Greek etiological theories for sickness (Entralgo 1970).

In all these groups, Mexican, Puerto-Rican, Southern White and Black, other fundamentalists, etc., religious healing is regarded as an appropriate remedy for supernaturally caused illness (cf. Hufford 1977; Harwood 1977; Fabrega 1974; Hillard 1978). While the cultural lexicon of these groups varies from place to place reflecting particular social and historical contexts, the cultural grammar which orders those elements seems to be quite similar if not isomorphic. So it is that we find different ethnic groups, Blacks and non-Puerto Rican Hispanics participating in Puerto Rican *espiritista* events (Harwood 1977), and seemingly distinct cultural groups falling victim to the same folk illnesses. An example of the latter is bewitchment among southern Blacks and Whites as well as other ethnic groups including Italians, Mexicans, Central and South Americans, Puerto Ricans and other Caribbean Hispanics at home and in America.[3]

In Protestant Europe's world view, the physicalist, empiricist tendencies find expression as the world of wonders is obliterated. Explanations are sought in the tangible, empirical world. As shown elsewhere (Gaines 1980), the Kraepelinian notion of a biological seat of mental disorders reflects the German cultural notion of social classification wherein the essential individual differences are thought to be biological. In this empiricist view of the classification of social actors, mental illness and cultural/ethnic identity have a common empirical, physical basis. (Townsend [1979] has recently noted the interrelation of explanations of ethnicity and mental disorder.) American biomedicine and the specialty of psychiatry are embedded within the cultural context of this Protestant European tradition.

The following section considers the notions of self which represent essential and fundamental expressions of the world views of the Great Traditions briefly sketched above.

Persons and Selves [4]

A recent paper by Vincent Crapanzano (1980) employs two useful terms, "indexical" and "referential", in creatively viewing the nature of encounter, discourse and the self in psychoanalytic therapy. These terms introduced by Pierce (1931–1958), are used to facilitate the presentation below, but not necessarily in the same way as used by Crapanzano.

The conception of the person held implicitly by Western psychiatrists is one which sees the individual, in Geertz's terms, as a

bounded, unique, more or less integrated motivational and cognitive universe, a dynamic center of awareness, emotion, judgment, and action organized into a distinctive whole and set contrastively both against other such wholes and against a social and natural background ... (1977:9).

Here the individual is seen as capable of instituting personal change, almost at will. One is capable of making himself or herself over, and may be expected to do so if problems in relationships or occupation develop. Change is viewed as positive, both as it relates to the individual and to other elements in the behavioral environment. Change is seen as occurring as one gains insight. Insight is gained through experience ("it was a learning experience"), reflection, exchanges with friends and, of course, forms of therapy. Talk and insight therapies are clearly based upon some notion of self as an alterable yet consistent and coherent entity which is self-reflective. The latter quality may be seen as a cultural elaboration of the self-awareness described by Hallowell (1955). Various intervention and therapeutic strategies in psychiatry, such as private therapy, reinforce this notion of individuality. These views of therapeutic change entail an implicit theory of existence and a conception of the person as an empirical being always in the process of becoming, or, for that matter, unbecoming. This "referential" conception of self has its basis in the Great Tradition of Protestant Europe.

In contrast with this "referential" conception of self, the notion of self common to Mediterranean groups, especially the Latin European groups, may be termed "indexical". The Latin, "indexical", self is not defined as an abstract entity independent of the social relations and contexts in which the self is presented in interaction. Notions of the self as a discrete, unique social entity are far less important as an explanatory construct used to interpret the behavior of persons across situations. Rather, the self is perceived as constituted or "indexed" by the contextual features of social interaction in diverse situations. (See Shweder and Bourne, this volume, for similar contrasts in American and Asian Indian person concepts.) For "indexical" notions of self, the presentation of quite diverse and contrastive sorts of behavior in different contexts may not be regarded as "inconsistent". The French self described here is typical of the Latin European self found in Mediterranean cultural traditions.

In France, the perception of situational contrasts in behavior is linked with a seemingly paradoxical concept of individual character and disposition as formed nearly at birth and not readily changed. One's initial character is immutable (cf. Wylie 1974; Turkle 1978). This concept of character, however, is not articulated in terms of a bundle of behavioral traits which are mutually consistent and expressed as a coherent whole in social interaction. Thus, divergent behaviors or attitudes are not seen as a sign of "change" or "inconsistency", only as expressions of variant facets of the same underlying being. Changes which American observers might think they perceive with respect to the actions of a French person would be seen by the French as simply realizations or manifestations of existing selfhood. These realizations are not, I hasten to add, thought of in the sense of becoming, but rather are conceived of as 're-cognition' of that which is and has always been. An individual expresses himself or herself variously, but it is the same self which is variously presented. Hence, there is no change seen. In this way André Malraux saw himself expressed uniformly through his political affiliations which, over the years, included Communism, Fascism, and Gaullism. François Mitterand, longtime head of the 'parti socialist' of France, and now recently elected as the President of France, for more than 20 years held various ministerial positions in conservative governments in France. And, Lévi-Strauss has maintained that he was "born" a structuralist.

Lutheran and Reformed (Calvinist) notions of religion predicated upon the tie between God and the individual are important for the Protestant European (referential) sense of self. The individual is not seen as an extension of another social entity, such as the family or the Church, as in the Latin Tradition. While the theory of the referential self is that of an empirical being always in the process of becoming (or unbecoming), the indexical self presupposes a constancy in 'being', but one that, in its expression, is created over and over again in interaction.

The mode of presentation of each sort of self conception is distinct. In the presentations of the indexical self, the self which is presented indexes a given time and place, a given interlocator, in short, a given encounter. Self is created and recreated in a dramatic production and varies from interaction to interaction. The Mediterranean self is created in interaction in terms of what I call "the rhetoric of complaint", at least in some encounters. This rhetoric entails communication about the self as moral being, moral in terms of an ideology which is contextual and situational. It portrays the individual as beset with problems and suffering. Often, the self is seen as ennobled by suffering and the rhetoric serves to communicate the self's ennoblement.

On the other hand, the referential self is presented in interaction in a referential framework. The person is seen, implicitly, as an empirical, real entity. Communications about the self are references to a concrete entity rather than a phenomenal encounter. While more or less of the empirical self may be revealed in a given encounter (measured revelation also serves as a means of impression management), the self presented is a coherent whole independent of the particular context of interaction. As a distinct, autonomous entity, facts about that entity become meaningful and relevant to clinical and other encounters.

But with the Latin indexical self, facts are insufficient to tell the "story" of the self, the woes and 'the trouble I've seen', which are essential to characterize, not describe, the self. Lee (1959c) vividly depicts this sort of self-portraiture found among Greeks and Greek-Americans. Or, as Laget (1980:137), a French historian of medicine says, "Documents just recite the facts ... " and facts are simply insufficient for telling the story of the human condition. It is not enough to merely describe, one must elaborate, expand upon mere facts as these facts cannot 'tell', cannot provide the appropriate characterization of the self. The indexical self may present problems for ethnographer and clinician alike. As in the case with informants' stories, which may vary during fieldwork (Eickelman 1978), so too may medical history vary (cf. Rubin and Jones 1979). For example, folk practitioners may present illusive biographies or explanations of practice (see Michaelson 1972).

As among the French, the indexical self is not the bounded, unique individual found among Protestant (non-fundamentalist) Americans. The Mediterranean self is a social self which is opposed to the notion of an autonomous, independent self. The self is in part constituted by external social elements, namely the family, as in France (cf. Métraux 1954; Wylie 1974). Individuals are who they are in part because of their family, a family that existed before the individual and will continue after the individual's demise (cf. Wylie 1970). The Protestant (excluding fundamentalist Protestant) American notion of the autonomous self contrasts sharply with the Latin self which is not seen as entirely unique. The Latin self is not set contrastively against the social, natural and spiritual environment. The social (and sometimes the spiritual domains) are seen as located within the self, as being a part of the self (cf. Turkle 1978 on Lacanian notions of the intrusion of society in the individual [also see Lacan 1968]).

The boundary of the Latin self is not drawn around a single biological unit, but around the 'foyer', The self consists in part of significant others, primarily family. Thus, the self is partly composed of elements over which the individual has no control. Hence the self is seen as controlled from without by the demands of kith and kin, of fate or elements of the spiritual world. This self stands in stark contrast with the bounded, autonomous and, therefore, self-regulated and self-reflective Protestant individual. Rather than reflecting upon or examining motives and causes in one's own behavior, forces outside of the individual are seen as causative of the behavior of self and other. These forces are both material and immaterial, of this world and the next. Thus, as with the Ojibwa studies by Hallowell (1955), the self is a cultural construct which includes elements of both the material and spiritual worlds. This conception, then, is not that of Protestant Europe and America, of the empirical self articulated by Geertz (1973). The unchanging and unchangeable self which is in part composed of seemingly external social and spiritual elements is the self of Lacan's French version of psychoanalysis (Lacan 1968), a system of therapy which seeks to more or less 'witness' patients' conflicts, to 'understand' (comprendre) and to 'listen' (écouter), but not to cure, or to alter that arrangement (Turkle 1978).

With the perspective provided by this material, we should look again at some of the clinical encounters discussed in the first part of this paper. As noted earlier, American biomedicine and the specialty of psychiatry are embedded in the Protestant European cultural tradition. The therapeutic strategies employed by both Dr Bonner and Dr Lauren reflect different aspects of the "referential" conception of self described above. While both residents differ in their definitions of the character and etiology of psychiatric disorder, they adhere to empiricist medical thinking which uses diagnostic categories to label pathogenic entities assumed to exist as an objective reality at a certain point in time which can be altered through appropriate therapeutic intervention. In each case, implicit assumptions about the person as a discrete and coherent entity which is alterable, yet continuous through time, underlies their attempts to focus treatment on the individual and transform him or her to a more desirable, healthy condition (whether through the alteration of psycho-biological states, or through self-reflection and "insight"). These definitions of mental illness and approaches to therapy are consistent with the "referential" conception of self which is represented as an abstract entity (an autonomous individual), characterized by discrete symptoms and behavioral traits. Thus, even though Dr Bonner and Dr Lauren employ distinctly different modes of diagnosis and treatment, both are consistent with some of the basic premises about personhood which underlie the culture of psychiatry and, hence, are regarded as meaningful and appropriate types of behavior in the context of the emergency room.

The patients involved in the cases described earlier do, however, reflect more variation in the cultural assumptions which guide their presentations of self and illness. The manic-depressive patient sought only to respond to questions put to him without elaboration. On the other hand, the female tourist from New Zealand who fought with her physician husband, tried very clearly to paint a portrait of herself, to communicate to those present that she was a decent, God-fearing and suffering woman. Her suffering should be borne and should not serve as a source of resentment or action which would terminate the relationship, even though much physical punishment was part of that union. Her beliefs (and her husband's) are not isolated. In similar fashion, the ramblings of the young woman concerning pregnancy also reflect the indexical self described here. While the young woman was greatly confused, her concern with pregnancy was, in part, her probable fear of that condition and her great desire for it in order that she begin to be a 'proper' wife to her young husband.

Further support for this account of modes of self presentation and implicit notions of self is reported elsewhere (Gaines 1982). In the above cases, patients employing the indexical mode are both female, one a Charismatic Catholic, the other a born-again Christian. In my other report (1982) I examined two Catholic males who employed the 'rhetoric of complaint' which in both instances confused the construction of clinical reality. This possible confusion of the nature of clinical reality is the chief significance of ethnographic descriptions of conceptions of person and self. These conceptions are of fundamental importance in determining the nature of interaction in clinical encounters. The exchanges and self-presentations in clinical encounters can produce problematic clinical realities and affect patient interpretations of clinical efficacy. Delineation of these conceptions of person, and the Great Traditions in the West of which they are a part, may provide for the improvement of comparative research as well.

Researchers such as Kleinman (1980b) have attempted to provide systematic comparisons in which one cultural group is contrasted with Americans. Problems arise in such comparisons, however, because of the impossibility of accommodating all of the different ethnic groups in a comparative scheme which treats them either as distinct entities, or lumps them together, implicitly equating ethnicity, culture and nationality. The scheme presented here attempts to avoid enumerating every group in American society on the one hand, or ignoring them all on the other. Recognizing broad cultural fundamentals common to a number of ethnic groups allows for the development of a contrast pair. This contrast pair of cultural traditions in the United States can be used to look at data generated from research in this country or to clarify comparisons which researchers have sought to make cross-culturally.

So it is in Kleinman's signal work that he attempts to contrast his Chinese patients with American patients in terms of their depressive illness experiences (e.g., 1980b:138–141), but finds that some Americans are like the Chinese while others are not. The groups which show affinities to Chinese patients are those of the Latin or Mediterranean Great Tradition outlined here. Often described as 'lower class', their same values may be recognized in urban middle and upper class persons of Mediterranean societies. These similarities indicate that the crucial variable is not class, but culture, and that the two variables are easily confounded. Thus, this paper may provide a corrective and clarification of potential cultural units in American society which may be compared differentially cross-culturally so as to provide sharper contrasts with other cultures.

CONCLUSION

This paper has drawn upon earlier research to show connections between psychiatric actors' definitions and their behavior in clinical contexts. Here, psychiatric residents' etiological models of mental disorder were shown to affect physician-patient interaction, determining the length of time a resident would spend with a patient before making an evaluation and a disposition. Divergent models were shown to exist and to produce different interactional styles in the emergency room. Divergent approaches of the residents were shown not to generate disharmony or skepticism among other residents or clinical colleagues because each approach is evaluated in terms of meaningful cultural assumptions, and not in terms of objective scientific criteria.

The third portion of the paper presented and sketched the outlines of two major "Great" cultural traditions in the West: Northern Protestant and Mediterranean European. Then two conceptions of the person, the indexical and the referential, were discussed. These conceptions are seen as expressions of divergent world views of the two Great Traditions. It was suggested that the distinction drawn between two cultural traditions may provide a modicum of improved clarity in research which uses, implicitly or explicitly, the West as a single cultural standard of comparison.

It is also suggested that while biomedicine and psychiatry, in particular, are embedded in the Northern (Protestant) European Tradition, their patients, especially since the advent of third-party payments, often come from the Latin or other Mediterranean Tradition. The recognition of differences in conceptions of person have implications for improved clarity of communication in and about clinical encounters and in the construction of appropriate clinical realities. In general, this paper argues for the cultural contextualization of clinical practice and for a person-centered, hermeneutic approach to illness and clinical care.

ACKNOWLEDGMENTS

My thanks to Drs Arthur Kleinman, Geoffrey White and Anthony Marsella for kind assistance in the revision of this paper.

NOTES

1. Kleinman (1980b) develops this tripartite model of health care systems.
2. Indeed, the same ideology appears in vastly different economic circumstances, among Mediterranean herdsmen in Greece (Campbell 1964), in urban areas in Italy (Belmonte 1979), in both town and country in Spain (Kenny 1966) and among certain segments (French and Alsatian Catholics) in urban France (Gaines n.d.) not to mention the persistence of Mediterranean culture in urban industrial America.
3. For Caribbean and American Black groups, it should be recognized that since Herskovitz (1941), it is accepted that there are many behavioral and cultural syncretisms with (West) African cultures. Many of these syncretic beliefs and practices may have incorporated compatible ideas from other, European traditions, Today, either from sharing or matching of beliefs, southern Black and White cultures share many features, including social organizational forms (extended families, fictive kinship), fundamentalist religious traditions, and medical beliefs and practices such as herbalism, witch beliefs, root work and the like (Mitchell 1978; Snow 1977; Hillard 1978). Mitchell (1978) has shown that Native American, Euro-American and Afro-American herbal traditions have mutually influenced one another and formed common traditions in the South. Because of long contact and sharing of religious ideology Black traditions show a very strong affinity, if not identity, with those deriving from the Mediterranean area. The influence of Islam in West Africa is also of very major importance.
4. My thanks to the Duke University Research Council for funding for a small research project aimed at elucidating notions of the person among American ethnic groups. Their kind support has allowed me to confirm the appropriateness of the contention expressed here that marked cultural similarities exist between distinct ethnic groups, i.e., the similarity of American Black and Latin ethnic groups' notion of person. Snow (1977) has also noted the similarity of medical beliefs and practices, including humoral pathology, between Blacks and Chicanos in the American southwest.

   Research in a southern setting with Black and White pain patients, in which I am now engaged, bears out my view expressed here. In administering a questionnaire to the patients as a means of pretesting, I've found that patients will talk at great length about each symptom they have had and elaborate such stories into characterizations of themselves, their families, close friends, pets and the like as well as the kind of life they have led.

REFERENCES

Abram, H. and C. Meador.
   1976 Introduction: the Patient, the Physician and the Psychiatrist. *In* Basic Psychiatry for the Primary Care Physician. H. Abram (ed.). Boston: Little, Brown and Company.
Arensberg, C.
   1963 The Old World Peoples: The Place of European Cultures in World Ethnography. Anthropological Quarterly 36(3): 75–99.

188 ATWOOD D. GAINES

Bailey, F.
    1971 Gifts and Poisons: the Politics of Reputation. New York: Schocken Books.
Bateson, G.
    1976 Naven. Stanford: Stanford University Press. (orig. 1936).
Belmonte, T.
    1979 The Broken Fountain. Chicago: University of Chicago Press.
Boehm, C.
    1980 Exposing the moral self in Montenegro. American Ethnologist 7:1–26.
Boissevain, J.
    1980 A Village in Malta. New York: Holt, Rinehart and Winston.
Bott, E.
    1971 Family and Social Network. London: Tavistock.
Bourguignon, E.
    1965 The Self, the Behavioral Environment, and the Theory of Spirit Possession.
          In Context and Meaning in Anthropology. M. Spiro (ed.). New York: Free
          Press.
Campbell, J.
    1964 Honour, Family and Patronage. Oxford: Oxford University Press.
Clark, M.
    1959 Health in the Mexican-American Culture. Berkeley: University of California
          Press.
Cohen, A.
    1948 On the Place of 'Themes' and Kindred Concepts in Social Theory. American
          Anthropologist 50:436–443.
Crapanzano, V.
    1980 The Subject as Object: The Phenomenology of Encounter. Paper presented at the
          24th Annual Meeting of the American Academy of Psychoanalysis: San Francisco,
          May.
DuBois, C.
    1936 The Wealth Concept as an Integrative Factor in Tolowa-Tututni Culture. In
          Essays in Anthropology Presented to A. L. Kroeber. R. Lowie (ed.). Berkeley:
          University of California Press.
    1955 The Dominant Value Profile of American Culture. American Anthropologist 47:
          1232–1239.
Ebeling, G.
    1970 Luther: An Introduction to His Thought. R. Wilson (trans.). Garden City, NY:
          Doubleday and Company.
Eickelman, D.
    1955 Moroccan Islam. Austin: University of Texas Press.
Entralgo, L.
    1970 The Therapy of the Word in Classical Antiquity. New Haven: Yale University
          Press.
Erickson, C.
    1976 The Medieval Vision: Essays in History and Perception. New York: Oxford
          University Press.
Fabrega, H.
    1974 Disease and Social Behavior. Cambridge: The MIT Press.
Foster, G.
    1953 Relationship Between Spanish and Spanish-American Folk Medicine. J. American
          Folklore 66:201–217.
Foulkes, E., et al.
    1977 The Italian Evil-Eye. Journal of Operational Psychiatry 8:28–34.

Friedl, E.
  1967 The Position of Women: Appearance and Reality. Anthropological Quarterly 40:97–108.
Gaines, A. D.
  1979a Psychiatry as a Cultural System. Invited Grand Rounds, Department of Psychiatry, John A. Burns School of Medicine. Honolulu, April.
  1979b Definitions and Diagnoses. Culture, Medicine and Psychiatry 3(4):381–418.
  1979c The Word and the Cross: Ascendant Alsatian Ethnicity and Religious Affiliation in Strasbourg, France. Ann Arbor: University Microfilms International.
  1980 Race and Culture as Cultural Systems: Ethnicity in Strasbourg. Paper presented at 79th Annual Meetings of the American Anthropological Association meeting, Washington, D.C., December 4–7, 1980.
  1981 Faith, Fashion and Family: Religious Aesthetics and Family Social Organization in Strasbourg. (In submission, Anthropological Quarterly).
  1982 Knowledge and Practice: Anthropological Ideas and Psychiatric Practice. In Clinically Applied Anthropology: Anthropologists in Health Science Settings. N. Chrisman and T. Maretzki (eds.). Dordrecht, Holland: D. Reidel (in press).
  n.d.   The Word and the Cross: Cultural Identities and Paradox in Alsace. Cambridge: Schenkman. (in submission).
Geertz, C.
  1973a Thick description: Toward an Interpretive Theory of Culture. In The Interpretation of Cultures. C. Geertz (ed.). New York: Basic Books.
  1973b Ethos, World View and the Analysis of Sacred Symbols. In The Interpretation of Cultures. C. Geertz (ed.). New York: Basic Books.
  1977 On the Nature of Anthropological Understanding. Annual Editions in Anthropology. Guilford, Connecticut: Dushkin.
Gilbert, D. and D. Levinson
  1958 Ideology, Personality and Institutional Policy in a Mental Hospital. American Journal of Abnormal and Social Psychology 53:263–371.
Good, B.
  1977 The Heart of What's the Matter: The Semantics of Illness in Iran. Culture, Medicine and Psychiatry 1:25–58.
Good, B. and M. DelVecchio Good
  1980 The Meaning of Symptoms: A Cultural Hermeneutic Model for Clinical Practice. In The Relevance of Social Science for Medicine. L. Eisenberg and A. Kleinman (eds.). Dordrecht, Holland: D. Reidel.
Hall, A. and P. Bourne
  1973 Indigenous Therapists in a Southern Black Urban Community. Archives of General Psychiatry 28:137–142.
Hallowell, A.
  1955 The Self and Its Behavioral Environment. In Culture and Experience. A. I. Hallowell (ed.). Philadelphia: University of Pennsylvania.
Harrison, B.
  1972 Meaning and Structure: An Essay in the Philosophy of Language. New York: Harper and Row.
Harwood. A.
  1977 Rx: Spiritist as Needed. New York: John Wiley.
Herskovitz, Melville J.
  1941 The Myth of the Negro Past. New York: Harper and Row.
Hillard, J. and W. Rockwell
  1978 Disesthesia, Witchcraft and Conversion Reaction. Journal of the American Medical Association 240(6):1742–1744.

Hufford, D.
   1977 Christian Religious Healing. Journal of Operational Psychiatry 8:22–27.
Kapferer, B.
   1979. Mind, Self, and Other in Demonic Illness. American Ethnologist 6:110–133.
Kenny, M.
   1966 A Spanish Tapestry. New York: Harper Colophon.
Kiev, A.
   1968 Curanderismo. New York: Free Press.
Kleinman, A.
   1977a Problems and Prospects in Comparative Cross-Cultural Medical and Psychiatric
         Studies. In Culture and Healing in Asian Societies. A. Kleinman et al. (eds.).
         Cambridge: Schenkman.
   1977b Rethinking the Social and Cultural Context of Psychopathology and Psychiatric
         Care. In Renewal in Psychiatry. T. Manschreck and A. Kleinman (eds.). Washing-
         ton, D. C.: Hempisphere Publishing Company.
   1980a Major Conceptual and Research Issues for Cultural (anthropological) Psychiatry.
         Culture, Medicine and Psychiatry 4(3):3–13.
   1980b Patients and Healers in the Context of Culture. Berkeley: University of California
         Press.
Kleinman, A., L. Eisenberg, and B. Good
   1978 Culture, Illness and Care: Clinical Lessons from Anthropological and Cross-
         Cultural Research. Annals of Internal Medicine 88:251–258.
Kluckhohn, F.
   1950 Dominant and Substitute Profiles of Cultural Orientation. Social Forces 28:376–
         393.
Lacan, J.
   1968 The Language of the Self. A. Wilden (trans.). Baltimore: Johns Hopkins
         Press.
Laget, M.
   1980 Childbirth in Seventeenth and Eighteenth Century France. In Medicine and
         Society in France: Selections from Annals, Vol. 6. R. Forster and O. Ranum
         (eds). Baltimore: Johns Hopkins University Press.
Lebra, T.
   1976 Japanese Patterns of Behavior. Honolulu: The University Press of Hawaii.
Lee, D.
   1959 Freedom and Culture. Englewood Cliffs, NJ: Prentice-Hall.
   1959a Personal Significance and Group Structure. In Freedom and Culture. D. Lee
         (ed.). Englewood Cliffs, New Jersey: Prentice-Hall.
   1959b The Conception of Self Among the Wintu. In Freedom and Culture. D. Lee (ed.).
         Englewood Cliffs, New Jersey: Prentice-Hall.
   1959c View of the Self in Greek Culture. In Freedom and Culture. D. Lee (ed.). Engle-
         wood Cliffs, New Jersey: Prentice-Hall.
Lefley, H.
   1979 Prevalence of Potential Falling-Out Cases Among the Black, Latin and Non-Latin
         White Population in the City of Miami. Social Science and Medicine 13B:113–
         114.
Light, D.
   1976 Work Styles Among American Psychiatric Residents. In Anthropology and Mental
         Health. J. Westermeyer (ed.). The Hague: Mouton.
Marsella, A. J., D. Kinzie, and P. Gordon.
   1973 Ethnic Variations in the Expression of Depression. Journal of Cross-Cultural
         Psychology 4:435–458.

Marsella, A. J.
  1979 Cross-Cultural Studies of Mental Disorder. *In* Perspectives on Cross-Cultural Psychology. A. J. Marsella et al. (eds.). New York: Academic Press.
Métraux, R.
  1954 Themes in French Culture. Palo Alto: Stanford University Press.
Michaelson, M.
  1972 Can a "Root Doctor" Actually Put A Hex On Or Is It All A Great Put-On? Today's Health, March, p. 39ff.
Mitchell, F.
  1978 Hoodoo Medicine. Read, Cannon and Johnson Co.
Murphy, H. B. M.
  1976 Notes for a Theory of Latah. *In* Culture-bound Syndromes, Ethnopsychiatry and Alternate Therapies. W. Lebra (ed.). Honolulu: University Press of Hawaii.
Opler, M.
  1945 Themes as Dynamic Forces in Culture. American Journal of Sociology 51:198–206.
Peristiany, J.
  1974 Honour and Shame: The Values of Mediterranean Society. Chicago: University of Chicago Press.
Pierce, C. S.
  1931– Collected Papers. Vols. 1–6. C. Hartshorne and P. Weiss (eds.). Vols. 7–8. A.
  1958 Burks (ed.). Cambridge: Harvard University Press.
Quinn, N.
  1979 A Cognitive Anthropologist Looks at American Marriage. Paper presented at the 78th Annual Meetings of the American Anthropological Association. Cincinnati, Ohio, November 28-December 1, 1979.
  n.d. A Folk Theory of Child Training. Manuscript. Duke University.
Rogers, S.
  1975 Female Forms of Power and the Myth of Male Dominance. American Ethnologist 2:727–756.
Rubel, A.
  1971 Across the Tracks: Mexican-Americans in a Texas City. Austin: University of Texas Press for the Hogg Foundation.
Rubin, J. and J. Jones
  1979 Falling-Out: A Clinical Study. Social Science and Medicine 13B:117–127.
Snow, L.
  1977 Popular Medicine in a Black Neighborhood. *In* Ethnic Medicine in the Southwest. E. Spicer (ed.). Tucson, Arizona: University of Arizona Press.
Stack, C.
  1974 All Our Kin. New York: Harper and Row.
Strauss, A.
  1977 Northern Cheyenne Ethnopsychology. Ethos 5:326–357.
Tanaka-Matsumi, J. and A. J. Marsella
  1976 Cross-culural Variations in the Phenomenological Experience: I. Word Association Studies. Journal of Cross-Cultural Psychology 7:379–396.
Townsend, J. M.
  1975 Cultural Conceptions and Mental Illness: A Controlled Comparison of Germany and America. Journal of Nervous and Mental Disease 160:409–421.
  1978 Cultural Conceptions and Mental Illness: A Comparison of Germany and America. Chicago: University of Chicago Press.
  1979 Stereotypes of Mental Illness: A Comparison with Ethnic Stereotypes. Culture, Medicine and Psychiatry 3(3):205–230.

Turkle, S.
  1978 Psychoanalytic Politics: Freud's French Revolution. New York: Basic Books.
Valentine, C.
  1963 Men of Anger and Men of Shame: Lakalai Ethnopsychology and Its Implications
        for Sociopsychological Theory. Ethnology 2:441–477.
Vogt, E.
  1951 Navaho Veterans: A Study of Changing Values. Peabody Museum of Harvard
        University, Vol. 41.
Wallace, D. T.
  1978 I Am A Drunk: Redefinition of the Self in Alcoholics Anonymous. Manuscript.
        San Francisco State University.
Weber, M.
  1954 The Sociology of Religion. E. Fischoff (trans.). Boston: Beacon Press.
Weidman, H.
  1979 Falling-Out. Social Science and Medicine 13B:95–112.
White, G.
  1978 Ambiguity and Ambivalence in A'ara Personality Descriptors. American Ethnol-
        ogist 5:334–360.
Wolf, E.
  1969 Society and Symbols in Latin Europe and the Islamic Near East. Anthropological
        Quarterly 42:287–301.
Wylie, L.
  1970 Les Francais. Englewood Cliffs, NJ: Prentice-Hall.
  1974 Village in the Vaucluse. Cambridge: Harvard University Press.
Yap, P. M.
  1969 The Culture-Bound Reaction Syndromes. In Mental Health in Asia and the
        Pacific. W. Caudill and T. Y. Lin (eds.). Honolulu: East-West Center Press.

7. SAMOAN FOLK KNOWLEDGE OF MENTAL DISORDERS

INTRODUCTION

The purpose of this paper is to describe Samoan folk knowledge of mental disorders and to examine how this body of knowledge articulates with other aspects of Samoan culture and society. Samoan folk knowledge provides descriptions of mental disorders and propositions about the causes and treatment of these problems.

The first section of the paper is devoted to an explicit presentation of the concept of folk knowledge and the related perspective that underlies the analysis of Samoan data given here. "Folk knowledge" is an extensive reconceptualization of the concept of "ethnoscience". Inspired by research findings from cognitive studies, this conceptualization analytically separates group knowledge from individual knowledge. The second section of the paper describes Samoan representations of mental disorders. The remaining three sections address the following questions: (1) What are the flexible aspects of Samoan knowledge about mental disorders? (2) What are the more basic aspects of this knowledge that integrate it with other areas of Samoan folk knowledge? (3) What is the situational relevance of these folk representations? (i.e., How are folk representations used by Samoans in their everyday lives?), and (4) What processes of change and maintenance seem to be affecting this body of Samoan knowledge? The answers to these questions reveal that the folk knowledge of mental disorders articulates with other areas of knowledge through cultural themes, that this folk knowledge is only loosely coupled to what individual Samoans do about mental disorders, and that social forces such as the Christian churches' drive for hegemony in matters of the supernatural, are impinging upon the body of folk knowledge.

FOLK KNOWLEDGE AND FOLK REPRESENTATIONS

Folk representations are expressions of the knowledge and affect that a group has about itself and its environment.[1] In a sense, folk representations are affect-laden "descriptions" of the environment provided by the group through artifacts (e.g., ceremonial objects, tools), through routinized discourse (e.g., folktales, myths, novels), through ritualized, routinized, and dramatized events (e.g., curing ceremonies, games, plays), through terminology systems (e.g., classifications of emotions), and through the statements and actions of authorities, specialists, and other culturally-defined spokespersons.

The concept of "folk knowledge" derives from the tradition of cognitive anthropology, and bears some resemblance to "ethnoscience". Sturtevant

A. J. Marsella and G. M. White (eds.), Cultural Conceptions of Mental Health and Therapy, 193–213.

(1964:99) describes ethnoscience as "the system of knowledge and cognition typical of a given culture", and rephrases "society's ethnoscience" as "its particular ways of classifying its material and social universe" (Sturtevant 1964:100). Although both are conceptualizations of group knowledge, the concept of folk knowledge departs from that of ethnoscience on three important counts: (1) the forms in which knowledge is represented, (2) the locus of group knowledge, and (3) the stress placed on the social significance of representations. A brief discussion of the reasons for reconceptualizing group knowledge as "folk knowledge" is presented below in order to illuminate the basis from which the Samoan data are analyzed.

The first difference concerns the form in which cultural knowledge is represented. Sturtevant's rephrasing of the concept of ethnoscience highlights the representation focused upon in most studies of ethnoscience: the indigenous *classification* system. A predominant focus on exclusively language-based forms of folk representations has encouraged too much emphasis on the analogous aspects of language and culture. The concept of folk knowledge guides one to search for representations of knowledge in a variety of forms – in rituals, in games, in folktales, and in artifacts, for example, as well as in terminology systems.

The material analyzed in the present paper does not in itself sufficiently broaden the representational forms studied. What is described of Samoan folk knowledge is primarily terminology and beliefs which are readily verbalized. However, representations of knowledge of mental disorders occur in at least one other major form: curing routines and rituals. Unfortunately, there are no extensive studies of these routines and rituals in Samoa.[2] Because this information is lacking, the present analysis is considered to be only a partial analysis of Samoan folk knowledge in this area.

A second and even more important distinction between ethnoscience and folk knowledge lies in the locus of group knowledge. In the approach taken by students of ethnoscience, attention is focused upon cultural competence – the mentally held principles and recipes that the individual has learned which allow him or her to behave in a culturally appropriate manner. From the ethnoscience perspective, culturally patterned behavior and artifacts are but epiphenomena of this competence. Group knowledge, then, is the aggregate of all the cultural competencies of the members of the group (see Goodenough 1971:41). In contrast with the position taken in studies of ethnoscience, *folk* knowledge is viewed as an aspect of the group. Folk representations, the means through which folk knowledge is expressed, are, in a sense, products of the institutionalized patterns of information processing and knowledge distribution within the group. The exposure and homogeneity of folk representations are controlled by these institutions. Some representations are widely exposed to large audiences while others are not as widely exposed. For example, compare American television coverage of football games to that given to ping-pong tournaments. In other cases, representations may not be exposed at all, such as social race terms in some desegregated schools (see Clement and Livesay 1979). Some representations are maintained at a high degree of homogeneity while others are allowed to be relatively heterogeneous (e.g., compare clothing styles of American men to the wider variety allowed American women).

Given this definition, folk knowledge cannot be equated with the aggregated knowledge of individuals. Folk knowledge both exceeds and is exceeded by the sum of the knowledge of the group's members. The sum of members' knowledge includes some content that is not incorporated into group knowledge. Individuals, for example, know representations of race that are not allowed in the desegregrated schools referred to above. On the other hand, folk knowledge includes some knowledge which is not reflected in the cultural competencies of its members. Although the ethnoscience perspective is based upon the idea that all cultural products are the result of individuals acting in accord with their mental blueprints for culturally appropriate behavior, it is clear that there are events for which adequate blueprints cannot be developed. One type of such events involves dynamic, open-ended interactions such as occur, for example, in the therapy sessions described in both W. Lebra's paper and that of the Goods in this volume. They describe sessions in which diagnosis and choice of treatment clearly result from the interaction between the curer and the client. A model of the curer's cultural knowledge of illnesses would not be sufficient for predicting the diagnosis that results in the session since the diagnosis is a product of the exchange that goes on between the curer and the client. Many folk representations such as certain types of games, meetings, and public encounters with "madpersons" are probably the result of similar dynamic interactions among participants. Since these representations are not reflected in the cultural competencies of individuals, it can be seen that there is more to folk knowledge than that proportion which individuals have the mental blueprints to produce.

As the reader may have already noticed, there are areas of group knowledge the content of which would be similarly described no matter whether it was approached from the ethnoscience perspective or from the folk knowledge perspective. Descriptions of segments of terminology and belief systems, for example, would be very similar. This point applies to a good portion of the material presented in this paper on the Samoan folk knowledge of mental disorders. The material could well have been collected for either type of analysis. What differs in these instances of overlap are the questions that are asked about the segment of group knowledge.

One question that should be easier to answer from the conceptual framework of folk knowledge concerns the degree to which group knowledge is integrated and how the integration is maintained. Cognitive anthropologists have progressed rapidly with the study of the cognitive structuring of cultural knowledge by individuals (e.g., D'Andrade 1976), but they have not contributed as much as might be expected to questions about the structuring and integration of group knowledge (but see Roberts (1964) and Harding and Clement (1980)). A related area is the long tradition in anthropology of comparing and assessing group knowledge on the basis of variables such as "open" versus "closed". Except for a few studies, such as that by Shweder (this volume), there have been almost no contributions by cognitive anthropologists to this area. If they were equipped with a strong sense of the distinction between group knowledge and individual knowledge which Boas (1911) pointed out many years ago, but which is still forgotten in some contemporary "modes of thought" approaches (see Cole and Scribner 1974:21), cognitive anthropologists should have a great deal to contribute to these questions.

The third and final distinction to be drawn between ethnoscience and folk knowledge concerns the stress placed on representations of knowledge as social phenomena. Originally, the ethnoscience perspective focused solely on the cultural aspects of behavior. The implicit assumption was that individuals use their knowledge to ensure that their behavior meets standards of cultural appropriateness. Situational factors were not incorporated into the perspective. In many cases, studies of ethnoscience gave the impression that representations occur simply as a result of referential meaning (see Lave et al. (1977) for discussion of this point). However, cognitive anthropologists have realized that just as individuals are sensitive to social context in constructing their linguistic behavior, so too are individuals sensitive to social context in the representations they choose (Frake 1977). This point guides a query posed in regard to Samoan folk knowledge of mental disorders: in what situations do individuals use these representations?

This introduction has provided a description of the conceptual framework which underlies the analysis to follow. The bulk of the data was collected using ethnosemantic techniques developed in the ethnoscience tradition. However, the data presented are not analyzed from the ethnoscience perspective, but rather from the folk knowledge perspective described briefly above. I do not take as my task the presentation of the data from the perspective of cultural competence. Rather, as indicated in the introduction, I am interested in questions suggested by treating the material as data on folk knowledge. Specifically, the questions that are asked are: What factors are operating to produce changes in Samoan folk knowledge of mental disorders? How is Samoan folk knowledge integrated? How is folk knowledge of mental disorders related to other areas of knowledge? How flexible is the knowledge of mental disorders? And in what sort of situations do individual Samoans use their knowledge of these representations of mental disorders?

SAMOAN FOLK REPRESENTATIONS OF MENTAL DISORDERS

The Study

As mentioned above, Samoan folk knowledge of mental disorders is primarily represented in the terminology system and in curing routines. The present study addresses the former – the ethnosemantics of mental disorders.

The data for this study were collected in the course of a broad study of Samoan folk knowledge of health problems and resources conducted in the spring and summer of 1972 by myself and Joe Harding. The larger study, which was contracted by the Department of Medical Services of the Government of American Samoa, is useful here in that it provides an indication of how Samoan folk knowledge relates mental disorders to other health problems, and in that it provides information on knowledge about specialists and their respective authorities in the domain of health problems.

Techniques and Data Collection

The methods employed included a variety of ethnosemantic techniques in combination with more traditional ethnographic methods. Traditional ethnographic approaches of participant observation and indepth interviewing were used for the purpose of gathering contextual data on the situations in which people use the representations of mental disorders and the reactions that Samoans have to individuals identified as suffering from mental disorders. Existing literature augmented this contextual data. Although there is only a limited literature on topics directly related to Samoan concepts of mental health and functioning (e.g., see Gerber 1975), there is extensive work on such topics as the nature of the descent groups, the political systems, the economic institutions of redistribution, and, to a lesser extent, Samoan prehistory. This material provides a basis for identifying the institutions that affect Samoan folk knowledge of mental disorders.

A description of the Samoan terminology for mental disorders was obtained through ethnosemantic techniques. A number of ethnosemantic techniques have been developed to elicit the terms, associated beliefs and values which structure specific domains of knowledge. In this study, four of these techniques were used: domain definitions, belief matrices, judged similarity interviews, and rankings. The first interviews, the domain definition interviews, consisted of open-ended questions heuristically structured so that the answers to the initial questions could be inserted into the subsequent questions. The remaining interview formats contained standardized questions constructed from the responses to the domain definition interviews. For background and description of the techniques used, see the overview presented by Black (1974). The particular combination of techniques and analyses reflected here grew out of work by Stefflre (1972) and Stefflre et al. (1971). Clement (1974) explains the techniques used in this study in much greater detail.

The interviews were conducted by trained Samoan interviewers during visits by the research team to a set of 14 villages on the island of Tutuila, American Samoa. The team which consisted of myself, Harding, and the interviewers was sometimes accompanied by a Samoan chief who made the necessary speeches on our behalf.

Samples

The sampling design called for non-random, quota samples. Respondents were chosen within specified categories by the chiefs and ministers who hosted our visits in the villages. For some of the small samples, the Samoan interviewers helped to recruit the respondents. The sample sizes ranged from seven for the pilot interviews on valued characteristics to 184 for the ranking interviews. Table I lists the sample sizes for the various interviews. Rationales for the different sizes of the samples plus descriptions of the sample characteristics and possible biases are given in Clement (1974:307–341).

TABLE I
Sample sizes by type of interview

Type of interview	Number of Respondents
Domain definition	
Mental disorders	13
Troublemakers	5
Health concerns	50
Samoa's future problems	26
'Āiga's future problems	20
Judged similarity-valued characteristics	7
Beliefs matrix	
Health concerns by resources	26
General concerns by resources/solutions	28
Rankings	
Health concerns	184
General concerns	184
Resources/solutions	184

Feature Versus Generative Models of Folk Knowledge

Roughly speaking, analyses of ethnosemantic data can be sorted into two types depending upon whether they produce a feature or a generative model of the data (D'Andrade, 1976). Feature models delineate pervasive underlying elements of meaning for a particular domain. They are static in that they are addressed neither to the process of how individuals use knowledge nor to those segments of the system which are likely to change. In contrast to feature models, genera- tive models devote attention to the process by which individuals cognitively generate culturally appropriate responses. Generative models are useful for identifying points of flexibility and patterns of change in the body of folk knowledge. Feature analysis, on the other hand, is advantageous for charting and anticipating constraints on the body of folk knowledge that promote continuity (see Harding and Clement, 1980:10–14). Interest in both the continuity and change of the Samoan folk knowledge system dictates that both types of analyses are relevant here. The next section on the terminology of mental disorders takes a generative approach, stressing key propositions about mental disorders. Following the description of mental disorders and related propositions, the focus shifts to the underlying features of meaning which relate mental disorders to other domains.

FOLK REPRESENTATIONS OF MENTAL DISORDERS AND ASSOCIATED PROPOSITIONS

Samoan terminology for mental disorders does not include a generic term that encompasses both psycho-social problems and the more severe mental sicknesses. The following discussion pertains to responses given to a question glossed in English as "What are the sicknesses or things that can be wrong with people's minds?" The characteristics of the illnesses, of the victims of these disorders, and of the appropriate treatments are those given in the interviews. (See Clement (1974) for more details.)

Samoan representations of mental disorders can be broken into three subsets which share similar causes, therapies, and symptoms: (1) *ma'i o le māfaufau* or conditions due to brain abnormalities; (2) *ma'i aitu* or conditions due to spirit possession; and (3) conditions caused by experiencing an excess of emotion. In talking about these disorders, there is a tendency to lump all conditions which are severe and apparently incurable under the general term *"ma'i valea"*. Conditions due to brain abnormalities are placed in this category. In the following, *ma'i valea* (including *ma'i o le māfaufau*) is discussed first, then *ma'i aitu*, and finally the mental problems caused by an excess of emotion.

Ma'i Valea

In Samoa, being a *tagata a'oa'oina*, which I will gloss as a "cultured person", is very important. To be a cultured person, one must at the very least have learned to behave appropriately toward others, to speak in a manner that is acceptable, to care for oneself properly, and to perform useful tasks and services. *Ma'i valea* is a mental condition characterized by either not having or not being able to demonstrate these minimal skills. According to informants, a person who has *ma'i valea* tends to walk around without purpose at strange times, talk without meaning, and behave without concern for etiquette patterns. He or she behaves in a stupid manner which benefits no one.[3]

It should be noted that although respondents used "*ma'i valea*" as a general term for severe mental disorders regardless of their etiology, on a more specific level, "*ma'i valea*" refers to conditions caused by an excess of emotion or an *aitu* (spirit). "*Ma'i o le māfaufau*" refers to problems with thinking that have come from an abnormality in the person's brain. Such an abnormality may have been present from birth, a result of a blow to the head, a by-product of using narcotics, or the result of illness in another part of the body.

When *ma'i valea* occurs without the presence of a brain abnormality, the person who was previously all right begins to act in a *valea* manner. A temporary condition of *valea* can result from acquiring too much knowledge, being overly concerned about something, jealous, or afraid of something; it also can result from the way a person is treated (disciplined) by his family or from an *aitu*. *Ma'i valea* which is not due to physical damage or congenital retardation is thought to pass if the afflicted person ceases to believe or decides not to believe that he is like those who have something wrong with their brains. Also, a temporary condition of *valea* caused by over-concern can be cured by removal of the person from the context that is stimulating concern (for example, if the *ma'i valea* is due to over-studying, the person should stop studying and go enjoy himself).

In the belief matrix interviews, severe mental disorders of longstanding were associated with a small set of sources of help: doctors, special doctors, the hospital, special hospitals, and the mental health program (at the hospital). There was doubt expressed that severe mental illness, including conditions of mental retardation, can be cured — especially if the condition is of long duration. Medical specialists are not thought to have yet found a means to cure these conditions.

Apart from Western-style doctors, pastors, and traditional curers, there are also home methods for the treatment of mental disorders. For sudden outbursts, the emphasis is upon bringing the person back under control by calming him down. If the person is thought to be capable of self-control, he or she may be hit or scolded or taken away from the situation. If the person cannot be restrained, he may be taken to the hospital.

Ma'i Aitu

Ma'i aitu (also referred to by some as *ma'i fasa*) is a term which refers to a mental illness that is disavowed by the Christian Congregational or London Missionary Society Church as well as the Catholic Church and the Church of Jesus Christ of Latter Day Saints. The traditional view is that a spirit may take possession of a person's body and cause the person to behave strangely. An *aitu*, for example, may cause a person to speak rudely to those he should speak to with respect (like the *matai* — the titled head of the extended family), to tell those above him (in rank, authority or age) what they are doing wrong, to physically assault other family members, and/or to physically injure himself. The churches teach that belief in spirit possession may be used by a person as an excuse for committing reprehensible acts toward members of his family.

The responses to behavior associated with *ma'i aitu* depend upon whether an *aitu* is thought to be the cause of the person's delirious behavior. An ancestral spirit may become angry at the misbehavior of *'āiga* (family) members and express dissatisfaction through possession of the erring person or another person through which the *aitu* speaks to members of the family. If it seems that a dead ancestor is possessing the person, then the person is treated with respect and his or her wishes heeded. If the message or grievance is unclear, the victim may be taken to a person who knows *vaiaitu* (traditional cures) or treatments for illnesses brought about by *aitu*, which include internally taken preparations.

Traditional Samoan priests were spirit mediums and healers (Freeman 1959). Today, some Samoan bush doctors called *fōma'i aitu* and *fōma'i vaiaitu* treat *ma'i aitu*.[4] The treatment involves, with the help of medicine administered to the victim, discovery of the identity of the *aitu*, the grievance, and the making of apologies or amends if the *aitu* is that of an ancestor. A home treatment used if the *aitu* is *not* thought to be a respected family ancestor, is to place the dirty covering from an outdoor oven on the afflicted so as to chase away the *aitu*.

Mental difficulties may also be caused by spirits associated with a particular village. Telesā of Lepea, Western Samoa, and Sa'uma'iafi of Sale'imoa, Western Samoa, who were *taupo* (princesses) in their respective villages have become perhaps the most well known of these spirits. These spirits have certain dislikes concerning clothing, hair styles, and etiquette patterns. Offensive or disliked behavior may draw a punishment from the spirit. Visitors may be warned to observe certain preferences of the spirit and to avoid certain areas and time periods of the day to avoid an encounter. If a person is afflicted by one of these spirits, he or she may go or be taken to someone in the village whom the spirit respects, such as a high chief, so that apologies can be made.

If a person's possession by an *aitu* is doubted, the person may be beaten in order to force him to drop the pretense. Because *aitu* beliefs have been criticized by the Church and because of increased exposure to Western education, especially in American Samoa, the idea that a mental condition may be due to *aitu* is acted upon only after other alternatives have proven ineffective. Although the Church has tried to dissuade people from believing in possession by *aitu*, some pastors will pray for the afflicted person to engage spiritual help to dispel the *aitu* and keep them away forever.

Mental Disorders Caused by an Excess of Emotion

The third type of mental disorder results from too much emotion and/or thinking. Due to some aggravating situation, the victim feels some emotion to excess. Depending upon the emotion, the afflicted either strikes out at those around him or her or else turns inward in a self-destructive manner. The general therapy is to remove the person from the aggravating situation.

1. *Ma'i popole, mafatia māfaufau i le popole.* There are a number of types of mental problems that fall into this subtype. *Ma'i popole* (worry sickness) is one that people ranked as an important health concern relative to the other mental disorders in the ranking interviews. *Ma'i popole* is a condition of depression, anxiety, and lack of confidence in which the person: (1) contemplates or anticipates losing something he values; (2) dreads being unable to avoid or circumvent unwanted pressures; or (3) feels overwhelmed by unending problems. Some possible situations which people gave as provoking depression and anxiety in a person are: when he is jealous of his girlfriend; when there is a problem that cannot be solved easily or immediately (like a family dispute over titles); when he might be censured by the council of chiefs about not obeying their orders; when there might be a disagreement with people in a village where he is going on *malaga* (a formal visit); when he is really happy about something that is going to happen; when she is dreading delivery of a baby; when he does not have enough money and he must contribute his share for *fa'alavelave* (family trouble).

The individual who is deeply involved with worrying (*mafatia māfaufau i le popole*) is despondent and depressed. He does not want to talk, to work, or do anything, and only stays in the house; he feels sad and can find no joy in diversions. He may lack confidence in himself, may feel nervous and agitated, and is unable to sleep. Worrying usually passes away when the situation about which the person has been concerned is resolved or left behind, by going somewhere else, or when his attention is attracted by something less problematic or worrisome. Sources of help for excessive worrying include friends and relatives, the pastors, and even the hospital. A condition of depression and anxiety which continues for an extended period may develop into a more severe problem or *ma'i valea.*

2. *Ma'i manatu, ma'i fa'anoanoa, ma'i alofa.* *Ma'i manatu, ma'i fa'anoanoa*, and *ma'i alofa* are terms which refer to strong feelings of depression and sadness caused by separation from a loved one either through physical separation, death, or emotional separation (in the case of *ma'i alofa*). *Ma'i manatu* was used in the responses to refer to all three conditions; *ma'i fa'anoanoa* was used specifically with death and with physical separation; *ma'i alofa* was used to refer only to emotional separation. The characteristics associated with *ma'i manatu* were sadness, poor appetite, inability to eat, little desire to talk to anyone or do anything but sleep (or, conversely, inability to rest), and being unhappy.

The suggested solutions for *ma'i manatu*, when it involves a child's feelings about an adult or vice versa, included reuniting the child with the parent or relative he misses. For "love-sickness" (*ma'i alofa*) or loss due to emotional separation from a person with whom one is in love, the remedies are getting involved with someone else, doing other things, or in some fashion trying to forget about the person. For *ma'i fa'anoanoa* (mourning sickness), the solutions offered were to read the Bible and to take time and try to forget.

3. *Ma'i Ita*. A person with *ma'i ita* has an angry outburst or a rage in which the person may break things or say bad words to someone else in the family or someone who is teasing him. These outbursts are sometimes like those exhibited by a person suffering from *ma'i aitu*, *ma'i valea*, or a condition like *ma'i fasa* except that it often occurs under the influence of alcohol. Alternatively, the anger may be turned inward, causing the person to get a headache. The pastor, the police, or someone in the family can be brought to try to calm the enraged person or discourage his behavior. *Ma'i ita* is thought to be controllable by the person himself, thus methods for helping the person include scolding or castigating him for lack of self-control. As with other conditions resulting from too much emotion, *ma'i ita* can become a permanent condition of *valea*.

In sum, the folk representations of mental disorders as expressed in the terminology system constitute a system that is open-ended at three points. Anything which causes brain abnormalities can be incorporated into the Samoan folk knowledge of mental disorders through the subset of beliefs about *ma'i o le māfaufau*. Mental disorder caused by drug abuse is a recent addition to this particular subset of mental illnesses. The concept of *ma'i aitu* is equally expandable to encompass any sort of *aitu*. The third subset, mental disorders caused by an excess of emotion, is also open-ended. Any emotion experienced to excess can result in a mental disorder.

The following section shifts focus from these open-ended components to features of the system which seem to be deeply embedded in the culture in that they cross a number of domains. The following section can also be compared to the present section on another basis. Generally speaking, the Samoan concepts of mental disorders tend to focus upon conditions that are brought about by external, adverse circumstances and outside forces (e.g., *aitu*) rather than non-organic abnormalities internal to the afflicted person. As will be seen in the following section, those having what Americans might refer to as personality problems are not seen as having mental problems but rather as being types of people who cause problems for others.

CRAZY PEOPLE, TROUBLEMAKERS, AND IMPORTANT PERSONS

Besides constituting a problematic condition, *ma'i valea* also serves as an identifying characteristic of a social identity or type of person called a *vale* or *tagata valea*. When asked in a domain definition interview about people who cause trouble for others, "*tagata valea*" (stupid or crazy person) was given along with a number of other types of troublemakers. The list along with English glosses are as follows: *fa'atupu fa'alavelave* (troublemaker); *tagata fa'aleagamea* (spoiler); *tagata fa'atupu misa* (quarrel maker); *tagata fa'alialia* (show-off); *tagata mimita* (boaster or conceited person); *tagata lēa'oa'oina* (uneducated person); *tagata leai ma se māfaufau* (senseless person); *tagata 'onana* (drunk); *moetolo* (nightcrawler – a type of rapist); *tagata gaoi* (robber); and *tagata fasioti tagata* (murderer).

With the exception of the murderer, the negatively valued behavioral traits of these troublemakers are *not* attributed to situational stress as are many of the mental disorders. They are, even in the case of a murderer, attributed to a lack of proper training. A person who is cultured, that is, well brought up, well trained in Samoan custom, is unlikely to have bad manners, to be overly aggressive in the wrong situations, to consider himself over his family, or to carelessly destroy the property of others. The flavor of how an uncultured person is thought of can be gained from descriptions of the uncultured or "uneducated person" and the "senseless person".

The *tagata lēa'oa'oina* is a person who is always doing improper things because he lacks training. Examples of behavior considered improper include talking at gatherings while standing or eating while walking along the road. The "uneducated person" has not learned enough to function well in society. He does improper things and is afraid to speak because he does not know anything. A person is described as not having had enough education if he did not listen to the *matai* (the head of the family) or go to church on Sunday, or if he always disobeyed his parents and acted in a disrespectful way toward them.

The *tagata leai ma se māfaufau* is a type of person who does not have the good sense to behave appropriately. He does not manage his behavior well. He is not sensitive to appropriate behavior. This type of person carelessly destroys other people's things and takes their property without considering their feelings. He speaks impolitely and rudely to people and about people. He is a person who was not properly trained because he did not go to the pastor's school; he does not go to church; he never listens to the wise people of the village; he never listens to the head of the family, and he never reads books.

In these interviews, *tagata valea* (stupid or crazy person) was described as an individual who does not know manners, know how to show respect, how to joke, or how to talk to others in an appropriate manner. The crazy person (*tagata valea*) behaves in an uncultured manner because of a brain abnormality or *ma'i valea*. The other types of troublemakers have the capacity to learn proper behavior, but for some reason did not take the opportunity to do so. All of these types of people are disvalued because, as a result of their uncultured behavior, they may interfere with the well-being of the family.

The feature of being cultured also appeared when Samoans were questioned about the characteristics necessary for holding important positions in Samoa. Key characteristics are being *poto* (wise), *atamai* (clever), *a'oa'oina* (cultured), *lelei* (good), *agava'a* (qualified), and *māfaufau* (sensible). Instead of causing quarrels, the valued characteristic is ability to settle quarrels; instead of not knowing how to talk, the valued characteristic is proper speech; instead of being uncultured, the valued characteristic is being cultured; instead of being insensitive to others, the valued characteristic is knowing how to manage social situations; and instead of stupidity, the valued characteristic is cleverness.[5]

From these characteristics, it can be seen that troublemakers are on opposite poles from valued persons. The madperson stands perhaps as a prototype for the kind of person that is not valued in Samoan society. A *tagata valea* is certainly not suited for the important positions in Samoan society and, in fact, does not even meet the minimum quality expected of a Samoan person, which is knowledge of appropriate behavior that would allow him or her to contribute to the family. The *vale* stands out as an exemplar of the class of troublemakers who embody a violation of what Samoans should be like. Those who are *tagata valea* of long standing with no apparent hope of recovery are often objects of scorn and derision. The affect their behavior elicits is associated with the fact that it reflects this negative prototype. These terms are used in a figurative sense in joking and in making insults because they carry a significant affective load useful for creating an effective image.

The first portion of the analysis drew attention to the representations of mental disorders with which Samoans are familiar. The analysis of these folk representations has revealed points at which the system is open-ended and may be easily expanded. The second thrust of the analysis has anchored the folk knowledge of mental disturbances in the broader domain of social identities. The *vale*, the madperson, constitutes an extreme type whose behavior is worthless and possibly embarrassing to his family. As such, the role stands out as a prototype constituting a standard against which other roles may be compared, an embodiment or representation of important cultural themes, and an image which is used in figurative speech for joking or teasing others.

THE SITUATIONAL RELEVANCE OF FOLK REPRESENTATIONS OF MENTAL DISORDERS

From the discussion of the terminology system, a description has been provided of the folk representations which are familiar to Samoans in their talk about mental disorders. In addition, the analysis has traced the open-ended nature of the system of folk representations and related mental disorders to important dimensions of the broad domain of social identities. Despite all this information, however, is it possible to predict what Samoans will do when they must make a decision about or respond to someone affected by a mental disorder? This question is especially reasonable in light of the argument that these folk representations are an aspect of group knowledge. No assumptions can be made as to when or under what conditions individuals will use these folk representations of mental disorders.

Ethnographic data on the use of folk representations of mental disorders in American Samoa, suggest that this knowledge is used in a variety of ways not all of which are predictable from a description of the representations themselves. Individuals do upon occasion rely upon folk knowledge to describe and explain the behavior of others. They also, however, use the representations in a figurative sense to make jokes and to insult one another. Referentially incorrect, but socially effective depictions are constructed through these metaphorical uses.

The situational relevance of folk representations of mental disorders can be illustrated with two examples.

A New Mental Health Program

The case of the newly introduced mental health program provided an interesting situation in which to analyze the use of the folk representations in individual behavior. A section of one of our interviews requested descriptions of ten of the programs run by the hospital. Seventy-two respondents were asked to complete this open-ended interview which included the mental health program as one of the items. The program had begun only five months before the study and people were generally unaware of its existence. However, the respondents agreed on what the program was probably like. They saw it as being for the treatment and cure of mental disorders and as being staffed by special doctors. Despite being able to describe these aspects of the program, many went ahead to voice perplexities about the rationality of the program. Applying Samoan folk knowledge to the feasibility of such a program would lead one to the conclusion that the program was not well conceived. Samoans believe that neither *ma'i o le māfaufau* nor *ma'i valea* of long standing can be cured. Additionally, some indicated doubt that doctors could treat the less severe mental disorders such as *ma'i manatu* because doctors do not know what these illnesses are. Samoans do see the hospital as a place to bring those who are recalcitrant to home treatment or who are uncontrollable; but they do not necessarily expect the person to be cured. The mental health program did not seem feasible as a source of effective treatment.

Despite the limited announcement of the program and despite the inappropriateness of the program as evaluated by the propositions of the Samoan folk knowledge system, the director/therapist was not at a loss for patients. Some were referred by medical personnel in the hospital and others requested treatment out of curiosity about whether the new program could help. Patients also continued to return despite the fact that they doubted whether the doctor was a special doctor (since he could not prescribe medicine) and despite the fact that they wondered when the doctor was going to quit talking and begin the treatment! Apparently, folk knowledge was being used in the construction of expectations about the program, but it was not being used as sufficient information upon which to decide whether to use or continue using the program.

Spirit Possession

A final point about the situational relevance of folk knowledge of mental disorders concerns *ma'i aitu*, the class of disorders caused by spirit possession. People know that *ma'i aitu* is disavowed by the churches in Samoa. As described in the previous section, in the eyes of church authorities, *ma'i aitu* is an illegitimate mental disorder. Supposedly, those wishing to show their allegiance to their church membership would, in church-related contexts, censor expression of beliefs they might have in the validity of the concept. Samoans are also aware that *papālagi* (people of European descent) do not believe in *aitu*. Again, Samoans who believe in *aitu*, but who wish to communicate an accommodating image to a *papālagi*, may omit any reference to *aitu*. Since *papālagi* were conducting the present study and since the Department of Medical Services was sponsoring the study, it is quite likely that our interviews were interpreted by some respondents as a situation in which it was inappropriate to reveal beliefs in *aitu*. In ranking sources of health care and assistance, the 184 respondents ranked Samoan treatment by Samoan medicines last out of 17 items and they ranked *ma'i aitu* as being significantly less important than the two other types of mental disorders included on the list of 16 health problems. They ranked worry-sickness, 8th, mental problem, 9th, and *ma'i aitu*, 15th.

The implications of these situational constraints on the display of knowledge about *ma'i aitu* are broader than their possible effects on the study. The case of *ma'i aitu* indicates a common tendency for large blocks of knowledge to be situationally bound by social convention. The other case given above reveals a second aspect of situational relevance. Although folk knowledge of mental disorders is part of the everyday life of Samoan people in such social activities as joking and interpreting illness, its use as an explanatory system in professional settings is more limited.

PROCESSES OF MAINTENANCE AND CHANGE IN SAMOAN FOLK KNOWLEDGE OF MENTAL DISORDERS

The previous section on individual uses of folk representations of mental disorders has foreshadowed the discussion of processes of maintenance and change in this body of folk knowledge. The individual patterns reflect processes of flux at the group level. Reference was made to two situations in which individuals may censor expression of beliefs about *ma'i aitu*. Although for different reasons, both the Samoan churches and people of European descent discredit the legitimacy of *ma'i aitu*. An additional consideration with regard to possible change has to do with the participation by Samoans in alternative institutions that utilize a different knowledge of mental disorders. While there is little evidence as yet that Western concepts of mental illness have been incorporated into the Samoan system, it is possible that Samoans will also become competent with Western folk and scientific representations as a result of utilizing the mental health program provided by the hospital. As was pointed out by respondents in the interviews on troublemakers, concepts of "criminals" from American television programs have been incorporated into Samoan folk knowledge. As will be elaborated below, both these trends of self-censorship and the utilization of alternative resources reveal the relationship of the processes of flux in the folk representations to the Samoan social structure.

The Role of Authority

The case of the church's position against *ma'i aitu* demonstrates a process of change that is probably quite common. Folk representations become objectified in the sense that they are seen as objects in the social environment and themselves associated with social and cultural meaning. These social meanings are then taken into account by individuals in their choice among alternative ways to behave or speak. Another, perhaps more familiar, description of this process is provided by sociolinguistics and by ethnographers of communication and cultural transmission. Both sociolinguists such as Labov (1972) and anthropologists interested in cultural transmission such as Goodenough (1971:16) and Gearing et al. (1979) have drawn attention to the property-like nature of knowledge. Beliefs, skills, knowledge, and ways of speaking become the property of or the markers of social identities such as church members. Another important point which is implicit in the writings of Labov, Gearing, and Goodenough is that the arbiters of the social meanings of these folk representations are those who hold positions of authority in the social structure. The meaning of folk representations such as *ma'i aitu*, in other words, is vulnerable to influence by those in positions of authority.

The role of authority figures as they affect the use and development of competence with alternative systems of knowledge must also be considered. Potential clients are not likely to present themselves to curers whom they believe lack the authority and power to cure, and as a result, these potential curers are less able to disseminate their knowledge. The attack of the churches on *ma'i aitu* indirectly attacks the authority of the *foma'i vaiaitu* (bush doctor) regarding mental disorders. If *ma'i aitu* is but a sham then the authority of the bush doctor is restricted in the eyes of potential clients. Other than this attempt to discredit *ma'i aitu* as a legitimate mental disorder, a struggle for authority in the area of mental disorders was not in evidence. The hospital's bid for expanded authority for mental health did not appear to be perceived as threatening by any of the alternative authorities – the pastors, or the bush doctors – to which Samoans look for assistance with various mental disorders.

The Social Functions of Folk Knowledge

Finally, before concluding the paper, I would like to speak briefly to the topic of the latent functions of the Samoan system for responding to mental disorders. It is obvious that the Samoan system of treating mental disorders benefits the Samoan social system. In the past, especially, the treatment routines associated with *ma'i aitu* included the making of a formal apology (*ifago*) on the part of the family to the offended *aitu*. Undoubtedly, the ritual had important social consequences for the family and possibly served as a safety valve for individuals frustrated by the abuse of power on the part of a family head. To some extent, "blowing up" at someone in authority now takes place under the influence of alcohol. The methods for ameliorating drunken expressions of anger and frustration are not routinized and do not have the beneficial effects of the process for treating *ma'i aitu*.

It is also possible that the Samoan system of treating mental disorders has been efficacious in preventing and reducing mental illness in Samoa. Walters (1977), for example, who served briefly as a director of the mental health program in American Samoa, suggests some benefits for the individual of the treatment regime associated with *ma'i aitu* and attributes some of the discrepancy between expected rates of mental illness and the low rate of actual cases to its efficacy. Walters addresses only the portion of the Samoan system that has to do with *ma'i aitu*, omitting those parts which concern problems of excessive emotion such as *ma'i manatu*. Home remedies for these problems may prevent the development of more serious problems. In any event, it is reasonable to suspect that the system is, or at least was, beneficial to both group and individual functioning.

These latent functions of the Samoan ethnopsychological system, of course, do not ensure its continuation. Samoans talk about the value of *fa'a Samoa* (Samoan custom) and see maintenance of it as an important problem facing Samoa (see Clement 1974:158). Despite the recognition of its importance, individuals cannot decide to keep or not to keep a body of custom. These latent consequences are worth mentioning here, not because they are directly affecting the processes of maintenance and change in the Samoan folk knowledge system, but rather because they should be taken into account in assessing the potential value of an alternative resource being considered for introduction.

CONCLUSION

The present study has addressed only a limited portion of Samoan folk knowledge of mental disorders, namely: language-based representations of types of mental disorders, their causes and cures. Although data on the expression of folk knowledge of mental disorders and treatments in curing routines and rituals is missing, a number of points have been made with regard to the Samoan folk knowledge of this domain.

Samoan knowledge of mental disorders includes three general causative propositions: (1) brain damage or brain abnormalities cause mental disorders; (2) *aitu* (spirits) cause mental disorders; and (3) too much of an emotion causes mental disorders. These propositions are abstract enough to generate explanations for new disorders. Drug abuse, for example, has recently been incorporated as a cause of the type of disorder related to brain abnormalities.

Not all aspects of the folk knowledge about mental disorders appear to be equally open or accommodating to new information. Some portions are firmly anchored in other areas of folk knowledge. Common themes connect folk knowledge of mental disorders, for example, with folk knowledge of social types. Severe mental disorders render an individual a type of person who is disvalued in Samoan society. Because madpersons fail to exhibit the important characteristic of being cultured (being educated in Samoan culture), they are disvalued. They, in effect, come to be living representations in themselves of what one should *not* be. In all likelihood, it would be difficult to change folk knowledge about victims of apparently permanent mental disorders without first changing folk knowledge about social types in general.

There are contemporary forces operating to change Samoan folk knowledge of mental disorders. One clearly challenged area is the general proposition and related beliefs that link *aitu* to mental disorders. Samoans know that ministers of the various Christian churches in Samoa have disavowed *ma'i aitu* as a legitimate mental disorder. Samoans also know that people of European descent do not believe in *aitu*. As a result, knowledge of *ma'i aitu* is situationally restricted. In situations where church membership is important, knowledge of *aitu*-caused problems is less likely to be expressed. The situational restriction of knowledge is probably a very common way through which bodies of folk knowledge change.

Use of folk knowledge of mental disorders by Samoans was considered in a discussion of their reaction to a new mental health program. Samoan clients presented themselves and family members for treatment despite the fact that the mental health program does not make sense if evaluated on the basis of Samoan folk knowledge of mental disorders. Individuals may be well versed in the relevant folk knowledge, but not rely upon it in particular situations.

Aside from the specific information presented on Samoan folk knowledge, this examination of Samoan folk representations of mental disorders has offered an opportunity to discuss a reconceptualization of group knowledge in cognitive anthropology. Traditional studies of ethnoscience are based upon an equation of group knowledge with the aggregated cultural knowledge of members of the group. This perspective highlights questions of individual cognition — generally, questions about cultural competence. In the case of Samoan folk knowledge of mental disorders, for example, the ethnoscience perspective would have guided the analyst to ask what must one know in order to be able to label mental disorders and talk about their causes and consequences in a manner that would be culturally appropriate to Samoans. Here, a reconceptualization of group knowledge has been offered which denies the equation of individual and group knowledge. This perspective guides the analyst to ask questions about characteristics and processes related to group knowledge as well as about individual knowledge. The perspective offered here is not meant to exclude the questions that the ethnoscience perspective has traditionally posed. Studies of cultural competence continue to be very important. However, it does seem to be time for cognitive anthropology to begin to develop a more general and powerful conceptual framework than that afforded by the ethnoscience perspective.

ACKNOWLEDGMENTS

This paper has profited from the efforts of a number of people. Some of the ideas on group knowledge came from discussions with Michael Livesay. He also read and commented on various drafts of the paper along with Jeff Boyer, Mari Clark, Joe Harding, Sylvia Polgar, Naomi Quinn, Joanne Taylor, and Geoff White. Andy Puletasi, a Samoan who helped with the original study, also helped with this paper by reviewing some of the analyses. Also helpful was the stimulation and comments on the paper from other participants in the East-West Center conference at which a draft of the paper was presented. Finally, I would like to thank the University Research Council of the University of North Carolina at Chapel Hill for their grant which supported the collection of some additional data.

NOTES

1. "Folk" is used in a broad sense to refer to any group of people participating in a cultural tradition. Cognitive anthropologists use "folk" in this broad sense to legitimate the study of indigenous classification systems in their own terms. Unfortunately, this use of "folk" may be confusing to those accustomed to the Redfieldian sense of the term. A means of avoiding "folk" would have been to employ the label "collective representations". This label, however, is solidly associated with the Durkheimian tradition. While there is overlap between the concepts of collective representation and folk representation, the difference between the assumptions and foci of the cognitive versus the Durkheimian approaches are sufficient to maintain a distinctive label.
2. Some information on curing practices is available in Moyle (1974), Epling and Siliga (1967), and McCuddin (1974).
3. Milner (1966:312) gives the meaning of *valea* as: 1. (Be) mad, insane. 2. (Be) stupid, dull-witted. According to informants, "*valevalea*", refers to senility where the old person tends to forget things and possibly gets angry a lot.
4. The term "*taulāitu*" can be used to refer to a spirit medium.
5. These preliminary data were collected by Joe Harding. He worked with an informant using a domain definition interview to elicit words for important kinds of people (e.g., pastors or chiefs), and the characteristics which qualify individuals for those positions. From this interview a list of 24 characteristics were compiled for a judged similarity interview which was administered to seven respondents.

REFERENCES

Black, M.
  1974 Belief Systems. *In* Handbook of Social and Cultural Anthropology. J. Honigmann (ed.). New York: Rand McNally.
Boas, F.
  1911 The Mind of Primitive Man. New York: Free Press.
Clement, D.
  1974 Samoan Concepts of Mental Illness and Treatment. Ph.D. Dissertation, School of Social Sciences, University of California, Irvine.
Clement, D. and M. Livesay
  1979 The Organization and Representation of Social Race Relations in Six Desegregated Schools. *In* When Schools are Desegregated. Murray L. Wax (ed.). Washington: National Institute of Education.

Cole, M. and S. Scribner
1974 Culture and Thought: A Psychological Introduction. New York: John Wiley & Sons, Inc.
D'Andrade, R.
1976 A Propositional Analysis of U.S. American Beliefs About Illness. *In* Meaning in Anthropology. Keith H. Basso and Henry A. Selby (eds.). Albuquerque: University of New Mexico Press.
Epling, P. and N. Siliga
1967 Notes on Infantile Diarrhea in American Samoa: A Sketch of Indigenous Theory. Journal of Tropical Pediatrics 13:139–149.
Frake, C.
1977 Plying Frames Can be Dangerous: Some Reflections on Methodology in Cognitive Anthropology. The Quarterly Newsletter of the Institute for Comparative Human Development 1:1–7.
Freeman, J. D.
1959 The Joe Gimlet or Siovili Cult. *In* Anthropology in the South Seas. J. D. Freeman and W. R. Geodes (eds.). New Plymouth: Avery.
Gearing, F., et al.
1979 Working Paper 6. *In* Toward a Cultural Theory of Education and Schooling. Frederick Gearing and Lucinda Sangree (eds.). The Hague: Mouton Publishers.
Gerber, E.
1975 The Cultural Patterning of Emotions in Samoa. Ph. D. Dissertation, University of California, San Diego.
Goodenough, Ward H.
1971 Culture, Language, and Society. An Addison-Wesley Module in Anthropology, No. 7. Reading, Mass.: Addison-Wesley Publishing Co., Inc.
Harding, J. and D. Clement
1980 Regularities in the Continuity and Change of Role Structures: The Ixil Maya. *In* Predicting Sociocultural Change. Susan Abbott and John van Willigen (eds.). Athens: University of Georgia Press.
Labov, W.
1972 On the Mechanism of Linguistic Change. *In* Directions in Sociolinguistics: The Ethnography of Communication. John J. Gumpers and Dell Hymes (eds.). New York: Holt, Rinehart and Winston, Inc.
Lave, J., A. Stepick, and L. Sailer
1977 Extending the Scope of Formal Analysis: A Technique for Integrating Analysis of Kinship Relations with Analysis of other Dyadic Relations. American Ethnologist 4:321–339.
McCuddin, C. R.
1974 Samoan Medical Plants and Their Usage. Pago Pago, American Samoa, Government of American Samoa, Department of Medical Services.
Milner, G. B.
1966 Samoan Dictionary. London: Oxford University Press.
Moyle, R.
1974 Samoan Medicinal Incantations. Journal of the Polynesian Society 83:155–179.
Roberts, J.
1964 The Self-Management of Cultures. *In* Explorations in Cultural Anthropology. Ward Goodenough (ed.). New York: McGraw-Hill.
Stefflre, V. J.
1972 Some Applications of Multidimensional Scaling to Social Science Problems. *In* Multidimensional Scaling: Theory and Applications in the Behavioral Sciences, Vol. 2: Applications. A. Kimball Romney et al. (eds.). New York: Seminar Press.

Stefflre, V. J., P. Reich, and M. McClaran-Stefflre
    1971 Some Eliciting and Computational Procedures for Descriptive Semantics. *In*
          Explorations in Mathematical Anthropology. Paul Kay (ed.). Cambridge, Mass.:
          MIT Press.
Sturtevant, W.
    1964 Studies in Ethnoscience. American Anthropologist 66:99–131.
Walters, W.
    1977 Community Psychiatry in Tutuila, American Samoa. American Journal of Psy-
          chiatry 134:917–919.

8. POPULAR CONCEPTIONS OF MENTAL HEALTH IN JAPAN

INTRODUCTION

This paper will examine briefly some of the traditional beliefs and medical practices used in East Asian medical systems.[1] The relationship of these beliefs to contemporary conceptions of mental health will then be examined by means of a semantic network analysis (Good 1977). These data will then be assessed for their implications for clinical care and the question of the incorporation of traditional medical systems into the official health care systems of large urbanized societies in general.[2]

In the closing sentences of his presidential address to the Fourth Congress of the International College of Psychosomatic Medicine held in Kyoto in 1977, Morton Reiser asked, as he put it, "a somewhat whimsical question" of the East Asians in the audience: "Does the idea of unity of mind and body pose the same implicit threat to you as I think it may to many of us (Westerners)?" He continued, "My question may even strike you as irrelevant or strange -- if it does, we still have much to learn from you." (Reiser 1979:322).

It is fashionable in the West to castigate ourselves about the impact that Cartesian dualism has had on our attitudes toward the natural world and towards the human organism. At the same time, there has been an assumption made that in East Asia such a mechanistic approach is unusual and, from a superficial acquaintance with traditional Eastern philosophy, the conclusion is often drawn that mind and body are always united and that monism is the prevalent way of envisioning the natural order. While there is undoubtedly some truth in such an assumption, many of the comparisons that are made are between ideas held by the ancient civilizations of Asia and those of contemporary Western society. It is important, therefore to try and establish how both professional groups and lay people in modern East Asia organize their ideas on this topic before useful comparisons can be made, and the subject of beliefs and behavior relating to health and illness in contemporary Japan is a useful starting point for such an exercise.

In 1973 and 1974, when I conducted research into the revival and practice of traditional East Asian medicine in urban Japan, I expected to find that traditional medicine was being practiced in what I regarded as a holistic fashion; that is, that patients' social, psychological and possibly, spiritual needs were being attended to with as much care as were the physical problems. My illusions were dispelled after my first day of interviewing in the clinical setting when I found that diagnosis and treatment procedures appeared to be reductionistic and directed almost exclusively to producing change at the somatic level.

215

A. J. Marsella and G. M. White (eds.), Cultural Conceptions of Mental Health and Therapy,
215–233.

In order to understand why this should be so, despite the apparently unifying and inductive approach taken in many traditional medical texts, it is necessary to analyze not only medical practice in historical and contemporary Japan, but also to study the domain of popular health care. The beliefs and practices used in any medical system are modified by the social organization of the society in question and by dominant cultural values. As Freidson puts it, even "scientific" medicine is *not*, after all, "an unchanging biological reality that is as independent of man as the realities of physics and chemistry" (Freidson 1970:206). In the clinical setting, there is constant interaction between professional medical ideas and lay, or popular, ideas that each practitioner/patient encounter, and healers themselves, of course, bring cultural values to their medical practice. Hence, while the contemporary practice of bio-medicine and traditional East-Asian medicine is changed on the basis of the results of experimental and empirical data, it is also modified in part as a result of the pressure of ideas, often only indirectly related to medicine, which are perpetuated and generated within the lay culture.

The Popular Health Care System

Before presenting this data, the notion of a popular health care system must be clarified. The popular health care system includes all those beliefs and practices which are carried out in a lay context without the participation of health care professionals or institutionalized advisors in such matters. It contains, as Kleinman puts it, several levels: "individual, family, social network and community beliefs and activities" (Kleinman 1980:50). Emphasis in the popular domain is upon health maintenance, but also included are ideas about the labeling and evaluation of an illness, selection of the appropriate action to take when ill, and judgments about efficacy of treatment procedures. Knowledge obtained during the early socialization process, from the educational system, the religious system and so on, are intimately related to and form part of the popular medical system. Philosophical ideas, such as beliefs about the nature of reality and the concept of self, are integral to the popular health care system, as are psychological concepts, such as the management of dependency, nurturance, aggression, sexuality and so on. Beliefs about healthy family functioning, interpersonal relationships of all kinds and of the role of society *vis-à-vis* individuals and families are also important. Some of the ideas in the popular system about the structure and mechanism of the human body and some of the lay therapeutic practices will be derived in part from the professional and folk medical systems of the society in question. In a highly literate society, such as Japan where there is a pluralistic medical system, ideas derived from science, from the traditional medical system and from the mass media can all be found coalesced into the popular health care system.

By analyzing the popular health care system, it is possible to gain some insight into the early stages of the management of illness and to understand why certain types of behavioural strategies, explanatory systems and sets of symptoms are stressed rather than others. Through the use of a semantic network analysis, one can elicit the shared cognitive assessment of what should be done to maintain health, and of how illness episodes are likely to be experienced.

The historical roots of this popular system will be considered first through an examination of traditional East Asian medical concepts about health and illness.

CONCEPTIONS OF HEALTH AND ILLNESS IN TRADITIONAL EAST ASIAN MEDICINE

Chinese medicine, known in Japan as *kanpō* (the Chinese method) was first brought to Japan in the fifth and sixth centuries, and its early propagation was closely associated with the acceptance and spread of Buddhism. The philosophical foundations of this medical system were originally derived from Taoism and Confucianism, but at certain historical periods, ideas derived from Buddhist thought have made important contributions to the theoretical approach used in East Asian medicine.

Yin and Yang

In the East Asian medical system, the explanation for the functioning of the cosmos and everything in it is one based on the concept of the continuous interaction of the complex entities of yin and yang.[3] Man, as part of the cosmos, and hence possessing yin and yang qualities, is therefore viewed dynamically. Within the healthy human body, a physiological and psychological equilibrium should exist: social relationships should take the form of harmonious exchange and one's relationship with nature in all its forms should be one of adjustment to the continuous cycle of change. Illness occurs when balance is not maintained with the total environment. The nature of things, however, including man's body, is one of homeostasis; that is, there is an inherent tendency, up to a point, for a balance to be restored gradually and without outside intervention.

The application of this dynamic concept to actual medical practice encourages an attitude of viewing the patient as a whole person; it is difficult to conceptualize either the parts of the body in isolation or the human being as an individual machine-like organism relatively uninfluenced by the environment.

Ki

The concept of *ki* (a hypothetical system of energy similar to that of the Greek *pneuma*) is thought to form a means of communication between the body parts and is also visualized as occurring outside the body in various related forms in the macrocosm. It is postulated that there is a continual exchange of *ki* between the body and environment, thus enhancing the view of the human body as a microcosm.

In this system, illness is regarded as a process and is not seen predominantly either as a disruptive event or as an attack. Health and ill-health are part of a continuum; perfect health is a hypothetical state which can never actually be fully maintained, and in medicine, therefore, restoration of *perfect* health is not the ultimate goal of either doctor or patient. Moreover, during an illness episode, the state of the patient is viewed dynamically and as responding not only to-wards medication but also to environmental changes, both regular (for example, diurnal cyclical change) or irregular (for example, the social environment).

Therapy

The fundamental premise underlying therapy in East Asian medicine is that human beings are naturally healthy and able to live in harmony with their envi-ronment. At times, however, a push is needed to restore order when a number of factors have combined temporarily to upset the balance. Even then, the assumption is that the body will largely heal itself and that therapy should be used as a kind of catalyst to start the process. Therapeutic techniques are therefore characterized as "mild", "natural", and "slow". Therapy is designed to act on the whole body — removal of the main symptoms is not considered adequate, as all parts of the body are thought to be inter-dependent — in this sense, the model is holistic.

It is also acknowledged that in order to prevent recurrence of the problem, a search for original causes should be made. However, treatment is rarely focused on removing original causes unless they are physical in nature, such as diet, or due to climatic changes. It is believed that the functioning of mind and body is inseparable and that biochemical and physiological processes, which in turn depend upon climatic changes, diet, and hereditary constitution, as well as the social milieu, are constantly modifying emotional and subjective states. The reverse, that emotional states can affect general body functioning, is also accepted. However, in the practice of East Asian medicine in Japan today, it is usually agreed among both doctors and patients that it is easier to restore balance at some levels than others (Lock 1980a, b). In therapy, use is generally made of dietary changes, herbal medicine, acupuncture, moxibustion and massage, with the ultimate objective of bringing about a physiological change within the body leading to tension reduction and, incidentally, to a calmer emotional state.

REDUCTIONISM IN TRADITIONAL JAPANESE MEDICINE

The Shōkanron

Emphasis on a somatic approach to therapy has apparently been true from early times, because there is little mention in the classical medical texts of other types of therapy. The text which was most widely used in Japan, the *shōkanron*, is an extreme example of such a position. This text was compiled in about A.D. 200 in China and, although it has always been available in Japan, it was promoted particularly in the seventeenth century, in association with the rise of an important medical faction, the *kohōha*. Other medical texts of the time were regarded as too philosophical and speculative, and too closely associated with Neo-Confucian thinking. The shōkanron was hailed for its simplicity.

In this text, various diseases are named, their physical symptoms are described in minute detail and 113 prescriptions are included with which to treat the diseases. There is no theory of disease causation, no mention of preventive medicine or of a possible relationship between social and psychological systems and the physical system anywhere in the text. What the book does focus on is the dynamic nature of the human body and the change of symptoms with time, as a disease is modified by the body's natural defenses and by pharmacotherapics. It also focuses on the inter-relationship of the bodily parts one with another, and the impact of both illness and the then-known therapies on all of the body systems. There is, therefore, an emphasis on the unified nature of the human body, but *not* on the relationship of the body with external events; in this respect, the *shōkanron*, which has recently been reprinted and is still widely quoted in East Asian medical circles, is unusual as an East Asian medical text. Implicit in such an approach is the belief that restoration of order at the somatic level will induce psychological well-being and that this in turn will promote good social relationships between people.

Medical theories promoted in feudal Japan therefore encouraged a reductionistic approach to patient care, but such an approach was reinforced by cultural factors. According to Confucian tenets, status and roles are ascribed rather than achieved, and the needs of the individual should be subordinated to those of the group. A person succeeds in life as part of a group and group affiliation should be a life-long commitment — there is little room for social mobility and the individual, in order to succeed, should be compliant and flexible towards the group. It has been demonstrated by DeVos (1973) and Rohlen (1974b), among others, that such values are still prevalent in modern Japan. The assumption in East Asian medical practice, therefore, historically and in contemporary times, is that because someone must forego many of his or her individual needs as part of daily life, a lack of balance is inevitable at times, but that since the social order takes primacy over individuality, then medical treatment must be directed towards changing the individual. Stress imposed by group demands is acknowledged but unquestioned. The focus of attention in the East Asian medical system is therefore upon the individual as a biological unit, even though environmental and social origins of imbalance are accepted.

The Role of Buddhism

Buddhist concepts appear to play a dominant role in reinforcing the idea that treatment should be predominantly at the somatic level. There is a widespread belief, possibly due originally to Buddhist concepts of *karma*, that personality is a relatively fixed entity. Emotional states may change, but these changes are transient and do not produce a lasting effect on personality structure. Secondly, the Buddhist approach, and particularly that of the Zen sect, to learning and emotional insight, is to stress understanding through physical activity and actual experiential involvement in things and events. However, verbal analysis of problems is equated with too much rationality and is considered less effective than quiet inner reflection. Historically, many of the great East Asian doctors were experienced practitioners of Buddhism and this probably influenced their ideas, so that emphasis is placed upon bringing about change at the somatic level which in turn is thought to bring one's emotional state back into balance. The aim is to achieve adjustment to the reality of the phenomenal world and to try to accept certain things as given and unchangeable – the individual learns to bend to the social order and thus the vicious cycle (*akujunkan*) is broken.

It is believed even today in East Asian medical clinics that minor physiological imbalances and somatic changes can be detected in all patients, even those diagnosed as, for example, having functional disorders such as neurasthenia[4] (Lock 1980; Reynolds 1976). Consequently, few patients ever leave a traditional medical clinic without receiving some form of treatment directed towards the production of somatic change.

The results of work carried out independently by Kleinman (1976), Marsella et al. (1973), Tseng (1975a) and others, are of great interest in this connection. Their results show that both Chinese and Japanese patients tend to present somatic complaints rather than psychological complaints, when suffering from problems which would be labeled as predominantly in the domain of mental illness by biomedical practitioners, with much greater frequency than patients from Western cultures. For such patients their physical complaints are the "real" illness which should be cured. It appears, therefore, that medical theory and practice, cultural norms, and the individual experience and labeling of illness are in a mututally reinforcing feedback system.

In summary, therefore, there is no mind/body dichotomy in East Asian medicine and no concept of mental health as distinct from physical health, either historically or at the present time. Despite extensive contact with European ideas in recent years, Cartesian dualism appears to have made no mark on traditional medical thinking. There is, nevertheless, a reductionistic somato/psychic emphasis of long historical standing such that for all problems, even where social and psychological components in disease causation are readily acknowledged, the physical manifestations of an illness are the focus of treatment. This does not mean that stigma is necessarily attached to problems of mental health. While this was and is true of psychosis, (Hayashida 1975; Namihara and Sanches 1977; Yoshida 1972), less florid mental aberrations are not considered shameful, but rather as inevitable, at times. Such patients are merely at the extreme of a normal scale, and therefore deserving of careful attention, and the best type of care for such problems is thought to be treatment of the physical complaints.

It is possible to better understand some of the notions generated in the popular health care system, which will be presented next, in light of the foregoing analysis.

CONTEMPORARY POPULAR JAPANESE CONCEPTIONS OF MENTAL HEALTH AND ILLNESS

Parts of the ensuing discussion corroborate previous studies on Japanese family systems and values (e.g., DeVos 1973; Doi 1973; Lebra 1976 and Vogel 1968), but the implications of these findings for health care have not been extensively studied.

It is usually assumed that a popular medical system will be relatively hard to elicit and that it will be difficult to make generalizations from informants' statements. In this study, I found that the majority of the informants expressed their ideas readily and gave highly consistent responses. This is a result, in part, of sample selection (see footnote 2), but it is also due to a widespread promotion of certain ideas about health in the Japanese mass media, and to the fact that the notion of health is currently an extremely popular topic for discussion. There was between a 75% and 100% agreement on the meaning of the concepts discussed below.[5]

Concepts of Mental Health and its Preservation

It was agreed among the informants that the notion of mental health (*seishin kenkō*), as opposed to health in general (*kenkō*), was a new idea and that middle-class housewives in particular (that is, the informants) had the new-found freedom and time to think about such a concept. It was also agreed that mental (*seishinteki*) and physical (*nikutaiteki*) health were in actuality inseparable, that one should look after them both, and that care of one reinforced a healthy state in the other. There was 100% agreement that a popular saying "*yamai wa ki kara*" (illness comes from *ki*) is a valid statement and that this means that one's psychological state affects one's physiological system.

In answer to questions about the preservation of mental health, Japanized words from English, such as "rhythm", "balance", and "control" were most frequently used. Informants stated that it was important to lead an orderly and "balanced" life, for example, "*seikatsu no 'rizumu' o amari ni dasanai yoni*" (one should not depart too far from the rhythm of daily life). There are, of course, Japanese words for control, balance, and so on, but these key traditional concepts have been updated and revitalized with the help of the mass media over the course of the past 20 years. By adopting certain words from English, traditional ideas can be associated with modernization and science, and therefore continue to be positively valued. In context, the meanings of such Japanized words are usually quite different from the original English meanings, and take on a distinct Japanese flavour, as in the example cited above.

The most important ingredients in a balanced life, and hence for the preservation of mental health, are thought to be physical exercise, balanced diet, getting out of the house, having close friends, having a purpose in life (*ikigai*), and understanding the needs of one's husband and children.

Body Constitution and Personality Type

Informants agreed unanimously that everyone has a specific body constitution (*taishitsu*) which is genetically determined. This cannot be changed and endows one at birth with a certain physical type and makes one vulnerable towards certain illnesses and indispositions. This concept of biological inheritance is an old one, derived largely from East Asian medicine (Fujikawa 1974), but is now reinforced through the teaching of elementary genetics in the school system. Informants describe themselves readily as *hiesho* (a chilly type), *tsukareyasui* (easily tired), *allerugi taishitsu* (an allergic disposition), or even occasionally as *insei* (a yin type) or *yosei* (a yang type).

As a result partly of genetic inheritance, but largely due to early socialization experiences, a personality (*seikaku*) is developed. Informants stated that basic personality cannot be changed and, hence, early socialization and the general environment in which an infant is raised are considered crucial. The term "*seikaku*" for personality has only become widely used in Japanese relatively recently, but the importance of the early years has long been recognized and is made explicit in the old adage "*mitsugo no tamashii hyaku made*" (a three-year-old soul will last one hundred years). Therapy that aims, therefore, to change one's actual personality is not highly regarded. There is general agreement that much of one's personality is outwardly expressed in public. In the important distinction between *uchi* and *soto* (see Lebra 1976:112), that is, between the concept of inside, internal and private, and outside, external and public, most of one's personality belongs to *soto*. It is the fixed style or character type that one has to work with throughout life. One can have a "strong", "weak", "assertive", "retiring" personality, and so on. One can excuse certain types of behaviour by attributing it to one's personality which can't be changed: "*Seikaku dakara dōmo shikataganai*." (It's my/his/her personality and therefore can't be helped.)

Emotional States and the Concept of Self

The concept of self (*jibun*) has been frequently analyzed by many scholars and novelists and remains a popular topic for discussion in Japan. It was agreed among the informants in this study that they have an awareness of their public presentation of self as being somewhat separate and different from their private, inner selves, and that this inner self (*jibun*) should not be exposed to others, including family members. It was also agreed that verbalization of ideas about one's inner self is an inadequate form of expression, because this concept is intimately associated with feeling states, rather than with cognitive awareness. Nevertheless, with some difficulty, ideas about emotional states and the concept of self (*jibun*) can be elicited. It is noteworthy that, whereas in a discussion on personality, body type, physical ailments, familial relationships and so on, informants give many unsolicited personal examples, in the case of ideas associated with "the self", no such examples are forthcoming.

One's inner self is something which can and should be cultivated and developed throughout one's life and the fruits of such a cultivation are evident through one's bearing and ability to lead a balanced and hence, healthy life. The terms *seishin* (mentality), *kokoro* (one's physical and emotional center) and *ki* are central here. Informants were in general agreement that *seishin* and *kokoro* are overlapping domains, but *seishin* is a translation from the Western concept of psychological mentality, whereas *kokoro* is a very old Japanese word, for which the ideogram for "heart" is used. Rohlen has this to say of *kokoro* and *ki*:

> There is little justification for labelling *ki* and *kokoro* as concepts, since that would imply a narrowness of definition and a precision of logic that is not to be found. Rather, these nouns are so common that they are at once simple and yet impenetrable, if our intention is direct translation. They have an extraordinary density of association and in order to learn about Japanese culture, it is crucial to develop a deep empathy for just such words. We must recognize at the outset that daily life is so saturated with their mention that both the unconscious minutiae and the deeply considered ambitions of life are anchored in these words and their meaning derives from this fact. Rather than axioms at the base of a psychological system, we find in them an extraordinary world condensed. Simply to say *kokoro* is to evoke a profound value (Rohlen 1974a:1−2).

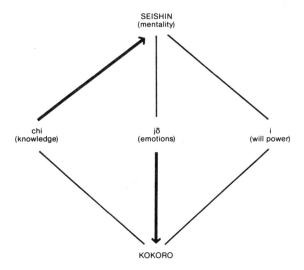

Fig. 1. The relationship of *Seishin* and *Kokoro* in the popular domain. Both are composed of 'knowledge', 'emotions' and 'will power', but *seishin* has a large component of 'knowledge' (*chi*) whereas *kokoro* has a large component of 'emotion' (*jō*).

Both *seishin* and *kokoro* are thought to be composed of three components: *chi* (knowledge), *jō* (emotion), and *i* (willpower). However, seishin is visualized as having a larger component of *chi*; one can have, for example, a "scientific *seishin*" or a "patriotic *seishin*". *Kokoro*, on the other hand, is more closely associated with one's emotions, but is cultivated and tempered by knowledge and willpower. *Kokoro* is a state and not subject to rapid change; it does not have an other-worldly component, although its cultivation, through meditation and related activities, among other things, can be associated with spiritual development. One informant described it thus: "*kokoro to iu no wa, jibun jishin no honto no sugata desu*" (*kokoro* is the real form of one's self). There are numerous daily expressions in Japanese which make use of this term. *Kokoro* can, for example, be strong or gentle; it can be purified, strengthened, or in a state of worry or care for others.

Kokoro is intimately linked with *ki*, but is a larger, more profound idea. *Ki* is associated very clearly with feeling states (*jō*) alone. There are also numerous everyday Japanese expressions in which *ki* appears, but almost all of them express transitional emotional states (for example, *ki ga fusagu*, to be gloomy or depressed; *ki ga chiisai*, to be timid or faint-hearted). The changeable nature of *ki* cannot be eliminated; it is a natural response to external events, but one should learn how to adjust to and deal with such changes, which are regarded as transient, and the martial arts, the tea ceremony, and flower arranging are examples of training techniques which enhance a sensitivity to one's inner state. Simple *hansei* (self-reflection) is also valued.

While *seishin* is located completely in the head region by all informants and is associated predominantly with brain functioning and cognitive processes, *kokoro* is not so clearly situated and is associated with both the head and the chest region. *Ki* is even more diffuse and is associated with both the head, chest, and abdomen. While *kokoro* has a small cognitive component, *ki* does not, unless one deliberately brings it into cognitive awareness. Informants do not regard any of these concepts as concrete entities, but as linguistic terms used to express conditions and states which are uniquely human. The use of *ki* has changed somewhat in the popular sphere. In East Asian medicine and in the martial arts, the existence of *ki* in both the macro- and microcosm is a basic postulate. In contemporary popular thinking, *ki*, though influenced by external events, is confined to the human body and the experience and control of *ki* is equated with control of one's emotional states. Such control, in the popular sphere, is thought to enhance health, whereas in the martial arts, for example, it is used in order to enhance one's power over an opponent, and the promotion of health is somewhat incidental. Despite these differences, the existance of *ki* and *kokoro* both encourage an awareness of the inter-relationship of somatic and psychic variables in the popular domain.

Stress and Anxiety

"Stress" is a word which is now included in the vocabulary of all Japanese speakers, and informants label physical stress and mental stress as two separate entities. Physical stressors, such as excessive exercise, climatic conditions and certain types of industrial pollution, act directly at the somatic level, with no intervention of psychological factors. Mental stress, on the other hand, can be caused by many factors, but those which are cited most are maintenance of good human relationships, repression of one's individual needs, and concern about completing tasks at work or school. These factors lead to a state of anxiety (*fuan*), which is experienced as a change of *ki*. This in turn, if not controlled, can be a threat both to one's mental state and to one's physical body. The postulated mechanism of this psychosomatic reaction will be considered by examining another central concept in the popular care system, that of *hara*.

Hara – The Center of the Body

It is well known that Japanese people suffer inordinately from stomach problems and that when cancer is contracted, it is frequently in the stomach. Diet certainly is a contributing factor to this problem, and so, possibly, is genetics, but there are other points to consider. The abdomen, *hara*, in Japanese, has long occupied the place corresponding to the heart in Western culture (see also T. Lebra, this volume).

Historically, yoga-derived breathing techniques were brought by Buddhist priests from India to China, where they were fused with similar Taoist beliefs. There breathing techniques were used both in meditation and as part of East Asian medical therapy, the principle in both cases being to sit in a relaxed way, concentrate on a spot (*tanden*) two inches below the navel and perform abdominal breathing. *Tanden* is thought to be the center of gravity of the body, and when breathing and concentration are performed correctly, it is a source of great strength, and the flow of *ki* will be at its best. Both *tanden* and the whole abdominal region, known as *hara*, thus came to be of central importance to the Japanese.

During the Edo period, with its emphasis on the role of the samurai and a fostering of the martial arts, the cultivation of *hara* was further developed. A good samurai practiced the art of talking from his abdomen, and his true emotions were also believed to originate there. The position in which a warrior or a soldier was thought to be most prepared for action was in a stance with abdomen out and shoulders unobtrusive – the reverse of Western ideas. It was believed that a man with *hara* could transcend his physical limitations (Durckheim 1975). At this time, *seppuku*, or in vulgar terminology, *harakiri* (the art of cutting the belly), as a means of suicide reached its peak. The equivalent act in the West would be to tear out one's heart to demonstrate the depth and sincerity of one's emotion.

As with the concepts of *ki* and *kokoro*, so with *hara*, many everyday terms related to the expression of emotion are used in the Japanese language. For example, the literal translation of *hara ga tatsu* is "*hara* stands up", which means "to be angry"; similarly, *hara no okii* translates literally as "*hara* is big" and means "to be generous"; *hara o kimeru*, literally "*hara* is decided", has the meaning "to make up one's mind". Some expressions that convey the idea that *hara* is the emotional center of the body are as follows: "He is an honest man in his *hara*", that is "at heart" (*kare wa hara no naka wa shojiki na hito desu*); "his mouth and his *hara* are different", which means "he says one thing and means another" (*kare no kuchi to hara to wa chigau*); to have a black *hara* means "to be black-hearted", "evil", or "wicked" (*haraguroi hito*).

Every informant stressed a connection between one's emotional state and the abdominal region, where anxiety becomes physically manifest, and which is equated today with the anatomical stomach (*i*). Most informants try to use simplified scientific concepts to account for this connection. However, apart from those concerning the stomach, there was no general agreement on psychosomatic connections. Some informants related mental stress to shoulder stiffness, others stated that a "heavy head" was psychosomatic, but not a headache with pain, which was thought to be purely physical. Some informants mentioned asthma, skin complaints and heart problems, as being related to mental stress. It was agreed that it depended upon one's *taishitsu* (physical constitution) as to where psychosomatic problems become manifest, and it was also stated that many diseases have nothing to do with one's psychological state.

Ideas derived from recent popular science have wide dissemination in Japan and apparently influence concepts of psychosomatic medicine, but the traditional emotional concern with *hara* remains central. Moreover, mild, recurrent symptoms, characteristic for each individual, such as shoulder stiffness or a heavy head, act as a signal that psychological or social factors could be involved, and that adjustments should be made at these levels (Lock 1980a). Early socialization practices enhance great sensitivity to mild somatic changes, which are regarded as important warning signs of early illness and of psycho/social stress (Caudill 1976). When somato/psychic connections are perceived, however, since disharmony at the social level is greatly feared, and since individual needs are subordinated for the welfare of the group, resolution of such problems is usually sought by manipulation of the somatic level. This may take the form of bathing, massage, moxibustion or medication (Lock 1980b). It is only *because* there has never been a dualistic approach to mind and body that such an attitude can prevail. However, the solution is reductionistic and appears to be partly responsible for the widespread abuse of medication in modern Japan, a problem that is known as *yakugai*, or "drug pollution" (Reich and Kao 1978). Oral gratification is central in early socialization in Japan and probably contributes to the value placed on the ingestion of medication. Moreover, herbal medicine is classified, as it always has been, as a type of food, and one "drinks" rather than "takes" such medicine. But the belief that oral medication of all kinds helps one's psychological, as well as physical, state exacerbates this situation and leads to a heavy reliance on medication for all kinds of disorders (Lock 1980b).

Stress and the Social Order

There is complete agreement among informants that the social organization of modern Japan is a stress-inducing system, and among the middle classes, particularly so for men and children. Businessmen are out of the house, on an average, 14 hours a day, and most of that time is spent commuting or at work. Overtime on Saturday is usual. The well-known examination hell (Vogel 1968) which children must endure, continues to be a source of great anxiety for both parents and children and a high proportion (22 out of 48 of the families sampled) go to a *juku* (a school for cramming) each day after regular school. But there is also agreement among informants that it is useless to try to deal with stress by imagining that one can change the social organization. Possibly in the future there may be radical policy changes, but stress and illness are personal and immediate events and a realistic attitude is to adjust to the given social order.

In a similar vein, within the family, it was agreed that a considerable source of stress originates around relationships with husbands, but only one informant out of 25 questioned on this subject, tries to talk problems over with her husband. For most wives, the very idea causes surprise and mirth. The accepted method of dealing with anxiety and frustration is to be patient (*gaman*) as long as possible and, at difficult times, to relieve some tension through physical exercise or by playing a musical instrument. Some women talk to close friends, but the majority use the traditional methods of repression of the feelings (that is, they try to control their *ki*). There may be non-verbal manipulatory devices employed in order to induce behavioral changes in a husband, but the initial and most-valued strategy is to try and adjust to the situation. Traditional values, therefore, still predominate: firstly, the belief that one's negative *ki* state will be transient and that one should simply endure the situation; secondly that stress and hence, an enhanced risk of becoming ill, are an inevitable part of life; and thirdly, an antipathy to verbal analysis of problems in human relations, which is seen as disruptive to a harmonious social life.

Informants believe that the stability and health of the wife is the most important among family members. Middle-class women see themselves as the focal point of the family, they see their modernized lives as relaxed compared with other members of their family, and they regard their new-found "free time" as a time for development of *kokoro*, something which their mothers and grandmothers could never do. They can therefore act as a kind of centered spiritual force, around which their family members gravitate and on which they can lean freely (see Doi 1973). They are explicit in stating that their poor health would be reflected in other family members since, if a wife is preoccupied with her own problems and cannot show care, then those she should look after are likely to become stressed, have accidents, and fall ill.

Some Case Examples

A case study is furnished by Mrs Honda, who is 30 years old, and lives in an Osaka suburb with her husband, their ten-month-old baby, and her mother-in-law. Her friends describe her life situation as old-fashioned and somewhat of a trial for her. Her mother-in-law is a retired teacher of *ikebana* (flower arrangement), and she supervises Mrs Honda's life and work very closely. Mrs Honda does all the housework, but she is not allowed to make any choices about the selection of meals or the selection of furnishings for the house, which belongs to her mother-in-law. Mrs Honda's husband leaves for work in an insurance company at 7.30 a.m. each day and arrives home each night to be tended to by the women of the house. His mother is most concerned that he should get a good night's sleep to cope with his long day at the office, and she complains bitterly if the baby cries in the night and wakes his father up. As a result, the moment the baby stirs, Mrs Honda starts to feed him, and the baby has settled readily into the habit of waking up regularly five or six times each night to nurse. Mrs Honda is tense and exhausted, and the baby has been diagnosed by his family as *kan no mushi* (that is, having a nervous and irritable temperament). Mrs Honda gives the baby patent medicine powders regularly, but also takes him to a temple, 30 miles away in Kyoto, for regular moxibustion treatments. She enjoys the expeditions enormously, for they give her a chance to have half a day out of the house, and she says that both she and her baby are relaxed for a few days after each treatment. Mrs Honda is well aware that the problem is basically one of social relationships and feels that her mother-in-law's attitude is really to blame. She does not believe that there is anything really wrong with her baby and does not think of him as ill. But she cannot even voice these ideas except with one close female friend of her own age, and cannot see any alternative way of handling the problem.

A second example is furnished by the case of Mrs Ito, who is 30 years old. When she married at 24, she moved from her home in Tokyo to live with her husband in a high-rise apartment near Osaka. She was excited at first, to be independent and to have some privacy in her life. But she found very quickly that she could not develop real friendships with her neighbors, and that her husband was absent from home for, an average, 14 hours a day and six days a week. She rapidly became bored in the tiny apartment, and gradually developed insomnia and mild stomach pains. Her family in Tokyo, her husband, and she herself, all labeled her problem as *danchi noiroze* (neurosis from living in a high-rise apartment), a recent, but common complaint among young Japanese housewives. She visited a doctor, who gave her medication but offered no suggestions for any changes in her lifestyle. Her family hinted strongly that pregnancy would solve her problem, but Mrs Ito was unable to become pregnant. After about 18 months of simply taking medication, Mrs Ito finally persuaded her husband to accompany her for a fertility examination. The report stated that there was nothing physically wrong with either partner. At this point, Mrs Ito went to several meetings of P. L. Kyōdan (a new religious group) but felt uncomfortable there. She had no further plans for resolving her dilemma and was unable to discuss her problem satisfactorily with her husband throughout the entire time. After nearly three years, the issue was settled by the transfer of Mr Ito back to his company's office in Tokyo. Mrs Ito re-established close contact with her extended family and old school friends, and became pregnant shortly after the move.

Many informants in this study expressed considerable ambivalence towards living in a nuclear family, which they believe can be a lonely existence, in which a woman is left with too much responsibility, and which can encourage self-ishness. For the maintenance of a healthy emotional state, it is acknowledged that it is essential to develop extra-familial relationships and to escape from structured family life at times, where repression of self is required. But such channels of escape for middle-class women are not yet built into the social system. Although, recently, more women are joining voluntary group organizations, many others remain, as Kiefer (1976) has shown, bored, isolated and lonely. Because the social order is rarely questioned, problems such as those of Mrs Honda and Mrs Ito are readily classified as medical and dealt with primarily at the somatic level.

IMPLICATIONS OF THE STUDY OF POPULAR MEDICINE FOR HEALTH CARE

Japanese education today, in all branches of science, is among the best in the world, and children in school learn a scientific approach to the body and hygiene. Nevertheless, it is clear from this study that popular ideas relating to health remain distinctly Japanese and that, although many terms and explanations sound familiar to Western ears and are influenced by scientific ideas, their seman-tic meaning and implications for health-related behavior have to be carefully interpreted.

Since maintenance of harmonious family relationships remains as a core value in middle-class life and can be a source of great tension, it might be assumed that the development of family therapy would be appropriate in Japan. I believe, however, that because the traditional values of avoidance of verbal analysis of psychological problems and the desire to protect one's inner self from exposure are believed to be important, family therapy could induce so much guilt and anxiety that it would not be beneficial. (Tseng (1975b) has made a similar suggestion regarding the use of psychotherapy in Taiwan.) Group therapy with peer groups might be more successful, since verbal expression is easier in such a situation. Indigenous Japanese therapies in which meditation techniques (*Naikan* therapy) are used and in which a diary is kept (*Morita* therapy) are more appropriate. Similarly, because of popular ideas regarding personality as a fixed entity, therapies which seek to change personality structure are not likely to meet with success.

It is also apparent that treatment at the physical level is likely to be regarded favourably by patients, and that disregard on the part of therapists of mild, somatized symptoms would be inappropriate. Traditional practitioners in Japan are very sensitive in this regard and in bio-medicine today, the use of yoga, biofeedback techniques, and so on, is enjoying great popularity. Ikemi and Ishikawa (1979) have stated why they believe somato-psychic therapy to be more valuable than verbal psychotherapy:

> The stimulation of somatic awareness can clearly elicit psychic awareness, which may prove to be a more powerful process than the reverse process, commonly known as "psychosomatic". According to Oriental thought, self-identification is a process that is based upon an awareness of body feeling which is directly in touch with nature and under its command. Such a self-identification helps the maintenance of lucid sensory awareness and an actual feeling of the law of nature in one's own body, an understanding which is qualitatively different from conceptual understanding . . . Oriental people used to consider it the higest virtue to obey natural law in a way parallel to that of the worship of God in Western culture. This attitude does not contradict the concepts of natural science in a broad sense (Ikemi and Ishikawa 1979:326).

Despite the apparent suitability of such an approach in Japan, such sensitivity to "the laws of Nature in one's own body" is usually only obtained after many years of training, most often in conjunction with Zen Buddhist ideas. A complete somatopsychic approach can rather easily take on the elitism that psychoanalysis is associated with in the West -- in order to take part fully, one needs time, and a philosophical approach to life which is the product of a certain type of upbringing. For most doctors and patients this approach can rather easily be reduced to the mechanical insertion of a few acupuncture needles, a prescription of herbal medicine, or a session of autogenic training. I believe that, while a somatopsychic approach offers great therapeutic promise in Japan, if it is not administered in conjunction with appropriate social services and counseling of a very practical nature, then its potential will not be fulfilled.

CONCLUSION

In conclusion, therefore, the Japanese case indicates that traditional medical ideas and the popular health care system continue to be intricately bound to each other, despite long exposure to bio-medicine. These data confirm work in other parts of the world which demonstrates that it is good adaptive strategy to support the services offered by traditional practitioners, for the sake of the psychological well-being of patients, as well as for economic reasons. However, each medical system must be carefully analyzed for its biases; it cannot be assumed that traditional medicine is necessarily holistic, nor that it has adapted and modernized to meet the needs of rapidly changing social systems and organizations.

NOTES

1. The term East Asian medical system is used to refer to the medical beliefs which were dominant, until the nineteenth century, among the literate populations of China, Korea, and Japan, and which are usually referred to in the literature as classical Chinese medicine or Oriental medicine.
2. The field-work upon which this data is based was carried out in Kyoto from 1973 to 1974. Twelve clinics in which East Asian medicine is practiced were the focus of study. Fifteen medical practitioners and 200 patients were interviewed concerning their medical beliefs and practices. Five of the practitioners are M.D.s, the rest obtained a license to practice East Asian medicine by attending a two-and-a-half-year college course. In addition, 50 urban, middle-income families were interviewed in their homes regarding their health beliefs and practices. A follow-up study was carried out in 1980 when 25 Japanese housewives, between the ages of 28 and 38 years old, two-year college or high school graduates, and all married to middle-income businessmen, were asked to take part in small discussion groups in order to focus on the topic of beliefs about menal health and illness.
3. A classification system, in which all objects and phenomena are assigned either a predominantly yin or yang quality; yin and yang being two polar extremities symbolizing such contrasting pairs as night and day, female and male, the moon and sun, hot and cold (see Porkert, 1974:9ff for full details).
4. Neurasthenia (*shinkeishitsushō*) is a diagnostic category used frequently in medical settings of all kinds in Japan.
5. The conceptions analyzed in this section were selected on the basis of their high frequency of use in open-ended interviews conducted with patients and practitioners in the clinical setting. The semantic network analysis associated with these concepts was generated in small-group settings, in which informants were asked to explain the meaning and use of the concepts in their daily life.

REFERENCES

Caudill, W.
    1976 Everyday Health and Illness in Japan and America. *In* Asian Medical Systems. C. Leslie (ed.), pp. 159–177. Berkeley and Los Angeles: University of California Press.
DeVos, G. A.
    1973 Socialization for Achievement: Essays on the Cultural Psychology of the Japanese. Berkeley and Los Angeles: University of California Press.
Doi, T.
    1973 The Anatomy of Dependence. Tokyo: Kodansha International Ltd.
Durckheim, K.
    1975 Hara: The Vital Center of Man. New York: Samuel Weiser.
Freidson, E.
    1970 Profession of Medicine. New York: Dodd, Mead.
Fujikawa, Y.
    1974 An Outline of Japanese Medical History. Tokyo: Heibonsha, I. (Japanese text).
Good, B. J.
    1977 The Heart of What's the Matter: The Semantics of Illness in Iran. Culture, Medicine and Psychiatry 11:25–58.
Hayashida, C. T.
    1975 The Koshinjo and Tanteisha. Institutionalized Ascription as a Response to Modernization and Stress in Japan. *In* Modernization and Stress in Japan. T. Fuse (ed.), pp. 84–94. Leiden: E. J. Brill.

Ikemi, Y. and H. Ishikawa.
  1979 Integration of Occidental and Oriental Psychosomatic Treatments. Psychotherapy
         and Psychosomatic Medicine 31:324–333.
Kiefer, C. W.
  1976 The Danchi Zoku and the Evolution of Metropolitan Mind. *In* Japan: The Paradox
         of Progress. L. Austin (ed.), pp. 279–300.
Kleinman, A.
  1980 Depression, Somatization and the 'New Cross-Cultural Psychiatry'. *In* Social
         Science and Medicine 11:3–9.
Kleinman, A.
  1980 Patients and Healers in the Context of Culture: An Exploration of the Borderland
         between Anthropology, Medicine and Psychiatry. Berkeley and Los Angeles:
         University of California Press.
Lebra, T. S.
  1976 Japanese Patterns of Behavior. Honolulu: The University Press of Hawaii.
Lock, M.
  1980a East Asian Medicine in Urban Japan: Varieties of Medical Experience. Berkeley:
         University of California Press.
  1980b An Examination of the Influence of Traditional Therapeutic Systems on the
         Practice of Cosmopolitan Medicine in Contemporary Japan. The American
         Journal of Chinese Medicine 8:221–229.
Marsella, A. J., D. Kinzie, and P. Gordon.
  1973 Ethnic Variations in the Expression of Depression. Journal of Cross-Cultural
         Psychology 4:435–458.
Namihara, E. and M. Sanches.
  1977 Hare, Ke and Kegare: Cognitive Categories of Socio-Cultural Experience. Paper
         read at the 76th annual meetings of the American Anthropological Association,
         Houston, Texas.
Needham, J.
  1962 Science and Civilization in China, 2. Cambridge: Cambridge University Press.
Otsuka, Y.
  1976 Chinese Traditional Medicine in Japan. *In* Asian Medical Systems. C. Leslie (ed.).
         Berkeley and Los Angeles: University of California Press.
Porkert, M.
  1974 The Theoretical Foundations of Chinese Medicine. MIT East Asian Science Series,
         3. Cambridge: MIT Press.
Reich, M. R. and Kao, J. J.
  1978 A Comparative View of Health and Medicine in Japan and America. New York:
         Japan Society, Inc. (Public Affairs Series 6).
Reiser, M. F.
  1979 Psychosomatic Medicine: a Meeting Ground for Oriental and Occidental Medical
         Theory and Practice. Psycotherapy and Psychosomatic Medicine 31:315–323.
Reynolds, D. K.
  1976 Morita Therapy. Berkeley and Los Angeles: University of California Press.
Rohlen, T.
  1974a Ki and Kokoro: Japanese Perspectives on the Nature of the Person. Paper Pre-
         sented at the Regional Seminar on Japanese Studies, Center for Japanese and
         Korean Studies, University of California, Berkeley.
  1974b For Harmony and Strength: Japanese White Collar Organization in Anthropo-
         logical Perspective. Berkeley and Los Angeles: University of California Press.
Tseng, W. S.
  1975a The Nature of Somatic Complaints among Psychiatric Patients: The Chinese Case.
         Comprehensive Psychiatry 16:237–245.

1975b Traditional and Modern Psychiatric Care in Taiwan. *In* Medicine in Chinese Cultures: Comparative Studies of Health Care in Chinese and other Societies. A. Kleinman et al. (eds.), pp. 177–194. Washington, D. C. U.S. Department of Health, Education, and Welfare, Public Health Service, National Institutes of Health, DHEW publication No. (NIH) 75–633.

Vogel, E.
    1968 Japan's New Middle Class: The Salary Man and his Family in a Tokyo Suburb. Berkeley and Los Angeles: University of California Press.

Yoshida, T.
    1972 Spirit Possession and Kinship System. East Asian Cultural Studies 11:44–57.

GANANATH OBEYESEKERE

9. SCIENCE AND PSYCHOLOGICAL MEDICINE IN THE AYURVEDIC TRADITION

INTRODUCTION

This paper presents a brief account of the theory of psychological medicine in the ancient Indian medical tradition of Ayurveda. In doing so, attention is drawn to the integration of medical belief and theory with cultural propositions about mind, bodily functioning and the environment. The application of Ayurvedic theory by medical practitioners is illustrated with case material derived from fieldwork carried out in Sri Lanka. In discussing the uses of theory in psychological and physical treatments, I suggest that experimentation and the generation of new ideas have had a continuing impact on the paradigm of Ayurvedic medicine.

In the social sciences and humanities there has been a tendency to see science as essentially a Western invention. Non-Western systems of thought and medicine have been presented by anthropologists, as "ethnosciences", radically at variance with the kind of science that developed out of Greek rationality. In *The Savage Mind*, Levi-Strauss also deals with the modes of knowledge of primitive and non-Western people. There, Levi-Strauss says that the primitive experimenter is a *bricoleur* and the experimental tradition that prevails in primitive societies, a kind of *bricolage*. Bricolage is the "experimentation" of the typical handyman of the West: it is putting things together from the available repertoire of practical knowledge. Thus, while the avowed intention of *The Savage Mind* is to show that all of us — primitive and civilized, Western and non-Western — think alike, the actual effect of the book is to show that genuine scientific thinking does not occur outside the West, and when it does, it is in the form of *ad hoc* experimentation or bricolage.

Is there anything more sophisticated than bricolage in the intellectual traditions of non-Western societies? I think there is, if not in preliterate societies, at least in the great traditions of the Middle East, China and India. None of these traditions developed anything analogous to the post-Renaissance science of the West, but they nevertheless produced, in several intellectual domains, forms of thought characterized by a notion of a theoretical system, clear-cut ideas of systematic experimentation, and the manipulation of the theoretical system to generate new information. Theoretical thinking or the manipulation of abstract concepts to account for empirical phenomena, rather than bricolage, characterizes the thought processes of practical scientists in these great traditions. I shall argue for the existence of this kind of scientific thought and experimentation for the Indian traditions which scholars have generally regarded as mystical and aesthetic and hostile to scientific rationality as known in the West.

235

A. J. Marsella and G. M. White (eds.), Cultural Conceptions of Mental Health and Therapy, 235–248.

In this paper, I shall illustrate the nature of scientific thinking in the ancient Indian medical tradition and its contemporary uses in Sri Lanka, focusing particularly on the theory of psychological medicine. Nevertheless, I do not believe that Indian medical theory *qua* theory is identical to scientific theories as we now understand them. The theoretical framework developed in Indian medicine constitutes a formal paradigm that has practially remained unchanged from the time of its founders — Susruta and Caraka — till our own time in the on-going operative medical traditions of India and Sri Lanka. Thus, one of the features of theoretical systems in South Asia is the absence, or rather infrequency, of paradigmatic change.

The medical tradition of Ayurveda represents the widest practical use put to theoretical, abstract and rational thinking in South Asian society, even more than Buddhism. The higher Buddhist rationality was, by and large, the intellectual preserve of monks, at least until very recent times. By contrast the Ayurvedic paradigm was held by practically every medical practitioner in the country. Even today the proportion of Ayurvedic physicians to Western doctors is overwhelming and all of the former hold, with varying degrees of sophistication, the classical paradigm. Moreover medicine, unlike Buddhism, has a greater practical and mundane relevance — the amelioration of illness and physical suffering. It is also basically secular unlike Buddhism where theoretical rationality is anchored in a larger religious world view and a metaphysical rationality. The views of body function and illness in Ayurveda are also held by non-specialists, though in non-technical and popular form, much as the germ-theory of disease is held by ordinary citizens in Western society. It is, therefore, a good example of a sophisticated non-Western theoretical system operative at various levels, by both specialists and laymen. It will help us to understand some crucial aspects of indigenous cultural creativity.

AYURVEDA: THE FORMAL PARADIGM

In this paper I cannot deal with the metaphysical base on which the Ayurvedic paradigm rests, but I can only direct the reader to it. Contemporary practitioners of Ayurveda see this base in Sāmkhya philosophy, one of the six orthodox systems of Indian philosophy, though it is likely that, in actual fact, the medical traditions antedated Sāmkhya, and that the direction of influence was from the Ayurveda to Sāmkhya. Sāmkhya is an extremely original, complex and unusual philosophical system, which cannot be adequately presented in a brief discussion. I refer the reader to Hiriyanna for a simple presentation of the main ideas of Sāmkhya and my earlier paper for a discussion of the relation between Ayurveda and Sāmkhya (Hiriyanna 1956; Obeyesekere 1977).

While both Yoga and Ayurveda were influenced by metaphysical ideas, such as that represented in Sāmkhya, Ayurveda took its own course and developed a theory of physiological function and dysfunction suited to its own needs as a system of medicine. Unlike Yoga, which had a symbolic view of the human body, Ayurveda had fairly clear notions of body physiology and functioning (Dasgupta 1968:273–346). It had highly detailed descriptions of human anatomy and physiology, much of which was based on observation. Yet, fundamental to the theory is not so much practical anatomy but the physiological theory of the three humours. The basic paradigm on which the theory of illness rests – the five *bhūtas* and three *doṣas* – has been unquestionably accepted right through the ages by all practitioners of Ayurveda. "Experimentation" could exist within the paradigmatic set of assumptions, so that controversy and debate could occur regarding the manner in which the *doṣas* operate to cause disease; or the efficacy of ingredients used in medical prescriptions. The paradigm itself remains unaltered to this day.

A highly sophisticated and aesthetically elegant theory has been constructed on the basis of these fundamental assumptions. The fundamental principles (*mūla dharma*) of Ayurveda include the doctrine of the five *bhūtas* or basic elements (atoms) of the universe, the *tridoṣa*, or three humours, and the seven *dhātus*, or components of the body. The five elements are ether (*ākāśa*), wind (*vāyu*), water (*ap*), earth (*prthvi*), and fire (*agni* or *tejas*). These elements are constituents of all life and as such also make up the three humours and the seven physical components of the body. As the five elements contained in food are "cooked" by fires in the body, they are converted into a fine portion (*āhara-prasāda*) and refuse (*kitta* or *mala*). The body elements are produced by successive transformation of the refined food substance into food juice (*rasa*), blood (*rakta*), flesh (*māmsa*), fat (*medas*), bone (*asthi*), marrow (*majja*) and semen (*śukra*). Semen is said to be the most highly refined element in this body, the "vital juice" that tones the whole organism (Filliozat 1964:27).

Physical health is maintained when the three humours are in harmonic balance, but when they are upset they become *doṣas*, or "troubles" of the organism. The universal element (*bhūta*) of wind appears in the body as a humour, also called wind (*vāyu*); fire appears as bile (*pitta*); and water as phlegm (*kapha* or *sleśman*). Illness is due to upsetting the homeostatic condition of these humours (*tridoṣa*). The more serious condition is one in which all three humours are upset (*sannipata*). When a *doṣa* is "angry" or excited it increases in proportion to the other humours. The aim of medication is to reduce or control this excess. The excited *doṣa* may also damage one or more *dhātu* (blood, flesh, fat, etc.) so that treatment must aim to restore the affected body substance.

These assumptions have several consequences: (a) If the five elements are found in nature, then nature itself can be a factor in the cause of disease and also in its cure. This has special relevance to the intake and consumption of foods. Thus, for example, an excessive consumption of heat-producing foods may lead to an excess of bile in the organism, thereby producing illness. In the case of a person with a congenitally heated body, the consumption of such foods may lead to serious consequences. He would be advised to avoid such foods and generally have a diet of cooling foods that can counter the congenital *pitta* (bile produced by heat) in his body. (b) If the five elements pervade all of nature, and if they are essential for curing and prophylaxis, then all substances are *ausada* (curative). This applies particularly to vegetable substances (herbs, roots, bark, flowers) which are specially used in Ayurvedic decoctions. (c) Flowing from the same logic is the view that both seasons and climates can have therapeutic or pathogenic effects. Thus Susruta has elaborate classifications of seasons and climates in terms of the *dosas/bhūtas* they contain. (d) Finally, there are several views of temperament in Ayurveda based on these assumptions, the most important pertaining to the relative preponderance of one of the three humours in the human body as a result of congenital factors (temperament). Prognosis and diagnosis of both mental and physical health may depend on temperament. For example, if a patient has temperamentally an excess of *pitta* (bile), he may be specially susceptible to physical illness as a result of this humour; he should be careful of heat-producing foods since they may raise the level of *pitta* in his body. Hence, Sustruta's maxim: "A physician should cooly deliberate upon the different types of temperament described herein and their characteristic features" (Susruta 1963:III, 158).

PSYCHOPATHOLOGY IN CLASSICAL AYURVEDA

It is not possible to study "mental illness" in any society unless we are aware of the indigenous definition of mind and its functions. Ayurveda derived its notion of mind from the same source as *sāmkhya* and *nyāya-vaiśeṣika* philosophy. Here mind functions very much like the ego of psychoanalytic theory, rather than the id or superego (Obeyesekere 1977:157). The impairment of these mental functions and consequent mental pathology are due to physiological factors. Practically all classical theorists of Ayurveda assert that the mind and self are located in the heart rather than in the brain. The only exception to this view in the whole of Sanskrit literature is Bhela, who considered the brain as the locus of mind (Dasgupta 1968:340). Mental illness arises when the heart does not function efficiently, because the ducts (*sirā*) and channels (*dhamani*) that carry the *dosas* (humours) and vital elements (*dhātus*) to that organ have failed to function satisfactorily. (It should be noted, however, that contemporary Ayurveda in Sri Lanka locates the mind primarily in the brain, and only secondarily in the heart.)

Thus, in classical Ayurvedic theory, the major cause of mental malfunctioning is the upsetting of the humours. The general theory explains all illnesses, mental as well as physical. The major cause of mental illness is somato-psychic, rather than psychosomatic. Logically there must be at least four basic types of mental illness; one for each of the major humours, and a fourth from the concatanation of all three humours. Susruta has a fifth type of illness which affects the mind as a result of sorrow or shock and a sixth due to the effects of poison. It is also possible to have subtypes based on various combinations of the three basic humours.

Caraka, the great Ayurvedic authority on medicine, defines *unmāda* (psychopathology, insanity, madness) as follows: "Insanity is to be known as the unsettled condition of the mind, understanding, consciousness, perception, memory, inclination, character, behavior and conduct" (Caraka 1949:267). He discusses the premonitory symptoms and the onset of full blown psychopathology. The causes of humoral upset are manifold and may include faintheartedness, mental shock, consumption of improper foods, wrongful bodily activity, or other diseases; or "those whose minds have been impaired by the attacks of lust, anger, greed, excitement, fear, infatuation, fatigue, grief, and also those that are injured by trauma" (Caraka 1949:267).

In a similar vein, sustruta discusses the premonitory symptoms of *unmāda* or madness:

Fits of unconsciousness, agitated state of mind, ringing of the ears, emaciation of the body, excessive energy of action, aversion to food, eating filthy things in dreams, perturbation due to *vāyu*, and vertigo or giddiness are the symptoms in a patient which forebode a speedy and impending attack of insanity (Susruta 1963:II, 387).

After presenting the general and premonitory symptoms, Susruta discusses the symptoms produced by each of the three humours and, finally, the fourth and incurable form of madness resulting from *sannipāta* or the upsetting of all three humours.

Note that the same causes can produce imbalance and bring about diseases which *do not* affect the mind. Psychopathology occurs when the upset humour (or humours) reaches the area of the heart, where the mind is located, and blocks the ducts (*sirā*) and channels (*dhamani*) that carry the *doṣas* and *dhātus*.

Susruta and particularly Caraka, have elaborate discussions of the symptoms of each type of insanity. They also have discussions of therapeutics. Basically, the principle of cure is the same in all diseases: the upset humour has to be controlled by ingredients that have the right counteractive properties. I shall discuss symptoms and therapeutics in more detail when I deal with the contemporary practice of Ayurvedic psychiatry. However, it is worth mentioning that the classic texts have harsh measures to control intractable and extreme cases of madness, such as threatening patients with flogging, piercing the patient with pointed instruments, or putting the patient in a dry well with a cover over it. Yet Susruta does have more humane treatment for those patients suffering from sorrow or shock. "In the case of the fifth kind of insanity, the cause of grief should be first removed." Also:

In all forms of insanity the restoration of serenity of mind should be first attempted. Mild and gentle forms of these remedies should be resorted to in the case of *mada* (preliminary stage of insanity) (Susruta 1963:II, 391).

The almost identical set of causes may produce both insanity (*unmāda*) and *apasmāra* (epilepsy). In both, the mind is affected by the blockage or malfunctioning of the ducts and channels leading to the heart. However, in *apasmāra* the upset humour results in unconsciousness rather than mental malfunction. In *apasmāra* the morbid humours lie dormant near the heart. When roused by a sudden, emotional shock like desire, anger, fear, greed, infatuation, excitement, grief, worry or anxiety, they block the channels of the heart and sense organs, thereby causing an epileptic fit (Caraka 1960:246–253).

We also noted that similar causes can produce different diseases: the crucial fact again is the *manner* in which the intervening humours are affected. In this sense Ayurveda recognizes strictly psychosomatic illnesses, though they do not receive conceptual formulation as such. Emotional conditions like sorrow and excitement can not only produce madness and epilepsy; they can also produce, through a radically different effect on the *doṣas* (humours), diseases which have nothing to do with mind, but are entirely organic or physical. These psychosomatic ailments are not treated as a special category; they are nevertheless referred to right through the whole corpus of Ayurveda. Let me give a few examples: fevers caused by grief and anxiety owing to an excess of heat finding lodgement in the *rasa* (food juice, lymph-chyle), one of the seven body elements; aversion to food owing to psychological causes can cause digestive ailments (*atisāra*); eczema (*kuṣṭha*) by suppression of bodily urges and sin (guilt?); and finally sexual incapacity and "mental impotency" owing to bitter thoughts arising in the mind or forced intercourse with a disagreeable woman (Susruta 1963:III, 357, 366, 346; II, 311). However, nowhere in Ayurveda is there a psychodynamic theory to explain these phenomena. By contrast, the somatic theory of the three *doṣas* is always systematically spelled out.

APPLICATIONS OF THE THEORY: A SRI LANKAN CASE STUDY

In this section I shall consider the application of the classic Sanskrit paradigm in the treatment of mental illness in contemporary Sri Lanka. I shall focus on Dr Indrasena de Alwis, a lay pupil of a famous Buddhist monk, now deceased, of Nilammahara. Nilammahara is a Buddhist temple about 20 miles from Colombo and a long-established center for a local tradition (*dēsiya cikitsa*) of Ayurvedic psychiatry. Dr Alwis is a highly-educated person thoroughly familiar with the Sanskrit as well as his own local (*dēsiya*) tradition. He has also a working knowledge of English. He is a dedicated physician with a high sense of duty and well-developed standards of professional ethics. He makes his own medicines and also dispenses them. He has no facilities for warding patients; but he has trained attendants who look after patients in their (the attendants') own homes.

The theory of illness in the Nilammahara tradition is based entirely on classic Ayurveda, which has been sketched earlier. I shall therefore deal with the local application of this theory in respect of nosology, diagnostics and therapy. The Nilammahara tradition is based on the following: (1) a medical text belonging to this tradition and written in Sinhala verse, (2) the practical experience of four or five generations of physicians, and (3) familiarity with Sanskrit and Sinhala medical texts.

Prescriptions from these texts are used for treating patients. The Nilammahara psychiatrists follow their own medical text with reference to classification and symptomatology. According to Nilammahara, there are 22 types of psychopathology, which they proudly consider to be an improvement on the four or five types mentioned in the classical literature. The Nilammahara list consists of: (a) three diseases caused by each of the humours; (b) three diseases caused by combinations of two humours; (c) *sannipāta* or the most virulent form of madness caused by the upsetting of all three humours; (d) two types of psychopathology caused by bad blood in conjunction with excess of *pitta* and *vāta*; (e) 13 miscellaneous mental illnesses as a result of complications arising from other diseases – from TB, asthma, high fever (delirium), childbirth psychosis caused by the womb's impurities, menorraghia, bodily debility, mental shock, epilepsy, hemorrhoids, action of demons, excess consumption of alcohol, poison and rabies, and from paralysis.

For purposes of this paper I shall describe the causes of illness arising from the upsetting of each of the three humours.

1. *Vāta Unmāda: Madness from "Wind"* (*vāta, vāyu*)

Consumption of bad foods, indigestible foods, revulsive foods, and also lack of adequate food intake may all lead to madness from wind. Extremely "cool" foods are also bad; as are conditions that can weaken the body like excessive work or exercise or excessive sexual intercourse. These cause *vāta* to be excited; and if the *vāta* affects the brain and heart, *vāta unmāda* may develop.

The patient sees dreams and illusions: serpents, elephants, non-humans, horses, royal officials. He hears the sound of flutes and of fire-arms. Some patients shout in fear, or try to scare people. Others try to run away, or abuse people. Very often they wake up in fright.

Foods that have the property of wind are generally dry and hard to digest like most cereals and dried meats. When food is ill-digested (it cannot get "cooked" in the stomach) it forms a "vapour" (i.e., wind). Stomach gas is one symptom of this condition. Even excessively cool foods may produce *vāta* since they are often difficult to digest, producing flatus. Some kinds of foods have excess of both wind and phlegm and as a result of bad digestion can produce excess wind (*vāta*) in the body. Piping-hot foods also produce *vāta* perhaps through the vapour they exude. The major effect of *vāta* is edema as well as diseases involving pains and swelling of the joints as a result of trapped air. *Vāta* affects the mind when the upward moving currents of air hit the brain and heart.

The symptoms are clearly based on Sanskrit texts. In interviews, the doctor pointed out some of the connections between theory and symptoms. *Vāta* (wind) is the principle of movement; thus, when *vāta* increases, the patient becomes hyperactive or manic. Such symptoms as shouting, abusing, attempting to run away clearly indicate the effect of *vāta*. The patient's dreams are also of animals and royal officials in movement such as pursuit. When elephants appear in dreams they are seen as breaking or shaking trees and branches. *Vāta*-based mental illnesses are always serious.

2. *Pit-unmāda. Madness from Pitta (bile)*

Madness from bile may be caused by eating sour and harsh (*kaṭuka*) foods to excess or by an excess of foods with *giniguna* (the property of heat); sleepless nights and irregular food habits can also cause this condition.

The premonitory symptoms are the following: the patient attempts to run away; he may experience great anger; his face may turn yellow and eyes red. When full blown illness develops the patient experiences sleeplessness and a gnawing hunger. His hands and feet "burn" and his mind hankers after cool things. Behavioral symptoms include obstinancy and attempts to frighten those around him.

Here the relationship between causes and symptoms with the upset *pitta* or bile is even clearer: sour, harsh foods contain excess of the element of heat (fire). This increases the bile in the body, and could cause any type of *pitta* disease. Factors like a weak mind or temperament, or a physiological factor like a current of air in the body, may force the *pitta* upwards towards the brain (and heart), thereby producing madness.

The symptoms of excess heat are also clear. Heat=red=rage is one symbolic equation. Thus the patient has red eyes and sees red, causing fright in others. When the body is heated there is a craving for cool things. Burning sensations in the hands and feet are also clearly related to heat or *pitta*. So is hunger since heat "cooks" the food in the digestive system, giving rise to the need for more and more food. Some symptoms, such as attempts to run are not immediately related to *pitta*. In general such symptoms are due to "wind". But emotional heat produces impatience and can cause motor activity also.

3. *Sem-unmāda: Madness from Phlegm*

The most important cause of madness from phlegm is due to excess consumption of "nutritious" foods. When this is combined with little exercise, the patient becomes a candidate for phlegm (*sema*) diseases, including those affecting the brain. The symptoms are a distaste for food and an aversion for "cool" things including water. Excess phlegm oozes from the nose and mouth. The patient cannot sleep; he has rigid, fixated body movements. He also has an excessive desire for sex.

Here as elsewhere, the local texts lay more emphasis on symptoms than causes, as befits their purpose as handbooks of practical medicine. However, even here the importance of food in the etiology of disease is clear. According to Ayurvedic thinking, the most nutritious foods are those containing the cooling principle. Thus, sweet foods are invariably cooling and invariably nutritions, and phlegm-producing. Therefore, too much good food and lack of exercise lead to excess phlegm. If and when phlegm clogs up the passages to the brain and heart, you have madness from phlegm.

Most of the symptoms are once again clearly related to the cause of the disease. If wind causes movement, then water (phlegm) is the static principle. Thus, rigid, lethargic, lazy behavior is the result of madness from phlegm. The excess of phlegm also leads to a natural bodily aversion for cool things. It also produces symptoms of excess phlegm like coughs, colds, sneezing, hypersalivation and expectoration. Furthermore, sweet, cooling foods have aphrodisiacal properties (*vājikarana*); they increase semen (*śukra dhātu*) and stimulate the sex drive.

Ayurvedic therapy is directly related to its theory of disease. In classical Sanskrit as well as in Sinhala, humoural disequilibrium is referred to as "excitement" or "anger" of the *dosas*. Another technical term in Sanskrit is *dosa vaisamya*, "disturbance of the *dosas*"; its opposite is *sāmya*, which is rendered in current Sinhala as *samanaya*. Thus *dos samanaya* is the goal of therapy: "the calming of the *dosas*", "the evening out of the *dosas*", "the restoration of the balance or equilibrium of the *dosas*". All therapy of somato-psychic diseases are directed to this goal. In psycho-somatic diseases (like diarrhea caused by emotional factors) emotional therapy (generally consolation) must be accompanied by medication to restore humoural balance.

To effect humoural homeostasis in *unmāda* the following therapies are essential: (1) *hisa kudicci*: Head packs containing cooling substances which the patient keeps on his head for several hours. (2) *nasna*: Nasal draining where certain ingredients (e.g., $1\frac{1}{2}$ seeds of *mī*, bassia/latifolia, 6 seeds of white pepper ground together with a little breast milk) are blown into the nostrils of the patient through a forked funnel (*nasnāyuda*). The use of these techniques are very popular all over Sri Lanka and is based on the (Buddhist) view that the mind is located in the brain rather than the heart. If so mental illness is caused by the passages to the brain being blocked or impeded by one or more of the humours, particularly phlegm which then dries up due to the action of excess heat. Head packs and nasal draining help to loosen and expectorate the phlegm. (3) *kasāya*: decoction. Since Ayurvedic experimentation occurs primarily in relation to decoctions, I shall deal with them here in some length.

Decoctions are essential for the cure of all diseases in Ayurveda, including *unmāda*. The vegetable ingredients used have certain *guna*, "essential properties", and *vipāka* or effects. *Guna* generally refers to the preponderance of the five elements in each ingredient, particularly wind, water and heat. The *vipāka* is the effect of the *guna* on the body. Thus the ingredient "dried grapes" has the *guna* or property of "coolness" (water); its effect or *vipāka* is to calm excess bile or *pitta* (heat): i.e., *pitta samanaya* in Sinhala. In general, the property of heat counters excess cold (phlegm) and renders the latter *samanaya*, and vice-versa. The problem becomes more complicated in the case of excess wind (*vāta*) since there is no binary opposite involved here. Sinhala doctors have several ingredients that have the property of calming (*samanaya*) excess of wind. Furthermore, an excess humour can not only be calmed (*samanaya*) but totally destroyed (*nāśtaka*) by certain ingredients. Such ingredients muct be carefully used, and matched with others in order to counter the drastic effects of the former. The careful "matching" of the various ingredients used in any particular decoction is known as *samyōga*, a critical word in the vocabulary of Ayurvedic therapy. The *samyōga* or matching or combination of properties in any decoction can be quite complicated, and depends on the nature of the disease. Let us say that a certain ingredient "*x*" may have the property of "coolness" and also some "heat"; if the patient suffers from excess of bile (heat) then this ingredient may only be partially successful, since the property of "coolness" may be nullified by the "heat" in the same ingredient. In which case the *samyōga* requires another ingredient "*y*" in the prescription to counteract the "heat" in ingredient "*x*". The contraindication of certain ingredients in known as *viruddha* (opposition). But, as we noted, a particular *samyōga* (matching or combination of ingredients) neutralizes an otherwise contraindicated ingredient. Neutralization of ingredients often results in *sama-sītōṣna*, "balanced hot-cold". Thus, when you have a high fever you are often given coriander which is "cool" combined with "ginger" which is "hot". The combination of the two (i.e., its *samyōga*) renders it neither hot nor cold, i.e., *sama-sītōṣna*, which is good for the fever which has to be brought to normal.

All ingredients are measured in terms of *kalam* (k) and *mancādi* (m), the seed of the *Adenanthera pavonia*. Each m is about $1\frac{1}{4}$ grains: $20\ m = 1\ k$. In general the ingredients used in one decoction must add up to $12\ k$; in the case of a decoction containing an unusually large number of ingredients $24\ k$ can be used. These ingredients are generally boiled in water which is measured in terms of *pata*, each *pata* containing about nine ounces of water. In general all decoctions are reduced to $\frac{1}{8}$ of the original volume by boiling.

I shall now illustrate the Ayurvedic idea of *samyōga*, combination and balancing of ingredients and its therapeutic principles by examining a prescription for two decoctions (*kasāya*) for mental illness caused by the upsetting of wind (*vāta*). The first prescription is given in Table I.

Dosage: $1\ k$ of each ingredient; boiled in 8 *pata* of water; reduced to 1 *pata*; two times daily for 3—4 days; honey and sugar added as sweetening.

Vāta unmāda is caused by an excess of "wind" rising to the top and affecting the heart and brain. It may seem therefore that the remedy should be to correct the excess *vāta* and restore normal humoral function. But illness in Ayurveda is more complicated than this for the following reasons: (1) All *unmāda* is "hot" and results in excess *pitta*. Thus, *pitta* control is always essential to therapy. (2) An upset humour will affect other body functions. Excess *vāta* may affect the blood and increase its pressure (*lēgamana* "blood movement"). Thus, purification of the blood is essential. (3) Upset humours also affect bowel, kidney and bladder functions. As a result, impurities will collect there. These impurities must be flushed out and cleansed. There are standard ingredients for this purpose (specially ingredients No. 5 and No. 12) which are popularly used as home remedies.

TABLE I

Prescription No. 1 for *vāta unmāda* (madness from "wind")

Name of ingredient	Botanical Term	Vipāka or effect
1. välmadaṭa	*Rubia cordifolia*	Purifies the blood
2. galkūra	*Melochia corchorifolia*	Cleanses the bladder (*mutrabokka*).
3. dried grapes		Phlegm is loosened and expelled. Also body vitality is enhanced.
4. hātāvāriya	*Asparagus falcatus* and *Asparagus sarmentosus*	*pitta* is controlled and evened out by its cooling properties. (It also fosters semen, i.e., strength but this is not the reason for prescribing it here.)
5. irivēriya	*Plectranthus zeylanicus*	Flushes kidneys; in combination (*samyōga*) with others it controls *pitta*.
6. sävändara roots	*Andropogan muricatus*	Control of *pitta* by its cooling properties.
7. mī flowers	*Bassiva latifolia*	Controls *vāta*; possesses intrinsic *vāta* control properties.
8. filaments of the blue lotus (*nelun*)	*Nelumbius speciosum*	Control of *pitta*.
9. suduhandun (white sandal wood)	*Santalum album*	Control of *pitta*.
10. mānel flowers (blue lotus)	*Nymphaea stellata*	Control of *pitta*.
11. väl mī (liquorice)	*Glycyrrhiza glabra*	Loosening and expulsion of phlegm.
12. iramusa (Indian sarsaparilla)	*Hemidesmus indicus*	For cleansing blood; very popularly consumed as a tea.

The total *samyōga balaya* ("power of *samyōga*") is to restore vital organ functioning and control *vāta* and *pitta*. By *pitta* control one refers to ingredients with cool properties that can reduce the *pitta* level; in the case of *vāta* there are special ingredients that either control or destroy it.

After this another decoction may be given to directly control *vāta* and *pitta*, as shown in Table II. In addition to the decoctions, *hisa kudicci* (head packs) and *nasna* (phlegm draining) are also given.

TABLE II

Prescription No. 2 for *vāta unmāda* (madness from "wind")

Name of ingredient	Botanical term	Vipāka or effect
1. hātāvāriya	*Asparagus fulcatus, Asparagus sarmentosas*	6 k of this; *pitta* control by virtue of its cooling properties.
2. beli roots	*Eagle marmelos*	The rest of the ingredients must total 6 k (i.e., 12 m each).
3. toṭila roots	*Oroxylum indicum*	This part of the decoction (ingredients 2–11) is known as the *dasa mul ganaya*: "the ten root group". The whole effect is to destroy *vāta*. But the 10 roots can also destroy *sema*; this destroying effect is neutralized by the heavy dose of *hātāvāriya*, which is cool and phlegm fostering. The total *samyōga* therefore is *samasitōṣna*, "balanced hot-cold".
4. grape roots		
5. palol roots	*Stereospermum suaveolens*	
6. ätdemaṭa roots	*Gmelina arborea*	
7. asvänna roots	*Alyssicarpus vaginalis*	
8. pol palā roots	?	
9. elabaṭu roots	*Solanum xanthocarpum*	
10. kaṭuväl baṭu roots	*Solanum jacquini*	
11. hīn gokaṭu roots	*Pedalium murex*	

THE USES OF THEORY: SAMYŌGIC EXPERIMENTATION

The Ayurvedic paradigm sketched above helps physicians to understand the causes of illness, interpret symptoms, prescribe medications, and give a general prognosis (prediction) as to outcome — all in terms of the general theory. It is superior to contemporary Western medicine as a theoretical system *per se*, i.e., in terms of its simplicity and aesthetic elegance, its capacity to explain all illnesses in terms of the theory (except those caused by supernatural beings) and above all its predictive value. In the more practically effective, and experimentally based Western system, such theoretical elegance is an end yet to be achieved. The latter contains several theoretical systems which have not yet been integrated into a general theory. This is inevitable because the development of an experimental tradition in Western medicine broke up the formal Medieval (Hippocratic) paradigm that prevailed till then, and introduced new conceptions of body function (e.g., circulation of the blood, genetics) and disease causation (e.g., germ theory, viruses, psychosomatic medicine) which cannot be accommodated into a single formally-elegant paradigm. As a result of the more "open" ideology of Western science, one can have a cure which is unrelated or poorly related to the theory of disease causation. For example, a surgeon may be totally ignorant of the cause of cancer but nonetheless perform an operation to remove the growth and "cure" the patient. In Ayurveda, by contrast, there is a systematic attempt to connect the cure to the theory of illness. Western medicine illustrates what Kuhn has ably shown — that new experimental knowledge must eventually shatter the old paradigms, sometimes with a bang but more often with a whimper.

Nevertheless, we have to address ourselves to the question as to the relationship between the formally elegant paradigm and the generation of new knowledge and information. The problem with the Ayurvedic paradigm when we compare it with Western medical theories is its very virtue — it is too abstract, too removed from everyday phenomenal reality. It cannot be easily manipulated to generate new theoretical knowledge through the formulation of hypotheses, or at least there are severe limitations to these procedures. Yet this does not mean that experimentation cannot occur or that new empirical information cannot be incorporated into the system. Let me examine these two issues separately.

Consider the two prescriptions devised by Nilammahara specialists for the cure of madness from an excess of *vāta* or "wind". This is their own prescription, devised through clinical experience with mental patients. It is also based on practical experimentation — putting ingredients together in terms of their essential properties, meeting an excess in one ingredient with its counteractive effect in another. The prescription was not invented by *apriori* reasoning; rather it was a product of trial and error and practical application in the clinics. It may be presumed that the prescription was not formulated in a day. On the contrary it is a product of experimenting with different ingredients, their clinical application to patients, observation of patient responses and disease prognosis and the eventual production of the present formula. The operations being performed here, irrespective of their "objective" efficacy, are of a genuinely experimental nature, even though these physicians lack the technical sophistication, the expensive gadgetry and expressive paraphernalia of modern medical science. Several experimenters in Ayurveda whom I interviewed recently, are spurred by a genuine intellectual and scientific curiosity.

Experimentation here is not considered in an *ad hoc* manner. The Ayurvedic paradigm itself provides the theoretical framework necessary for experimentation. Otherwise what emerges would be *ad hoc* experimentation, or Levi Strauss' notion of *bricolage*, rather than a genuine experimental tradition. Instead, we have here a form of experimentation guided by theory, helping to generate new knowledge. For what of a better term I label it *samyōgic* experimentation.

I have highlighted one example of experimentation within the framework of Ayurvedic theory. My current investigations show that this form of experimentation is extremely widespread. The reputations of well known Ayurvedic physicians rest on the "efficiacy" of their cures, and these cures have generally been the product of *samyōgic* experimentation. For example, some of the most famous physicians in Sri Lanka have specialized in diseases like asthma, sinuses and other allergies. In practially all of these cases the prescriptions have been devised through *samyōgic* experimentation. The Ayurvedic paradigm not only fosters an experimental tradition but it can incorporate existing empirically-verified knowledge into a scientific framework and thereby validate it.

CONCLUSION

This paper has sketched basic elements in the Ayurvedic theory of psychological medicine. The discussion outlined points at which the propositions of medical theory are integrated with metaphysical assumptions about mind, bodily functioning and the phenomenal world. Although explanatory models in Ayurvedic medicine contain elements familiar to Western psychiatry (such as psychosomatic illness), it is only bodily elements which receive consistent and explicit formulation as causative agents in the theory of Ayurveda. I have also argued that the Ayurvedic tradition has produced an abstract and "aesthetic" theory of psychological medicine which may be manipulated for the purposes of experimentation and the generation of new information.

REFERENCES

Caraka.
  1949 Caraka Samhita, V. Jamnagar. India: Shree Gulbkunverba Ayurvedic Society.
Dasgupta, S.
  1963 The Kapila and Patanjali Samkhya. *In* A History of Indian Philosophy Vol. 1. London: Routledge.
  1968 Speculation in the Medical Schools. *In* A History of Indian Philosophy. Vol. 2. London: Routledge.
Filliozat, J.
  1964 The Classical Doctrine of Indian Medicine, Trans, Dev. Raj Channa. Delhi: Munshiran Manoharlal.
Hiriyanna, M.
  1956 The Essentials of Indian Philosophy. London: George Allen and Unwin.
Levi-Strauss, C.
  1966 The Savage Mind. Chicago: University of Chicago Press.
Obeyesekere, Gananath.
  1977 The Theory and Practice of Psychological Medicine in the Ayurvedic Tradition. Culture, Medicine and Psychiatry. 1(2):155–181.
Susruta.
  1963 Susrita Samhita. K. L. Bhisagratne, (Ed. trans.) Vols. II, III. Varanasi: Chowkamba Sanskrit Series.

SECTION III

CULTURAL CONCEPTIONS OF THERAPY

LINDA CONNOR

10. THE UNBOUNDED SELF: BALINESE THERAPY IN THEORY AND PRACTICE

INTRODUCTION

Michel Foucault (1971) amongst other social and medical historians (e.g., see Ellenberger 1970; Szasz 1973), has located the development of psychiatry and institutions of medical custody in the historical epoch associated with the secularization of scientific inquiry and with the emergence of new ideologies of self and society which accompanied the onslaught of the Industrial Revolution in Europe.[1] This paper poses a question of anthropological relevance: If the concepts and practice of psychiatry are so culturally and historically embedded, how far can they take us in the exploration of self and other, madness[2] and "sanity" in societies which until recently were peripheral to these developments?

These concerns form the background to this paper, which focuses on Balinese indigenous therapies and healers called *balian*.[3] Balians thrive in Bali in response to popular demand for their services. In the district where I worked, one of eight on the island (which forms a province of Indonesia), there were 250–300 *balians* practicing publicly[4] in a population of approximately 151,000. I will discuss several case studies to illustrate therapeutic responses of *balians*, clients and families, and to show how the ideas which *balians* and their clients invoke about madness and other disturbances integrate with broader notions about health, human personality and the influence of the supernatural in worldly affairs. To this end I present in the latter part of the paper a cultural phenomenology of 'person' in Bali.[5] I contend that a crucial component of therapeutic processes is communication about the key symbols which operate in the conceptualization of 'person'.

BALINESE VIEWS OF MADNESS

Medieval Europeans viewed madness quite differently from their descendants of today. Foucault, in *Madness and Civilization*, writes:

In the Middle Ages and until the Renaissance, man's dispute with madness was a dramatic debate in which he confronted the secret powers of the world; the experience of madness was clouded by images of the fall and the Will of God, of the Beast and the Metamorphosis, and of all the marvelous secrets of Knowledge (Foucault 1971:xii).

In Bali, too, madness is potentially at least an inspired and not a degraded state. The phenomenon almost invariably leads out of the mundane world, and in many instances is perceived to give humans intimations of the divine. Such madness is basically beyond human comprehension as the causes are

251

A. J. Marsella and G. M. White (eds.), Cultural Conceptions of Mental Health and Therapy, 251–267.

other-worldly. Therapy takes place within the frameworks of ritual, pilgrimage, prayer and blessing, as well as by more somatic ministrations such as massage and medicinal herbs.

Balinese classifications of madness are not rigid and there is a consistent difference in the distribution of knowledge about symptomatology and etiology between laypersons and *balians*, as well as within these categories of people (Kleinman 1980:83). Laypersons generally name madness in terms of the dominant behavioral manifestations, or refer to the affliction by the generic term (*buduh*), while specialists are consulted to find out the cause. Some of the terms used to describe the symptoms of disturbance are: 'dizzy', 'confused', 'disoriented' (*inguh, pusing, paling, lengeh*); 'running amok' (*ngamuk*); 'apathetic', 'dazed' (*bengong, samun*); 'raving', 'incoherent speech', 'talking to oneself' (*ngumikmik, omong kosong*); 'frightened', 'excessively timid' (*nyeh*); 'running away', 'resisting restraint' (*malumbar*); and 'wandering' (*ngumbang*). When referring to their own state, subjects almost invariably use the terms for 'dizzy' and 'disoriented', sometimes associated with terms to describe 'anger' (*gedeg, duka*) and 'heat' (*kebus, panes*) but find it difficult to articulate these further.

There are several refinements of the generic label for madness which balians utilize. Incidence of use varies with the 'diagnostic style' (see Gaines, this volume) of each practitioner, which is in part attributable to the different diagnostic and therapeutic techniques they emphasize.[6] Semantically, all these terms have etiological implications. The most common are: madness (*buduh*), due to inherited factors (*uli keturunan*); congenital influences (*uli pemetuan*); the grace of the gods (*kedewandewan*); and ancestral or divine curse (*keponggor*). The labels for other varieties refer to bewitchment through either the application of spells and mantras (*kena papasengan*); or the introduction of small live creatures (*babai*) into the victim's body (*babainan*) (See also Thong 1976; Tugby et al. 1976). Few of these categories are mutually exclusive, nor do they differ from the range of etiologies for many other illnesses and misfortunes. For example, an ancestral curse may lead to the withdrawal of supernatural protection over a family, and thereby render the victim more vulnerable to affliction by witchcraft. Diagnosis may change many times in the course of an episode or episodes.

When the madness is said to be caused by ancestral or divine curse, the precipitating factors are usually attributed to the neglect of important ritual by the family, or mistakes in ritual already completed. Blame is typically diffused or diverted. In the case of bewitchment, the victims or their kin have usually done something to arouse anger or jealousy in others, thus provoking covert expressions of hostility. In long-term cases, the final diagnosis is more likely to stress inherited or congenital factors. When such disorders are reputed to be inherited, this often includes the concept of an inherited curse.

The Balinese specialist closely integrates physical and mental dimensions of illness by relating both to concepts of spiritual well-being, and by attributing the behaviour of the individual to supernatural and other forces beyond the immediate control of clients.

THREE CASE HISTORIES OF DIAGNOSIS AND TREATMENT

The following three case histories illustrate some of the prevalent patterns of diagnosis and treatment. The first (Putu's) and the third (Sinta's) concern individuals who typify most victims of madness in Bali. The mental hospital rarely has any contact with such people. They recover as a result of the *balians*' treatment,[7] for other reasons less easy to specify except as contingent changes in life circumstances or 'spontaneous remission', or from positive public endorsement of their experience such as recognition as a healer. The second case exemplifies a situation of breakdown in interpersonal relations between kinsmen. They receive successful 'counseling' by the traditional practitioner Gusti Nyoman Tapakan, in a Balinese variant of the family-oriented therapy endorsed in the West by those psychiatrists who recognize the broader social context of the disturbances they treat. While the effects of such therapy are often positive, I do not mean to imply that *balians* subscribe to models of illness and therapy which are more secular or which systematically vary from those of their clients. They are distinguished rather by their developed interpersonal skills and by their position as mediators between humans and the supernatural. This latter role, which allows some degree of coercive elicitation, facilitates information flow and emotional catharsis in a way seldom replicated in everyday contexts.

As part of these therapies, relatives may participate in the preparation of elaborate rituals of propitiation, exorcism and purification. In some cases, pilgrimages are made to distant shrines, removing family members temporarily from stressful daily circumstances. At the houses of spirit mediums, groups of relatives engage in dialogue about their problems with the spirits of their ancestors. The more skillful practitioners are able to initiate discussion of issues which may be causing conflict. By these means, the healer may be instrumental in creating a temporary or permanent restructuring in problematic patterns of social interaction amongst the participants, especially where *balian*-client contact is long term or recurrent.

A Case Example of Witchcraft

Putu's experience typifies many cases which are treated successfully by the *balians* with no psychiatric intervention. Like many Medieval madpersons, Putu was considered to be the victim of witchcraft.

One afternoon, she and her brother walked into the houseyard of a healer I knew very well. She looked about twenty years old, and was unmarried. They were from a village where Jero, the healer, was well respected and had many clients. Putu, who remained silent, appeared dazed, vacant-eyed and deaf to any questions addressed to her. She sobbed quietly most of the time, while sitting immobile in a corner. Her brother said she had been like this for several weeks. They had taken her to the local general nurse about ten days previously and he had given her a multi-vitamin injection for general lassitude. When this was ineffective the nurse had confirmed the family's suspicion that her complaint was 'Balinese' and encouraged them in seeking the help of a *balian*.

Jero massaged the girl's neck. Beneath the jawbone she found the seat of the trouble —
babai. She laid my finger there and I could feel a small pulsation. 'They are living there,' she
said. She found another just behind the armpit. Jero said these were a special sort of *babai*
— 'wind babai' (*babai angin*), which can't be seen except by people with great magical
powers (*sakti*). 'The main danger with this sort of *babai*', said Jero, 'is that they can travel
throughout the body. If they go to the ears, the victim may become deaf; whilst if they go
to the brain, the victim may become violent and run amok.' She prepared some medicine
to prevent them moving around and ordered the family to return in two days, with the
ingredients for an exorcism ceremony. She told me that a rejected lover of the girl's was the
perpetrator. He had been incensed to hear of her engagement to another boy. The girl
stayed with Jero, and the family returned in two days for the exorcism ceremony. The main
part of it was a 'smoking' ritual (*madusdus*) to drive out the *babai*. Two small human effigies,
a male and a female, were made out of cooked rice (*nasi wongwongan*) and were set on the
ground to the south of the girl. When the *babai* were driven out of the victim's body by the
light smoking, they would be attracted to these effiges which would then be discarded,
explained Jero. The girl stood up draped only in a loose sarong, with an earthenware pot
full of the magical ingredients between her legs. The contents of the pot were set burning,
and the girl was slowly 'smoked' for about forty minutes. Then the effigies were removed,
and the girl was purified with holy water. During the course of the afternoon, her condition
visibly improved. She participated a little in the conversation of those around her. She
stayed at the house of the *balian* for a couple of weeks in all, and improved in response to
further strengthening and purificatory ceremonies for which she herself made most of the
preparations.

Such ceremonies are primarily directed to the *kanda mpat*, the four spiritual
siblings which guard every human being. These life-giving forces are believed
to be withdrawn by sorcerers as part of their manipulations, and much of the
balians' ritual manistrations focus on the reintroduction and fortifying of the
kanda mpat. By actively participating in these procedures, the patient is again
drawn into everyday work routines.

I found out later that there had been some conflict in Putu's home about
marriage arrangements that threatened her own preference for a husband. This
was no doubt coupled with the ambivalence sometimes expressed by females
of marriageable age at the prospect of leaving their natal houseyard to live
patrivirilocally.

Buduh babainan such as Putu suffered is usually treated successfully by the
traditional healers. It most often afflicts adolescents and is attributed to the
wrath of rejected lovers, although in the case of older victims other motivations
may be ascribed to the perpetrator.

In this case, no stigma was attached to the episode. Putu was under someone's
magical spell, which fact alone is considered to account for her behavior. In
cases such as these the family need only find a healer with more powerful magic
than the perpetrator to expel the foreign bodies within her. The drama of illness
and curing is played out without the individual ego becoming closely implicated.
This is so in most episodes of madness where supernatural causes are diagnosed.
These are beyond the patient's control most of the time. The victim may suffer
from the effects of ancestral wrath which others, including dead persons one or
two generations removed, have generated through neglect of ritual. Collective

responsibility is assumed by the kin group in such circumstances. If witchcraft is the cause, as in Putu's case, the perpetrator is considered blameworthy in that it is he or she who has succumbed to such passions as anger, jealously or lust. The victim shares no blame for having provoked such unruly passions.[8] Thus, when suffering the effects of such evil manipulations, she herself may release violent, pent-up emotions in uncontrolled behavior without having to take any direct personal responsibility. Emotional displays of this type are strongly repressed in everyday contexts in this culture (Belo 1960; Bateson and Mead 1942; Connor 1979).

In many cases I encountered in the *balians'* care, the patient recovered after only a short course of traditional treatment. Unlike psychiatric techniques, the diagnosis orients directly to the culturally construed cause of the disorder, while alleviating symptoms by therapy which is sensitive to underlying and culturally unarticulated psychosocial stressors in the clients' environment. Healing rituals are performed under the guidance of the *balian*, with the family helping in all stages of preparation and performance.

A Case Example of Social Stress and Strain

In some circumstances, relatives may consult a medium about a state of stress and tension in the family. Sometimes, as in the case outlined below, there is one member whose behaviour is sufficiently deviant to warrant the description 'eccentric', 'unpredictable', 'confused', without the designation 'mad' (*buduh*) being firmly applied. At other times, a general atmosphere of strain and frequent quarrels among various family members may be sufficient to prompt the decision to consult a *balian*. The practitioner chosen may be one skilled in divination, Balinese astrology or, as in the case described here, a spirit medium.

A group of relatives entered the house of the medium Gusti Nyoman Tapakan on the morning of the June full moon. They included a husband and wife in their early thirties, the husband's youngest brother, the wife's mother, and the wife's brother. The two brothers worked in government offices in the nearby town. The offerings they carried revealed little about the purpose of their visit.

Early in the first trance the medium, possessed by a guardian houseyard deity, tentatively diagnosed illness. When the clients responded negatively the diagnosis shifted to arguments and strife in the family, especially amongst the women. The elder brother, as the chief petitioner, confirmed this suggestion.

The medium proceeded to outline the symptoms in some detail: squabbling between the two wives, sulking, and laziness in performing household chores. The younger brother revealed that his wife's behaviour was so erratic she appeared to be going mad (*mamuduh*). The elder brother's wife declared that all the tension in the house was affecting the children, who frequently quarreled, cried, and were performing unsatisfactorily at school. The medium also suggested that many things were misplaced around the home. The members of the family agreed.

During a series of three trances, each followed by a discussion between the medium (out of trance) and his clients, it emerged that the brothers had originally come from Denpasar, but several years before had moved to the town where they now worked. During the shift, they had failed to make the necessary offerings at their houseyard temple of origin. The deity also accused them of never making enough offerings in the equivalent temple of their new house. Further divine wrath was to descend on them. The wife had interpreted a worm in the salad the husband was eating as a sign of sorcery. She threw the creature away, but the deity in bringing the matter to light, proclaimed that it was in fact an auspicious supernatural omen.

During the second trance, the spirit of the brothers' dead father possessed the medium, and accused the family of failing to divide up the inheritance correctly. In response to a question from the spirit of the dead father, the elder brother revealed that the younger brother and his wife still did not have their own kitchen, and therefore had not achieved full adult independent status which most couples are granted on marriage. At the time of the father's death, the youngest brother of the five (the one now residing in the nearby town with his elder brother) was still unmarried, and the inheritance had been divided up between the four married brothers. On his marriage he still had not received his share, and this was causing a lot of friction in the house, especially between the wives who had actually come to blows on occasions. Out of trance, a lengthy and meandering conversation ensued, in which the medium reminded the brothers of the perils of wives sharing a kitchen, and relevant anecdotes from the experience of friends and relatives were cited.

In between the second and third trances, the elder brother's wife informed me that her sister-in-law had in fact wanted to marry the elder brother, but had been passed over in favour of herself. She said that even when there were no actual arguments, the atmosphere in the houseyard was very tense.

The spirit of the dead father chided both the brothers for not making enough offerings to their ancestors at the house temple, and suggested that separate living quarters should now be built for the younger brother, as he had been married for some time, and had children.

In the third trance, the father's spirit informed the sons that the immediate reason for the younger brother's wife's strange behaviour was the introduction of a black magic spell into the houseyard by a jealous neighbour. He named the night of the event, two weeks previously. Earth from the cemetery, empowered by verbal spells, had been sprinkled onto the feet of the husband and wife while they were sleeping. The medium, out of trance, asked the client if in fact his feet had felt rather hot and itchy on that particular night. The husband agreed that it had been the case, and that the wife's behaviour had become worse since that time. The medium reiterated the dangers of neglecting offerings to ancestors, who could withdraw their protection from their descendants in response, and increase the potency of harmful spells.

'The clients left the houseyard with prescriptions for propitiatory offerings to appease the ancestors and instructions for an exorcism ceremony to remove the spell which afflicted the wife. They also came away with a supernaturally validated recommendation to commence the ritually and socially delicate process of setting up an independent living establishment, and thereby to complete the division of the inheritance.

Space prohibits detailed discussion of the multiple strategies this very astute medium uses as part of his therapeutic techniques. There are many similarities cross-culturally, and excellent treatment of this topic in other settings may be found in Kleinman (1980) and other papers in this volume.

When I visited the family two weeks later, they reported that the situation in the home had improved since the visit to Gusti Nyoman Tapakan. They had carried out all the ceremonies prescribed and were in the process of planning the household move which had been suggested at the seance. It is indeed unusual and highly stressful for wives of co-resident brothers to share a kitchen, although married brothers commonly use the same houseyard and temple. In this case, apart from endorsing the new living arrangements, the medium's utterances had indicated an external cause for the family strife especially in the case of the younger brother's wife, who had been diagnosed as suffering from a sorcerer's spell. In this way, blame and guilt were diffused and there was no stigma attached to the wife's behavior. The more equitable sharing of the inheritance, and the move to a new house, promised to ease the women's antagonism towards each other.

A Case Example of Blessed Madness

For a minority of people, madness is an inspired condition and not one necessitating 'treatment' in the usual sense of the word. Foucault (1971:xii ff), writing of Medieval Europe, asserts that the condition was a means of access to higher knowledge unavailable to other mortals. In Bali, too, madness can be a blessed state preceding initiation as a healer or priest. In this case the symptoms are distinctive, including encounters with the divine, wandering in sacred places, praying and meditation, and wearing ceremonial clothes on ordinary occasions. The violent behaviour often associated with other forms of madness is lacking.

There is the possibility that many cases of disturbance in the early stages will be interpreted in this way. Episodes of psychological dissociation in public ritual settings are common and highly valued in the culture. Priestly and healing roles often incorporate ritual trance states. An episode of madness may precede one's consecration as a healer or priest and is an opportunity to learn the skills of dissociation. Many people, during such a disturbed period in their lives, experience their first trance, which is later interpreted as possession by ancestor or deity. Some become spirit mediums and use their skills in the service of the community (Belo 1960).

The term for this madness – *buduh kedewandewan* – literally translated is 'madness from the gods'. I shall refer to it here as 'blessed madness'. Blessed madness is often experienced outside the physical margins of settled society. The madperson seeks isolation from relatives and friends by wandering in lonely places – the mountains, little used roads and tracks or wilderness areas.

Sinta, who lives in an isolated cottage in the mountains told me the story of how he became a spirit medium. He is about 40 years old, and lives with his wife and three sons. They are very poor, owning only a small orchard on barren land. He said that for three years before becoming a *balian* he roamed around in the mountain forest. He was in his late teens, still unmarried. He did not feel confused or sick for most of that time, but he had the desire to wander and to live an ascetic life. He would stay away from home for a few days at a stretch, and ask for rice at strangers' places, or pick fruit from the trees. Most of the significant events of this time seem to have happened at a small sacred grove with a shrine, not far from his home. He said that after wandering for a long time he discovered this grove where, as he put it, he 'died' for a few hours. He felt very weak and hungry from his wanderings and everything went dark all of a sudden.

Then a small white-skinned creature approached. This being was no bigger than a child, and had pointed ears. Sinta said it was a deity-like personage. It ordered him to a nearby clump of bamboo to wait for an omen. He obeyed, but after half a day nothing happened. He felt that it was stupid of him to be waiting around in the bush for he knew not what, so he decided to go home. But when he tried to leave, he felt as if his arms were tied and he could not get up. He resisted in vain. Again the voice came to him and it was the small creature which instructed him to look for a small bush to the north of the clump of bamboo. He was told to search for a sweet orange just to the northeast of this bush. He found the fruit and ate it, putting the skins in his pocket. Then he felt his normal self, and anxious about things at home, so he set off. But the creature came again, and told him he would receive a sacred charm which obliged the owner to help particular people without taking profit. After the creature disappeared, he felt in his pocket for the orange peel, which had changed into some ceremonial coins. Around this time he also found some sacred stones while wandering in the area.

He could not understand these strange happenings, and had no desire to follow the instructions of the little deity and become a healer. Several months later he was alone in his houseyard when suddenly he heard a voice (*suara angin*) telling him that he must try out the magical and curative powers of these objects. After that, he was dazed and disoriented for about one month, 'like a madperson,' he said. He kept hearing voices telling him to try out the powers of the sacred objects, but he was afraid to do so.

One day a person who was sick arrived from a nearby settlement — a woman who had suffered for many years from a 'weak heart' (*jantung lemah*). Her husband had dreamed that his wife might be cured by Sinta, who felt he had no choice but to attempt to treat the woman. He made some holy water by dipping the sacred objects in pure spring water, which the woman drank. Within half-an-hour she reported feeling better! The news of his powers spread, and people came from all around for advice and cure.

During this time Sinta first experienced possession trance. Neither he nor his relatives defined the periods of dissociation with accompanying visions and voices, whilst wandering in the forest, as ritual trance. Three days after the initial healing act, a man came to him who was troubled over inheritance quarrels in his family. He asked Sinta to present some offerings on his behalf, in an attempt to resolve the problem. Sinta did so and suddenly became possessed by one of the man's ancestors. He was able to advise the family members on their problems. Ever since then, people have been coming to request his services as a medium. After becoming a *balian* and undergoing the consecration ceremonies he never again suffered any serious illness, nor any more bouts of 'blessed madness', which he, his family and fellow hamlet members now identify as the cause of his earlier deivant behaviour.

This is a straightforward case, and many of the balians whom I interviewed had been through a similar period in their lives prior to practicing their skills. Such autobiographical accounts are, of course, cultural constructs *par excellence* and thereby an important means of validating aspirations to the role of healer. The episode which is labelled as blessed madness is often associated with the hardships of dire poverty coupled with more contingent misfortunes such as death of close kin and marital problems. There is usually no recurrence of symptoms after the purification and consecration ceremonies, which family and co-villagers support.

In all the cases cited, patients and families understand the fundamentals of traditional therapies, and comprehend the significance of the major symbols invoked in healing ritual. The importance of such client involvement raises questions about the efficacy of psychiatric treatments in cross-cultural settings, where concepts of personality organization and basic cosmological principles differ fundamentally, especially when such treatment is supposed to subjectively involve the patient and family.

To understand the above case histories, we need to examine the way Balinese conceptualize 'person'. The concluding section outlines a construct of the dimensions of 'person' in Balinese culture. I stress that the account draws on multiple 'theories' of personality which are implicitly held, with variations of emphasis, among *balians* and clients, and which are encoded in many of the classical texts only in schematic form.

PERSONHOOD IN BALINESE CULTURE

Medieval Europeans bequeathed to posterity a rich literature of religious tracts and treatises on witchcraft from which can be deduced the outlines of a psychology of personality. Balinese have an equally venerable literary heritage that elaborates a formal conceptualization of self (or, as may be more appropriate in their case, selves). The texts which encode these ideas are inscriptions on palm-leaf (*lontar, rontal*) and have passed from one generation to another within a small scholarly elite that adheres to a variant tradition of Hinduism, emphasizing its esoteric Tantric forms.

Over many centuries, Balinese variants of these philosophies have also absorbed inspiration from pre-Hindu animistic and ancestral cults which continue to exercise a profound influence on beliefs and rituals in villages today. *Balians* and priests consult and simplify the contents of the manuscripts for an illiterate population. The majority of experts interpret the solutions they recommend in magico-religious terms, effecting their remedies by ritual means. Healers who can dramatically manipulate the key symbols in Hindu-Balinese cosmology, as part of their interpersonal skills, have the greatest efficacy.

Balinese Microcosm and Macrocosm

Balinese texts[9] eschew the mind-body dualism which has pervaded much of Western philosophy and which has been central to European medical and psychological theory. A more fundamental ordering is of Sanskrit origin: the distinction between *buana alit* (literally: 'small world' — the microcosmos) and *buana agung* (literally: 'great world' — the macrocosmos). Each feature of the microcosmos has a counterpart in the macrocosmos (e.g., the hair on the body corresponds with the trees and plants of the earth; sweat and other somatic fluids with dew drops, rain and river waters). The two systems constantly interact and modify each other. The direction of causation is not predetermined. Ecological and technologically wrought changes are thought to be able to affect the functioning of the microcosmos; conversely, persons with great spiritual powers (*kesaktian, kewisesan*) may be able to influence changes in the macrocosmos by the correct symbolic manipulation of spiritual forces within the body. Secular agency in both domains is relatively underplayed.

Kanda Mpat: 'Sibling' Spirits

The human being as well as replicating the macrocosmos in detail, is a receptacle within which several supernatural forces interact as integral components of the individual's personality. The most important of these are the personified spiritual forces referred to as the 'four siblings' – kanda mpat. Many of the most sacred [10] manuscripts are discourses on the nature, care and strengthening of the kanda mpat. Their protection and guidance is ritually enlisted in all important endeavours and they are referred to familiarly in everyday conversation as 'my siblings' (nyaman tiange – a phrase which does not differentiate between one's spiritual and human siblings, indicating perhaps that both categories are regarded with the same intimacy).[11]

In all life cycle rituals these spirits receive as much attention as their human vessel. The bodily self is the fifth and youngest sibling who incorporates the other four, and as I will later show, whose boundaries are conceived to be indeterminate, even infinite.

Like the human sibling, the kanda mpat are gradually socialized to be fit to participate in Balinese society; this process in the life of a child being marked by an elaborate series of childhood rites of passage (see Bateson and Mead 1942; Covarrubius 1973; Mershon 1971). Before birth, the kanda mpat protect and nurture the foetus (see Hooykaas 1974:98 ff). They start out after birth as demonlike forces associated with the pollution of birth, and inimical to the child's welfare if left unattended. Through ritual, the four spiritual siblings gradually become assimilated to their human sibling and assume a protective role as custodians of a well-balanced relationship between the physical, psychological and spiritual dimensions of the individual.

The physical manifestation of the kanda mpat at the time of birth are the placenta, blood, amniotic sac and amniotic fluid. Each sibling governs certain aspects of the functioning of the human body, and there are symbolic correspondences with elements of the macrocosmos as well.

Worldly foibles and talents of the individual are often attributed to the various strengths and weaknesses of the kanda mpat. In sickness they are usually considered to have been weakened through ritual neglect, and have to be fortified again by the healer. In magical manipulations they are withdrawn by the sorcerer and must be retrieved by more powerful counter-magic.

For example, an excerpt from one tract on the kanda mpat reads as follows:[12]

The third one has as his/her manifestation the amniotic sac. S/he is called the Great Demon Banas Pati Raja. S/he is the chief caretaker of the Death Temple (Pura Dalem), and in this role s/he goes by the name of The Sacred One Nyoman Pengadangan. In this form his/her supernatural power (sakti) is beyond compare. S/he is the deity of the Taksu spirit; the deity of the cemetery; the deity of rivers; the deity of river sprites (dete tonya) as well as of spirits; the deity of birds. S/he is the deity of the Taksu spirit, of all sorts of sacred dances. As well s/he is the inspiration of the puppeteer-priest (*dalang*); the inspiration of *balians*, those who follow the path of the left and of the right; the deity of literate medical specialists (*balian usada*); spirit mediums; and diviners, both those who use texts and those who do not use texts. Moreover it is s/he who can give people spiritual powers. In the body, s/he resides in the connecting tissues (*uwat*).[13] S/he is called their finest fibres. His/her symbol is *ang*, and has the form of holy water (*tirta*). His/her supernatural power (*sakti*) is such that it conquers all powers based on texts and mantras. S/he can make love spells, and turn an enemy into an admirer, or vice versa. S/he can bring rain, and repel it. S/he can prevent illness, as well as all sorts of natural disasters. S/he can make sacred symbols, and inspire *balians*. S/he can draw many customers for traders. S/he can transform him/herself so that s/he can't be seen by ordinary eyes. His/her offerings are rice cooked in a woven basket, in the form of a 'gong', with an egg and a roasted duck; the cleansing offerings are a small lump of cooked black rice (Tonjaya 1978:9, present author's translation).

Each sibling has symbolic concomitants, for instance in an aspect of physical birth, a part of the body, a symbol of the alphabet, a mantra sound, and physical elements of the macrocosmos such as rivers, texts, temples, dances. Such correspondences also operate between the siblings and the guardian deities of certain vocations, and other sorts of spiritual forces. This abbreviation of a theoretically unlimited list illustrates that in Balinese conceptualization, the individual, the supernatural and the macrocosmos fuse with one another and interpenetrate. In cases of illness, an intensive diagnosis by a balian will often specify one or another area controlled by one of the *kanda mpat*.

Illiterate *balians* too are capable of giving and supervising instructions for these rituals: they learn from observation of others' rituals, from discussion with literate *balians* and priests, as well as from the sacred dramatic performances held before the public on ritual occasions in local temples (Young 1980). This systematization of symbolic correspondences, and thus their incorporation in ritual, is variable both in the texts (e.g., Hooykaas 1974) and in the *balians'* practices.

Spirit Reincarnation

Another element of the personality is the reincarnating spirit of a deceased relative (*ane mahiyang, Sang Numadi*). Prominent character traits are sometimes related to the personality of the deceased where he or she is still recalled by descendants. Thus, in the houseyard where I lived, one five-year-old child was particularly prone to throw tantrums when he did not get his own way. The family was tolerant as he was said to have inherited this personality trait from his grandfather who had reincarnated in him.

Sickness and misfortune in this life may be related to sins from a former life which a reincarnating spirit has not yet redeemed. To guard against this eventuality, in many areas of Bali the relatives of a newborn baby consult a spirit medium (the consultation is referred to as *ngaluang, nyapatin*) 12 days after the child's birth, to identify the ancestor who has come down to 'ask for rice'. (Belo

(1960:239 ff) provides a detailed account of a ceremony of this type.) Relatives engage in conversation with their ancestors, who possess the medium, to discover if there are any ceremonies which have been overlooked, or as they put it, if they have any 'debts' to the deities and demons of the Death Temple (Pura Dalem) who release all the spirits which come back to this world. Parents are anxious to perform these ceremonies to ensure their child's health and well-being, and to securely anchor the reincarnating spirit.

The Soul

The soul (*atma*) which most closely corresponds to concepts of 'soul' in Western European Christian traditions is yet another, more ethereal component of the human. This microcosmic manifestation of the highest divinity, Sang Hyang Widi Wasa, is the focus of elaborate mortuary rites rather than meticulous attention in everyday ritual contexts. Cremation ceremonies release and purify the *atma* to the point where it may fuse again with the godhead. Some of my informants maintained that one of the primary functions of the *kanda mpat* is to protect the *atma*.

Taksu: Spirit Intermediaries

The final element I wish to consider in relation to conceptions of 'person' is the *taksu*. This notion in Balinese cosmology refers to an 'interpreter' or 'inter-mediary spirit' (e.g., Belo 1960:246) which facilitates the communication of messages from supernatural realms through consecrated spirit mediums and which facilitates successful, and even inspired performances in all varieties of ritual dramatic arts. Like the *kanda mpat*, the *taksu* has both microcosmic and macrocosmic manifestations.

As a macrocosmic entity, *taksu* is invoked as Bhagawan Taksu (Lord Taksu), and is conceived as a deified intermediary between gods and humans. One spirit medium, in attempting to explain the concept to me, said: "The *taksu* is like a telephone, it enables a connection to be made between the deity and me." In microcosmic form, *taksu* is a personalized spirit associated with an individual's talents. Beliefs about *taksu* vary, but some informants asserted that each person has a *taksu*, be it for spirit mediumship, for farming, for scholarship and so on. It represents the potential to perform well in one's vocation.

"Self" and Possession

In the Balinese view of personality, the symbolic action of the agents I have discussed defies the distinction many other cultures draw between self and the macrocosmos, between mind and body, and between the natural and super-natural realms. This conceptualization is inseparable from a cultural ideology of possession, which is invoked in the explanation of a large range of human behaviour.

The balanced interaction of the forces within the body may be upset by the magical introduction of harmful agents or substances. The case of Putu (see above) illustrates this point. Her symptoms were attributed to the presence of small live demon-like creatures (*babai*) in her body. Inanimate substances and harmful forces introduced into the body by ill-intentioned sorcerers may affect behavior in the same way. Adjustment is effected by exorcism of the offending agent, and then by a ritual realigning of the *kanda mpat* and other energies in the body. Countermagic too operates on the principle of the introduction of charms and sacred substances into the body.

But the more ephemeral contexts of possession are not always negatively viewed, and may be institutionalized as ritual possession trance. Balinese from all sectors of society show a great proclivity for states of dissociation which are often interpreted as ritual possession trance (Connor 1979). Deities and ancestors possess human vehicles and make their will known to their devotees — usually a congregation of a corporate group having a ritualized identity. During possession the vehicle's everyday personality becomes latent and behaviour may change radically. He or she usually denies any subsequent recollection of the event. Even where the ritual mediation of possession is minimal, the subject of divine edicts or benevolence renounces all responsibility and motivation is projected onto the external agent. For instance *balians* who suffer 'blessed madness' and other inspirational experiences as part of their initiation to the calling, uniformly deny any personal wish to enhance their status by becoming a *balian*. They are, as they put it, merely acquiescing in divine will (*ngiring pikahyunan*). Sinta's case (see above) is typical in this respect. He followed the instructions of his divine voices and visions, whilst all the time protesting that he himself did not want to become a healer. Eventually, as he tells it, it was the pressure from clients which forced him to practice his skills, at risk of misfortune to himself and his family if he failed to comply.

CONCLUSION

If we look at the practices of therapists in Bali, coupled with the elements of personality as articulated in classical medico-religious texts, as well as by informants, it appears that the Balinese 'person' is not an isolated, indivisible unit but is rather a nexus of interacting forces, macrocosmic and microcosmic, natural and supernatural, always in a delicate balance.

The above portrayal of personality is, of course, overwhelmingly cognitive and by virtue of this emphasizes the exotic at the expense of the more mundane cultural interpretation of human behavior. My justification for this is that it does indeed represent the contours of a cultural phenomenology of 'person' which is of crucial significance in understanding indigenous responses to personal breakdown and interpersonal stress such as I have described in the three case studies. My analysis ultimately needs to be complemented by a study of primary socialization and adult personality structure. Mead and Bateson's work in the 1930s has provided an excellent beginning to this task on Bali.

Attempts at cross-cultural generalization provide a corrective to the excesses of cultural relativism, without negating the significance of the latter. It is obvious that in some instances, notably in interpersonal crisis management, a consideration of 'exotic' and polyvalent symbols is of singular importance in understanding human behavior; but appreciation of their significance needs to be tempered with an appraisal of their role in the cultural mediation of universal human experience and the patterning of emotional life (Levy 1973; Connor 1979).

In this paper, I have neglected the latter enterprise in order to focus upon the cognitive constructs which Balinese invoke to conceptualize 'person'. Such an emphasis poses several imperative questions concerning a major problem in cross-cultural psychiatry and the intrusion of that enterprise into Balinese society. A brief reference to volcanic eruptions on the island illustrates the point. The anger of Balinese gods is held responsible by the populace for this frequently occurring phenomenon. This explanation warrants no attention from the science of vulcanology which analyzes and predicts such disasters. But surely madness is a different species of phenomenon? The subjective experience of self, coupled with Balinese belief in the manifold representations of the supernatural which pervade their lives, is analytically crucial to any explanation of why these people not only suffer from unbalanced psyches but also recover from such disturbances.

Hence, we must continue to ask whether Western psychodynamic theories can have heuristic value or offer real therapy in a culture which denies their basic conceptual foundation. There are some serious implications to the acceptance of the validity of psychotherapies tailored to specific non-Western cultural contexts (e.g., Kondo 1976; Murase, this volume), and of the increasingly widespread recognition of the value of traditional therapies. They provoke us to rethink the issues of whether psychiatric and psychological theorizing thereby becomes a species of ethnocentric reductionism when applied to other cultures; or whether on the other hand, the rejection of that enterprise condemns us to a variety of unproductive relativism.

ACKNOWLEDGMENTS

Fieldwork in Bali was carried out during the period November 1976 to November 1978, under the sponsorship of Lembaga Ilmu Pengetahuan Indonesia. Financial support was provided by an Australian Commonwealth Postgraduate Research Award, and by the Carlyle Greenwell Fund of the Anthropology Department, University of Sydney. This paper has benefited greatly from discussions with participants in the conference on 'Cultural Conceptions of Mental Health and Therapy', East-West Center, Hawaii, June 1980. I would also like to thank Anthony Forge, Arthur Kleinman, Ann McCauley, Moses Pounds, Anak Agung

Made Rai Rama, Adrian Vickers, Peter Worsley, Elizabeth Young and especially Douglas Miles for discussion of the ideas expressed here.

NOTES

1. That the old ideologies persisted alongside the new is argued by Gaines in this volume. To explore the consequences of this in the history of psychiatry is beyond the scope of this paper.
2. I use the term 'madness' without intending any pejorative overtones, as I prefer it to the more ethnocentric, and thus misleading term 'mental illness.'
3. *Balian*, like the Indonesian term *dukun*, is difficult to gloss in English with either word or phrase. The usual translation for both designations is 'traditional healer' and while I would argue that the functions of all *balians* are broadly therapeutic, they can be both flexibly 'modern' and far transcend the treatment of illness as it is understood in Western medicine. Broadly speaking, *balians* treat problems by their common function of mediating between the supernatural and human worlds.
4. For the purposes of formal surveys, there is a problem in defining what a *balian* is, given that their functions are varied and often diffuse, some are reluctant to label themselves as such, and some only operate in the confines of their own houseyard or kin group. For my purposes here I identify *balians* as those practitioners who receive clients for payment in cash, kind or labour, and who practice outside the confines of their own networks of close kin.
5. C. Geertz (1973) has presented a cultural phenomenology of 'person' using a different ethnographic data base. His concerns were not immediately with indigenous healers and therapies.
6. The functions of *balians* are loosely defined. Many rise on a wave of popularity and fall again. They may switch roles and take on new functions as their self-confidence and the endorsement of others increases. The supernatural power (*sakti*) which is considered necessary for these sorts of activities is of a generalized nature which may be turned to any one of a variety of vocations. Some named functions include: *balian usada* – literate specialists in reading and interpreting the lontar manuscripts; *balian manak* – village midwives; *balian uwut, balian apun, balian tulang* – experts in massage and the repair of broken bones; *balian tenung* – diviners; *balian paica* – those who heal by the use of sacred charms found in unusual circumstances; *balian tapakan, balian taksu, balian konteng* – spirit mediums.
7. 79.2% of mental hospital patients in my survey (Connor 1978) had previously consulted one or more *balians* prior to admittance. This may reflect an even larger number of cases who never consulted personnel at the mental hospitals. In none of the cases of breakdown and interpersonal stress which I encountered as first presentations at the houses of *balians*, was mental hospital treatment considered as an option, although in many chronic or recurrent cases, the patient had often been in and out of the mental hospital one or more times, or had received treatment as an outpatient, interspersed with *balians'* treatment.
8. However, adolescents and women, the most commonly afflicted, are considered to have 'weak' personalities which makes them more susceptible to such machinations.
9. In some areas, studies of traditional health care systems have been dominated by reliance on classical manuscripts. (For comments on this, see Lock, this volume.) In Bali, while such studies have been carried out, the textual material is relatively schematic, and I only resorted to it after two years of field study, when I was better able to appreciate its significance in relation to my ethnographic data. I discuss here only those concepts which became salient to my understanding in the observation of therapeutic interactions or discussing cases with *balians* and clients.

10. Many of these manuscripts were also secret up until recent decades. For a discussion of this, see Geertz (1964:297 ff).

11. Nor does this phrase differentiate gender. Some observers (e.g. Geertz 1973) have commented on the 'hermaphroditic' nature of Balinese sexual identity, based on their perceptions of a low level of sexual role differentiation. There is much contradictory evidence, but this observation is certainly borne out by the fact that females need not necessarily have all female spiritual siblings, and the same for men and, to foreshadow a later discussion, a reincarnating ancestor does not have to be of the same sex.

12. As the male and female aspects of deities are balanced and of equal importance, each becoming salient in different contexts, I have adhered to the rather clumsy construction 'his/her' in this translation. The Balinese language does not differentiate personal pronouns according to gender. The pronouns I have translated here are *ida* and *ia*.

13. *Uwat* (Indonesian *urat*) are the channels of the body thought to carry lifegiving fluids and to eliminate dangerous toxic substances. This includes but goes beyond the nerves, muscles and tendons.

   Space does not permit a discussion of humoral theories held by the Balinese in relation to bodily functioning. There is some discussion of this, based on lontar manuscripts, in Weck (1937).

REFERENCES

Bateson, G. and M. Mead
   1942 Balinese Character, A Photographic Analysis. New York: New York Academy of Sciences, Spec. Pub. No. 2.
Belo, J.
   1960 Trance in Bali. New York: Columbia University Press.
Connor, L. H.
   1978 Laporan Singkat Tentang Hasil Penelitian Pasien-Pasien Penyakit Jiwa di Bali. Majalah Psykiatri Jiwa (Indonesian Psychiatric Quarterly) 11:No. 4.
   1979 Corpse Abuse and Trance in Bali: The Cultural Mediation of Aggression. Mankind 12:104–118.
Covarrubius, M.
   1937 Island of Bali. New York: Alfred A. Knopf, Inc.
Ellenberger, H.
   1970 The Discovery of the Unconscious. London: Allen Lane.
Foucault, M.
   1971 Madness and Civilization: A History of Insanity in the Age of Reason. London: Tavistock.
Geertz, C.
   1964 Internal Conversion in Contemporary Bali. *In* Malayan and Indonesian Studies. J. Bastin and R. Roolvink (eds.). Oxford: Clarendon Press.
   1973 Person, Time and Conduct in Bali. *In* The Interpretation of Cultures. C. Geertz. New York: Basic Books.
Higginbotham, H. N.
   1979 Culture and the Delivery of Psychological Services in Developing Nations. Transcultural Psychiatric Research Review 16:7–27.
Hooykaas, C.
   1974 Cosmogony and Creation in Balinese Tradition. The Hague: M. Nijhoff.
Kleinman, A.
   1980 Patients and Healers in the Context of Culture. Berkeley: University of California Press.

Kondo, K.
  1976 The Origin of Morita Therapy. *In* Culture-Bound Syndromes, Ethno-Psychiatry, and Alternate Therapies. W. Lebra (Ed.). Honolulu: University Press of Hawaii.
Levy, R.
  1973 The Tahitians: Mind and Experience in the Society Islands. Chicago: University of Chicago Press.
Mershon, K.
  1971 Seven Plus Seven: Mysterious Life-Rituals in Bali. New York: Vantage Press.
Szasz, T. S.
  1973 The Manufacture of Madness. London: Paladin.
Thong, D.
  1976 Psychiatry in Bali. Australia and New Zealand Journal of Psychiatry 10:95–97.
Tonjaya, Ny. Gd. Bendesa K.
  1978 Kanda Patsari. Denpasar. Transcription from the Lontar.
Tugby, D., E. Tugby, and H. G. Law
  1976 The Attribution of Mental Illness by Rural Balinese. Australia and New Zealand Journal of Psychiatry 10:99–104.
Weck, W.
  1937 Heilkunde und Volkstum auf Bali. Stuttgart: F. Enke.
Young, E.
  1980 Topeng in Bali: Change and Continuity in a Traditional Drama Genre. Unpublished Ph.D. dissertation, University of California, San Diego.

11. SELF-RECONSTRUCTION IN JAPANESE RELIGIOUS PSYCHOTHERAPY

INTRODUCTION

Psychotherapy as a form of persuasion must satisfy two general conditions to achieve its efficacy. First, its repertoire of messages, whether in diagnosis or treatment, must be embedded in the culture of its client so that it can tap his memory stored through enculturation. Second, the therapeutic messages, while they should thus sound familiar, also need to offer something novel or even stunning to arouse their receiver's curiosity and to capture his imagination. One way of combining these two prerequisites is to single out, simplify, elaborate, or exaggerate a segment of the total cultural fund. Most of the religious cults in Japan, which are known for their claimed records of healing and deliverance of sufferers, utilize this method. This paper focuses on one of these cults and analyzes the experiences of its members with reference to their "self-reconstruction".

The therapeutic or "divine" messages of the cult, which are meant to induce self-reconstruction, are deeply embedded in Japanese culture, particularly in its moral values. At the same time, they hyperbolize what the average Japanese would believe and practice. This is why outsiders — non-member Japanese — tend to be ambivalent toward the cult: on the one hand, they are impressed with the strong faith and moral commitment exhibited by the cult members; but on the other, they find the member's behavior odd, eccentric, or even "insane". This hyperbole turns out, as we shall see, to involve a bias for feminine values.

Although data are drawn from this particular cult, it is assumed that what is presented here can hold for most other healing cults in terms of the underlying belief systems, if not specific therapeutic techniques and, to an extent, for non-religious ethnopsychotherapies as well.

THE CULT AND DATA GATHERING

The cult, which was introduced in my previous papers (Lebra 1974, 1976a, 1976b) as the Salvation Cult, is actually called *Gedatsukai*, meaning "a society for deliverance". Founded in 1929 by a former businessman, Gedatsukai (or simply Gedatsu hereafter) not only survived the disastrous Second World War but has expanded as one of hundreds of "new religions" under the religious hospitality of postwar Japan. According to its own report in 1975, its membership rose to nearly 200,000, with more than 400 "teachers" engaging in missionary work at some 360 churches or branches (Bunkacho 1976). The founder,

269

A. J. Marsella and G. M. White (eds.), Cultural Conceptions of Mental Health and Therapy,
269–283.

who died in 1948, is deified by his followers as "Sonja" (the most venerable one), or "Kongosama" derived from his posthumous name, "Gedatsu Kongo".

The Gedatsu is listed in the Shukyo Nenkan (yearbook of religions, published by Bunkacho, the Cultural Agency of the Japanese Government) as one of the Shingon Buddhist sects. The more amorphous sect called Shugendo, "the way of mastering magico-religious power" (Earhart 1970:ix), is also associated with Gedatsu's origins. According to Gedatsu superintendent Kishida (1964:56, and personal communication), the founder trained in the Shugendo and mastered magico-religious power, including that of healing. The Shugendo, supposedly started by a legendary figure called En no Ozunu in the late seventh century, represents a union of all religions — native and alien — with mystic emphasis. This eclectic legacy was fully inherited by the Gedatsu in that it accepts all conceivable supernatural entities as objects of worship. Gedatsu altars are occupied by imported Buddhas, native Shinto kami, dead humans, and the like. While national Shinto, as embodied by the Sun Goddess and her "descendants" (emperors), runs through its tenets, the Gedatsu is also faithful to local Shinto shrines which are generally identified as *ujigami*, and to the countless local *kami* (deities) associated with particular places or objects such as the water deity. Among animal deities, the fox and the snake are most often mentioned. Although the Gedatsu is preoccupied with the supernatural world and receptive to the mystic aspects of Taoism, the secular moral doctrine of Confucianism comprises an important part of Gedatsu teaching as well. Like all other Japanese cults, it manipulates the magical appeal of Chinese ideographs.

Most suggestive of its connection with the Shugendo and esoteric Shingon Buddhism is the possession ritual which is treasured as "unique" to the Gedatsu. In a dramatic setting in front of an altar, a leader, as a mediator between the spiritual and human worlds, invokes a spirit to enter a human host who is a member afflicted with illness or other disturbances and who seeks an explanation or treatment. Signaling its arrival by the sudden shaking of the hands of the host holding a charm, the spirit responds through the mouth of the host to the solicitous questions and requests of the mediator. The spirit thus discloses its identity — e.g., an ancestor, kami, or fox; male or female; its name, and so on. Oftentimes, as I observed, communication is facilitated by the mediator's offer of a binary choice of a yes or no answer as well as by sign communication allowed for a reticent spirit: the mediator may ask, "Are you an ancestor or kami? If you are a kami, raise your hands over your head; if an ancestor, stretch your hands straight forward." Once rapport is thus established, the spirit will reveal why its host is suffering from a particular problem, and give an instruction of what to do. When its message-providing mission is felt completed, the spirit is thanked and asked to return where it came from. If unwilling to leave, the spirit will receive *kundoki* (reproach) from the mediator. The whole ritual may be conducted by the mediator and host alone, but often is displayed like a theatrical performance in front of other members.

Intensive fieldwork was conducted during the summers of 1970 and 1971, centering around two ward branches of Eastern City, a provincial tourist town in central Japan. Membership of the two branches together was then estimated at about 200, each branch headed by an elderly woman. Young members were not totally absent — they were mostly children of the members — but a great majority was between the ages of 40 and 70.

The sex ratio of the participants varied depending upon the situations or activities. In registered membership, the number of women only doubled that of men (partly because some women still were in the habit of identifying themselves by the names of the househeads), but the attendance at branch meetings was in the ratio of about one to five in favor of female members; furthermore, in smaller, sub-branch gatherings and informal activities women were even more predominant. Conversely, "lecturers" sent from the cult's headquarters (*Honbu*) in Tokyo or from prefectual divisions were almost all male; so were the counsellors or teaching staff who were giving advice to the pilgrims at *Goreichi* (the cult's central shrine complex in Saitama Prefecture). The meeting at the headquarters which I observed, was attended by about 500 people with a ratio of one male to four females: the greater male representation here than at the local ward branches reflects the likelihood that more leaders attended the headquarters meetings. In short, it may be surmised that women are more predominant and active at a local level, in informal activities, or in the capacity of the rank and file; whereas their preponderance decreases at the center of the cult, in more formal, public activities, and is totally replaced by male predominance in central administration and teaching roles. It seems that males are motivated by chances for leadership to join or stay in the cult. Except for the central leadership, however, female predominance, in varying degrees, was observed in all situations and activities. This sex imbalance was a topic of discussion at a local meeting of ward "officers". The only male among 13 participants complained saying, "The most fundamental problem is that men do not attend. Whatever you say, after all it's men [who really count]. We must reflect upon our fault over this matter." The female officers agreed and admitted that male participation would be a measure of success of a ward branch.

Fieldwork included observations of meetings and rituals, participation in conversation with local members and leaders during intervals of formal activities, and interviews with 16 individuals (including two males). In addition, I observed activities at the headquarters and Goreichi, and interviewed several leaders and teachers stationed there. The cult's publications, especially members' autobiographical reports of their Gedatsu-inspired experiences which appear in every issue of the cult's monthly called Gedatsu,[1] were also consulted.

ASPECTS OF SELF-RECONSTRUCTION IN GEDATSU THERAPY

Self-Accusation

One of the primary messages which a Gedatsu inductee or member (female, unless otherwise specified) receives through her exposure to leaders, other members, meetings, rituals, or publications is that she blame herself for whatever plight she is experiencing. This pressure for self-accusation is deeply embedded in the Japanese moral system. DeVos found, in the TAT reponses by a sample of rural Japanese, self-blame as a major reaction to stress. For example: "A husband comes home very late at night; the wife thinks it is for her lack of her affection and tries hard; he finally reforms" (DeVos 1974:128); "An elder brother did something wrong and is examined by the policeman; he will be taken to the police station, but will return home and reform. The younger sister also thinks that she was wrong herself" (129). Sofue (1979:20) also delineates the Japanese "intropunitive" tendency on the basis of his sentence-completion-test results: in response to "I could not do it because . . . " the Japanese respondents tended to attribute the failure to the actor's fault such as "because I am not yet competent enough". The Japanese in general are socialized to reflect upon themselves (*hansei*) instead of accusing someone else suspected to be the source of frustration. A weekly hour of *hansei* used to be part of the school curriculum. *Hansei* is supposed to lead to guilt consciousness, remorsefulness, and apology. Lanham (1979:13) points out that a common ending of a story appearing in moral-education textbooks is a request for forgiveness or an apology, and that Little Red Riding Hood in a Japanese version has the fox tearfully ask for forgiveness.

As a step toward self-reconstruction, a Gedatsu member is persuaded not only to conform to this cultural norm of self-accusation but to go further in this direction. One's suffering is to be understood as a consequence of the sufferer's negligence of her duty as a daughter, wife, mother, descendant, or believer. A woman, suffering from whiplash of the neck vertebrae, learned from her acupuncturist, a member of the sect, that bone injury is caused by the victim's lack of gratitude to the gods. Furthermore, she was told that the location of the injured bone indicates what kind of virtue is deficient: injury above the neck means insufficiency of loyalty (*chu*), injury above the chest signifies that of filial piety (*ko*), injury above the abdomen is caused by the lack of benevolence (*jin*), and so on down to the foot, involving two more virtues — justice (*gi*) and courtesy (*reisetsu*).

Ego's fault causes others to suffer also. Put another way, one should blame oneself if someone else is in misery. In despair over her daughter who had been bedridden with an intestinal disease for 10 years, another informant consulted a Gedatsu teacher and was told that the mother was responsible for the child's illness. Thereupon, "I realized how wrong I had been, felt remorseful, and cried, kneeling to my sleeping daughter so that my head would touch her spirit." The daughter soon recovered, which convinced the mother that a parent's moral defect *is* transferred to the child. The informant's guilt turned out to involve her own responsibility as a daughter and sister: her elder brother, childless, wanted to adopt her as a daughter[2] and lavished fatherly love on her (including giving a bath for her); her father, too, expected her, in order to perpetuate the *ie*, the stem-family household, to stay on with the family as successor to her brother and bring in an adopted husband to marry, instead of her marrying out. Ignoring their wishes, she moved out of her natal house to marry. Her lack of filial devotion (*oya-fuko*) was the cause of her child's affliction, she persuaded herself.

Interpersonal conflicts, as in marital relationships, tend to be attributed to an undesirable characteristic of a member, i.e., a strong ego, greed, aggressiveness, hostility, grudge and the like. She would be told that whatever she saw in her husband, such as his promiscuity, was only a reflection of her own disposition, that her suffering was an indication of the return of a noxious element originally emitted from herself. A victim of someone's aggression, then, should be awakened to her own aggression. This logic I called "the repercussion postulate" in a previous paper (Lebra 1974). Even when wrongdoing is clearly attributed to another person, it is still ego who must apologize for "allowing the person to commit sin" (*tsumi o tsukuraseta*).

Self-accusation is sometimes displayed in the possession ritual. The following exchange took place, as I observed, between a local leader as a mediator and a member (retired schoolteacher) as a spirit host. (Note that during the ritual the mediator plays two combined roles: a mediator and the unpossessed half of the host as a substitute since the host herself performs the role of the possessing spirit.)

Mediator: Please show us how you are related to the *bontai* (secular body, namely, the host).
Spirit: Listen, I am the guardian spirit [of the *bontai*]! (This was said in an authoritative, masculine tone.)
Mediator: Thank you, sir, for using me daily. Thank you for your help. Would you like to give me any instruction or request?
Spirit: This is my command to be taken seriously. Do whatever with a strong conviction. Get ready with your belly.[3] I am still displeased with you. You never finish what you start. I am displeased. You are the worst kind. I hate you.
Mediator: I apologize. Please beat me with a whip and use me.

As soon as the ritual was over, the mediator resumed a leader's role which had been suppressed during the ritual, and reinforced the spirit message by telling the *bontai*, the message receiver, that her guardian spirit was really upset by her.

The hyperbolic self-blame is a common theme cutting across most healing cults. A ritual song of Tenrikyo to be chanted daily, for example, includes a passage like "Suffering is rooted in your own mind, blame not others, the fault is yours" (Thomsen 1963:47).

Allocentric Attribution

Paradoxical though it may sound, Japanese morality, along with self-directed aggression, stresses allocentric commitment involving the desirability of sensitivity to other people's feelings. One's experience is to be evaluated from another person's point of view (*aite no tachiba ni naru*): ego is supposed to be sensitive to the harm he may have done to alter. Such allocentricity further involves crediting alter, instead of ego, for a favorable consequence. This is where the ethic of *on* (beneficence) plays a crucial role to sensitize ego as a recipient of *on*. One's achievement should thus be attributed to a countless number of benefactors, known and unknown, alive and dead; every individual is born with an overwhelming debt to his forebears, to begin with (Benedict 1946; Lebra 1974, 1976c:101—107). Japanese guilt is anchored in this sense of indebtedness (Lebra 1971).

The causal agent is thus reversed from ego to alter. Self is no longer a subject but an object of action. This ties in with the general passivity and obscurity characterizing the Japanese self. Linguistically, the Japanese speaker often uses the "passive" or the "passive causative" as in "[I] was caused to think ... " instead of "I thought". Such expressions are not necessarily morally relevant; in fact they could serve as a means of attributing unpleasant outcomes to others as demonstrated by Niyekawa-Howard. In an attempt to establish a correlation between the grammatical options for the "adversative and passive causative" on the one hand and the sense of responsibility, Niyekawa-Howard discovered that "Japanese consistently showed a greater tendency to attribute responsibility to others than any other group tested [German, American, ethnic American]" (Niyekawa-Howard 1968:5).

Allocentric attribution and ego's passivity are elaborated in the Gedatsu, again, to an excessive degree. First, the Gedatsu follower is sensitized to her debts to all conceivable supernatural beings, forebears, people, and natural objects. Particularly important is the *on* owed to Sonja, leaders, fellow-members, especially those who brought one into the Gedatsu. Misfortune is often attributed to a lack of gratitude (*kansha*) as well as to a lack of remorsefulness (*zange*). Urami (*grudge*) then must be converted into *kansha* and *zange*.

Gratitude is owed not only for a beneficial experience but for an adversity without which one would remain blind to the "truth". So thanks are expressed to a promiscuous husband, a rebellious son, a mean mother-in-law for awakening ego to her oversight, egocentrism, godlessness, and so on; marital disharmony is to be accepted with gratitude as providing an opportunity to discipline oneself, and a child's sickness as a message from the supernatural world which eventually will benefit ego.

Passivity is exaggerated in causative-passive-polite-grateful forms, as such expressions innundate the members' speech and writings. *"Ikiru"* (live) becomes *"ikasasete itadaku"* (am caused to live by [gods'] benevolence). One would be told: "Don't think you are living (*ikiru*) by yourself, but be grateful for *ikasasete itadaku*." One of the autobiographical reports, picked up by chance, happens to use this grammatical form 28 times within four pages (*Gedatsu*, March 1973:54—57).[4] "I learn" (*manabu*) or "I realize" (*kizuku*) is rephrased, without exception, as *manabasete itadaku* or *kizukasete itadaku*. Even a leg injury was experienced as *ashi o orasete itadaku* (was caused to break my leg by [divine] benevolence).

Passivity of self as an object, further, takes the form of possession or being controlled by a supernatural being. Illness and other misfortunes, while they are imputed to ego's fault as discussed above, also turn out to be signs of supernatural influence which have nothing to do with ego's volition. The sufferer is "caused to realize" that her suffering is due to a spirit that is, by means of the suffering, giving her some instruction or appealing for her help. Such a spirit, which is usually recruited from among ancestors, dead humans, dead infants and fetuses (miscarried), or animal spirits representing "guardian spirits", is wandering and suffering because it has not attained Buddhahood or has lost a divine status (*shinkaku*), and is thus seeking human help for its own salvation. An infant's spirit may cause breast pain or cancer in its mother as a way of notifying its helplessness. Mental disorder or "the head disease", as an informant puts it, is most likely to be caused by an angry spirit of a fox or snake.

Self-reconstruction here involves self as an *on*-debtor, a receiver of supernatural messages, and an object of solicitation and reliance. Passivity ultimately reaches the point where self is no longer self. Again, this is nothing unique to the Gedatsu. In Tenrikyo such passivity is articulated in the doctrine of *kashimono-karimono* (things lent and borrowed) according to which everything that a human being possesses, including his body, has been lent by God the Parent (Thomsen 1963:52).

Identity Interchange

There appears to be a logical contradition between self-accusation and allocentric attribution in that one involves interiorization and the other exteriorization of the cause of illness. But for Gedatsu followers these two are consistent and complementary. What makes them compatible is the belief that there is no clear-cut demarcation line between self and other. The identity of self is actually interchangeable with that of another. Identity interchange is acceptable and morally plausible in Japanese culture insofar as identity is framed within the concept of social role. The ability or willingness to play another person's role, to act as if one were someone's parent (*oyagawari*), for example, is looked upon as a consequence of normal socialization. Furthermore, the cultural stress on solidarity and togetherness makes one susceptible to *ittaikan* (feeling of oneness) with another where one's self loses its boundary and melts into another's self. Identity interchange is also embedded in the Buddhist notion of *innen*, karmic bond of affinity, whereby one's identity is destined to replicate another's.[5] The *innen* usually, though not exclusively, connects two persons who are consanguineally related, such as parent and child, ancestor and descendant.

The Gedatsu psychotherapy manipulates this culturally acceptable identity interchange to, again, an extreme degree. First, one's behavior or suffering is often interpreted as a replica or "mirror reflection" of that of another. A "lecturer" tried to enlighten me by saying, "My wife's illness is mine; I am just borrowing her body. You really can't tell whose illness it is." More often, this kind of identity interchange involves a spirit: a daughter's disappearance from home is a replication of the behavior of her great-grandmother who led an unsettled life; one cries because an ancestor is crying; a daughter bleeds to near death because her great-grandfather (or great-grand uncle? the informant is not sure), drafted in the Sino-Japanese War (1894—95), is still bleeding.

Influence, furthermore, is mutually felt and exerted. If one's illness is a reflection of an ancestor's illness, the former, in turn, is reflected back onto the latter's mirror. A descendant's happiness then brings happiness for an ancestor, which then returns to the descendant, and so on, as if two mirrors were reflecting one another. Mutual reflection boils down to a complete overlap or fusion of two or more identities: "My ancestors, I, and my descendants — we are one and the same"; "Ancestor worship means self-worship." Underlying this reasoning is the assumption of the *innen* bond. Allocentric attribution, then, overlaps self-accusation in that as long as suffering lasts the sufferer should realize that an ancestor (or another spirit) is also suffering and she, the living sufferer, has been unable to alleviate the ancestor's suffering. That is not all. The sufferer must also blame herself for this negative *innen* to be inherited by her innocent children.

More elaborated in the Gedatsu beliefs and practices is identity interchange through role substitution. The spirit does not always cause suffering for the person for whom its message is meant, but may select another person as a substitute because the latter is more vulnerable, more responsive, more helpful, more attached to, or more strongly *innen*-bonded. A dead woman who has lost her way tries to draw attention from her son and daughter-in-law by causing mental disorder in her grandson simply because the latter is smarter than the parents. (This bright grandson, to the parents' astonishment, fell sudden victim to school phobia and joined a group of "hippies" on a mountain, but later returned home after the mother's "sincere" compliance with Gedatsu instructions.)

The substitutive role further involves the role of the vicarious sinner. The spirit which causes suffering for the living often turns out to have committed *tsumi* (sin) while it was in this world. A variety of *tsumi* is mentioned including homicide (usually by samurai ancestors), suicide (most often the unreciprocated love suicide by women), polluting a god-governed place with blood (for this reason any kind of bleeding is considered *tsumi*), power and greed with which the poor were exploited. What stands out among my informants is *shikijo no tsumi*, sin of sexual emotion, which takes various forms — adultery, rape, love suicide, divorce, remarriage, abortion, miscarriage, menstruation (killing eggs as well as polluting), and the like. The sinner is punished by an enraged god (or gods) and thus prevented from salvation. The sufferer in this world then turns out to be vicariously punished for the sin committed by a spirit: "Whenever I encounter trouble, I decide one of my ancestors committed a sin." The sexual sin by an ancestor is manifested in a variety of punishments for a descendant: gynecological disorders, uterine or breast cancer, sterility, miscarriage, unhappy marriage, concubinage, repeated divorce and remarriage, involuntary celibacy, and the like. Interestingly, interviews reveal that punishment may take the form of impotence or frigidity. Note that there is partial overlap between the sin and its punishment; miscarriage, for example, is both sin and punishment. This makes sense because the "real sinner" and the vicarious sinner are linked by *shikijo no innen* (*innen* of sexual emotion) which makes one replicate the other.

To redeem sin, the vicarious sinner and sufferer must repent and offer apologies to gods, usually stationed in one of *ujigami* or other local shrines, again as a substitute for the sinner. *Owabi* (apology) offering in such a substitutive capacity is a major part of the discipline and rituals of Gedatsu. In front of the shrine, *owabi* is made with a vocal statement like "I apologize from the bottom of my heart as a substitute (*narikawatte*) for my ten-generation old ancestor, Matsuda Taro, for his *tsumi* in lacking respectfulness, faithfulness, and virtuousness. Please kindly forgive me." This vocal apology is reinforced by a written apology on a piece of paper (*wabijo*) submitted to the shrine. *Owabi* further involves *ohyakudo* (hundred times), meaning walking up and down to and from the shrine a hundred times to demonstrate the sincerity of the *owabi*-maker: "stepping *ohyakudo*" for Gedatsu means *owabi* offering. The shrine visit for *owabi* is repeated for as many days and as early in the moring (e.g., before dawn) as prescribed by the spirit through the possession ritual. Usually the spirit accompanies its substitute, but is so helpless that all initiative is taken by the substitute.

When the apology ritual is completed, the spirit may reappear in a possession ritual to inform its attainment of salvation and express its gratitude. The spirit is now ready to accept *kuyo* (nurturance through sutra, food, and special tea called *amacha*). The vicarious sinner is now able to take the role of a nurturant caretaker for the spirit.

Identity interchange thus involves a devotee to slip in and out of different identities, to assume multiple roles, and to split one identify into two. Indeed, some of the observed possession rituals revealed a vacillation between two levels of communication — spiritual and mundane — symbolized by formal and informal speech styles as well as high and low vocal pitches. In one such ritual, the host, after struggling hard to identify the possessing spirit, switched to her mundane role to confess, "I don't know". The mediator, irritated, became increasingly authoritative and insisted that the spirit be identified. On the basis of fragments of a sign message, the mediator finally worked out the information that the spirit was a seven-generation old male ancestor of the host. But of which household, the host's husband's or her natal one? The mediator began to ask, "Are you of the Yoshida House or", but could not recall the other name. Lowering her voice, and in a casual speech style, she asked the host, "What is your natal family's name?" This mundane question was answered immediately: "It's Watanabe". The pair then restored formality to resume spiritual conversation. The whole drama reminded me of ventriloquy.

The Gedatsu offers a special ritual which symbolizes identity-split in an unequivocal form. Every individual is believed, at least potentially, to carry his/her personal guardian spirit and assume its status. The status of the guardian spirit is promoted through its training at Goreichi. This is done by holding a sending-off ritual at a local shrine where some other members also participate. Upon completion of the training which lasts three weeks or so, the spirit returns to the same local shrine where the host and fellow-members gather to welcome the trainee back. During the spirit's absence, the host is supposed to go through the same kind of ascetic discipline at home as does the spirit at Goreichi. The returnee spirit, now accorded with a higher status, promotes the status of its host. The sending-off ritual and welcoming ritual seem to punctuate identity-split and identity-reunion.

Expurgation

Self-reconstruction through a hyperbolic version of self-accusation, allocentric attribution, and identity interchange, still remains incomplete without this final treatment — expurgation.[6] Purification constitutes the core of Shinto ritual, and the state of emptiness is a Buddhist ideal. The ultimate moral value in Japanese culture is represented by the pure heart, *magokoro* (true, sincere heart), *muga* (ego-lessness), or *mushin* (mind-lessness). What upsets the individual's health is the accumulation of impurities in him, which in turn are ingredients of ego itself. Removal of *ga* (ego) itself then is necessary for cure. Freedom from *ga* or attainment of *muga* or *mushin* entails a union of self with its environment or self's submission to nature.

The *Gedatsu*, like all other cults, stresses the need of abandoning *ga*, saying that obsessions with "I" are the cause of all troubles. Expurgatory rituals (*okiyome*) must be conducted to attain an empty self. Among such rituals is meditation which is required of every new convert. In the "right" sitting style (with legs folded under the torso), one joins one's hands at eye level with a charm held between the palms, eyes closed. The meditation ritual, either in a group or individually is repeated until purification is felt completed. Only after that is a convert entitled to host a spirit in the possession ritual. Otherwise the possession ritual could be as dangerous as "a madman carrying a knife".

Not only one's self but spirits must be cleansed for reasons made clear in the above analysis. In the logic of identity interchange, the expurgation of spirits means that of self, as well as vice versa. The spirits which are in need of purification are believed to hang on the *ihai* (mortuary tablets) which are placed in a pail at the alter of the household or the branch church. The expurgatory ritual for the spirits consists of repeatedly pouring *amacha* (the sacred tea) over the *ihai* while reciting a sutra. The Gedatsu goes to an extreme in expecting this ritual to take effect in a literal form: the spirits, under this *amacha* treatment, squeeze impurities out of themselves, which is verified by the defilement of the water: the muddier the water, the more purged and therefore "joyous" the spirits are. Gedatsu followers, thus, tell one another how thick their *amacha* has turned out. *Amacha* as a purgatory medium is also poured over whatever is believed to be a spirit's residence. Not only gravestones, but car tires also receive *amacha* treatment as they are regarded as causing traffic accidents because of polluted spirits hanging onto them.

Amacha turns out not just to wash away the pollutions on the surface of a spirit's body but to be consumed by the spirit, thereby purifying its internal system and expelling impurities out of the system. This belief is applied to human beings as well. *Amacha* is available for human consumption so that its drinker can clean up her physiological system − circulatory, digestive, eliminatory, etc. *Amacha* contains hydrangea which is evidently diuretic. Here is an equation between the spiritual and bodily expurgation, or between a metaphorical and literal meaning.

In addition to *amacha*, the cult prescribes "health foods", which are obtainable at the store run by the cult. A high rate of consumption of these foods can be inferred from the hyperactive trading observed at a local ward branch between the leader as a "middleman" and the followers buying them. When I visited the store, it had roughly 40 kinds of foods including a variety of tea, soybean products (bean paste, soy sauce), sesame seeds and oil, and seaweeds. All are supposed to be "natural foods" devoid of preservatives or other "artificial poisons". The most important among these seems to be *genmai*, unmilled brown rice. Again, its function is not so much nutritional as expurgatory. "Having a right diet," says a local member, "that is the shortest way to find yourself on the right track. *Genmai*, its germs in particular, has power to push everything filthy and harmful out of your body." The same belief apparently pertains to all other foods sold at the store. The business manager of the store stressed in the interview that all those foods are meant to cleanse the blood, to eliminate "poisons". In his view, clean blood and smooth elimination are essential to health maintenance.

The Gedatsu also runs its "health schools" and a "medical research institute". In an office of the latter, I was introduced to a machine whose vacuum glass balls, applied to the afflicted part of a patient's body, supposedly sucks poison out of his blood, as proven, said a "doctor", through the glass blackened and air fouled.

The expurgatory therapy, which runs across all aspects of Gedatsu beliefs and practices, is further based upon the assumption that everybody is clean and healthy as long as he is left in nature, that illness is a result of the entry of unnatural elements, such as drugs, into the body. What is important is to go along with the law of nature, to be united with nature, or to dissolve self into nature. "To purify yourself means to harmonize yourself with nature." This "naturalism" joins hands with the abandonment of egoistic self or attainment of *muga*.

CONCLUSION

This paper analyzed a type of psychotherapy developed and practiced by a

Japanese healing cult with a focus on self-reconstruction. Four aspects of self-reconstruction were delineated — self-accusation, allocentric attribution, identity interchange, and expurgation. It was noted that each of these is embedded in Japanese culture and is also exaggerated in the cult's teaching. All four aspects end up reinforcing in a hyperbolic manner the Japanese moral ideal of selflessness, self-denial, or self-abandonment.

Whether this kind of faith healing can be called "psychotherapy" or should be labeled "psychopathology", may be a matter of opinion. It should be reminded, however, that the above description of Gedatsu healing is not quite alien to some other non-religious ethnopsychotherapies which are perfectly respectable to professional psychiatrists. Naikan (Yoshimoto 1965; Okumura et al. 1972; Murase 1974, and this volume; Lebra 1976c:201—214), for example, concentrates on building up guilt in the client involving self-accusation and allocentric preoccupation. The acceptance of *arugamama* (things as they are) stressed in Morita therapy (Kora and Sato 1958; Morita 1960; Kora 1965; Kondo 1966; Lebra 1976c:215—231) overlaps Gedatsu therapy insofar as it recommends the acceptance of illness as fate, obedience to nature, and self-dissolution into nature. Yokoyama (1974), who was influenced by Morita and is practicing *seiza ryoho* (therapy by sitting), would sound familiar to Gedatsu followers when he recommends a renunciation of egocentric wishes, a replacement of one's mind with that of a baby, a development of infinite attachment to nature "as much as to be able to comprehend the language spoken by rice plants or wheat plants" (Yokoyama 1974:138). Further, both Naikan and Morita therapy in one phase intensify what might be regarded as pathological, as the Gedatsu does. If these therapies use the subsequent release of tension thus built up as a therapeutic leverage, so does the Gedatsu through confessions and expurgatory rituals and practice. The *innen* bond is recognized only to be nullified; the spirit is cared for only to become inactive. Naikan, Morita therapy, the Gedatsu and many other ethnopsychotherapies, religious and secular, all unite in stressing the renunciation of *ga* (ego — intellectual, emotional, or willful).

Despite these similarities, Gedatsu therapy is different from those mentioned above, most of all, in its manipulation of the supernatural hemisphere. Its therapeutic potentials may indeed derive from this difference since identity interchange with supernatural entities expands a spectrum of role options for self-reconstruction. If many psychiatric patients are driven by *amae* (dependency wish) as Doi (1974:146) claims about his patients, the option of taking the role of a helpless spirit may gratify the *amae* wish.

Another point of difference involves the feminine bias of the Gedatsu clientele. I speculate, as the final point of conclusion, on a link between the Gedatsu-inspired self-reconstruction and womanhood. It seems that female dispositions and/or expectations are played up in self-accusation, allocentric attribution, and identity interchange. Women are expected to be less self-assertive, less autonomous, more passive, and their identity more "relational" (Chodorow

1974). Motherhood in particular is exalted in the Gedatsu teaching and acted out in Gedatsu rituals. Maternal nurturance is symbolized by a member's care-taking ritual for an infant-like spirit; the woman's double identity of mother and child is acted out by her vicarious guilt and apology for the sake of a spirit.

A woman who is not feminine or maternal is, therefore, sanctioned against more severely than a male counterpart. A domineering wife is reminded of her place, and a voluntarily childless woman is accused of committing a grave sin. Traditional sex roles are thus imposed more upon females than males. The question remains whether this emphasis on femininity, motherhood, or female-role norms is peculiar to the Gedatsu and similar cults or whether the Japanese moral system tends to be skewed toward femininity which is only exaggerated by these cults. I prefer to leave the question open.

ACKNOWLEDGMENTS

I am indebted to H. Byron Earhart for correcting the errors which appeared in the original draft concerning the cult reported on here, and for making further suggestions. While some of his comments were incorporated, accountability for further errors and oversights is exclusively mine. I acknowledge the support from the National Institute of Mental Health (Grant MH-09243) for fieldwork on Gedatsukai, National Science Foundation (Grant BN76-11301) and Japan Society for the Promotion of Science for research on women, and University of Hawaii Japan Studies Endowment (funded by a grant from the Japanese Government) for the preparation of this manuscript. Thanks are also due to Linda Kimura and Freda Hellinger for their research assistance, editing, and typing.

NOTES

1. The two series of autobiographical testimonials are titled: *"Omoide"* (Recollections) and *"Yomigaetta jinsei"* (Revival).
2. Adoption of a younger sibling as a child and successor was not uncommon in prewar Japan.
3. The belly (*hara*) as the locus of the spiritual and bodily center is often referred to in Japanese speech particularly in the context of moral training.
4. See note 1.
5. The term *innen* is also used indiscriminately to refer to any kind of relationship, including a meeting of strangers.
6. The term "expurgation" is chosen, instead of the more common "purification", to convey the drastic nature of the cleansing process under discussion.

REFERENCES

Benedict, R.
    1946 The Chrysanthemum and the Sword: Patterns of Japanese Culture. Boston: Houghton Mifflin.

Bunkacho (National Cultural Agency).
  1976 Shukyo nenkan (Yearbook of Religion).
Chodorow, N.
  1974 Family Structure and Feminine Personality. *In* Woman, Culture and Society.
       M. S. Rosaldo and L. Lamphere (eds.). Stanford: Stanford University Press.
DeVos, G.
  1974 The Relation of Guilt Toward Parents to Achievement and Arranged Marriage
       among the Japanese. *In* Japanese Culture and Behavior: Selected Readings. T. S.
       Lebra and W. P. Lebra (eds.). Honolulu: University Press of Hawaii.
Doi, L. T.
  1979 Amae: A Key Concept for Understanding Japanese Personality Structure. *In*
       Japanese Culture and Behavior: Selected Readings. T. S. Lebra and W. P. Lebra
       (eds.). Honolulu: University Press of Hawaii.
Earhart, H. B.
  1970 A Religious Study of the Mount Harugo Sect of Shugendo. Tokyo.
Kishida, E.
  1964 Gedatsu Kongo to sono kyogi (Gedatsu Founder and His Teaching). Tokyo:
       Gedatsukai.
Kondo, A.
  1966 Morita ryoho (Morita Therapy). Seishin Igaku (Clinical Psychiatry) 8:707–
       715.
Kora, T.
  1965 Morita Therapy. International Journal of Psychiatry 1:611–645.
Kora, T. and K. Sato
  1958 Morita Therapy: A Psychotherapy in the Way of Zen. Psychologia 1:219–225.
Lanham, G.
  1979 Ethics and Moral Precepts Taught in Schools of Japan and the United States.
       Ethos 7:1–18.
Lebra, T.
  1971 The Social Mechanism of Guilt and Shame: The Japanese Case. Anthropological
       Quarterly 44:241–255.
  1974 The Interactional Perspective of Suffering and Curing in a Japanese Cult. Inter-
       national Journal of Social Psychiatry 20:281–286.
  1976a Anchestral Influence on the Suffering of Descendents in a Japanese Cult. *In*
       Ancestors. W. H. Newell (ed.). The Hague: Mouton Publishers.
  1976b Taking the Role of the Supernatural 'Other': Spirit Possession in a Japanese
       Healing Cult. *In* Culture-Bound Syndromes, Ethnopsychiatry and Alternate
       Therapies. W. P. Lebra (ed.). Honolulu: University Press of Hawaii.
  1976c Japanese Patterns of Behavior. Honolulu: University Press of Hawaii.
Morita, S.
  1960 Shinkeishitsu no hontai to ryoho (The Essential Characteristics and Therapy of
       Shinkeishitsu). Tokyo: Hakuyosha.
Murase, T.
  1974 Naikan therapy. *In* Japanese Culture and Behavior: Selected Readings. T. S. Lebra
       and W. P. Lebra (eds.). Honolulu: University Press of Hawaii.
Niyekawa-Howard, A.
  1968 A Psycholinquistic study of the Whorfian Hypothesis Based on the Japanese
       Passive. Paper Presented at the 13th Annual National Conference on Linguistics.
       New York.
Okumura, N., K. Sato, and H. Yamamoto, eds.
  1972 Naikan ryoho (Naikan Therapy). Tokyo: Igaku Shoin.

Sofue, T.
  1979 Aspects of the Personality of Japanese, Americans, Italians, and Eskimos: Comparisons Using the Sentence Completion Test. The Journal of Psychological Anthropology 2:11–52.
Thomsen, H.
  1963 The New Religions of Japan. Tokyo: Charles E. Tuttle Co.
Yokoyama, K.
  1974 Seiza ryoho (Therapy by Sitting). Osaka: Sogensha.
Yoshimoto, I.
  1965 Naikan yonjunen (Forty Years of Naikan). Tokyo: Shunjusha.

DAVID Y. H. WU

12. PSYCHOTHERAPY AND EMOTION IN TRADITIONAL CHINESE MEDICINE

INTRODUCTION

The purpose of this paper is to examine the role of emotion constructs and psychotherapy in the conceptualization of mental health in traditional Chinese medicine. The discussion makes suggestions for possible future studies of cultural resources which might prove useful for the improvement of mental health care both in Chinese society as well as in comparative, cross-cultural psychiatry.

Traditional Chinese medicine is perceived by scholars as deficient in psychological treatment. Western ethnomedical studies view Chinese medicine as lacking psychotherapy in its healing procedures, although psychiatric conceptualization in terms of Western models can be found in classical literatures of Chinese medicine (Tseng 1973). Tseng points out that for instance, as late as the turn of this century, Chinese treatment of insanity was by and large herb-oriented in spite of a growing knowledge of psychiatric concepts (Tseng 1973:572). Treatment of psychological and physical disorders in Chinese medicine was through acupuncture, moxibustion, and other measures intended to restore internal harmony (Croizier 1968:19, quoted in Dunn 1976:146). Contemporary examples of these treatment methods can be found in Lock's recent ethnographic studies (Lock 1980) of traditional Chinese medicine in Japan. Ethnomedical studies carried out in Taiwan and in overseas Chinese communities often mention that Chinese mental patients distrust 'talk therapy" (Kleinman 1977:8; 1980:95; Kleinman and Lin 1980). Somatization of psychological problems is characteristic of Chinese patients according to recent psychiatric findings (Tseng 1975; Kleinman 1977; Lin and Lin 1980). Indeed, Chinese patients to this day are described as only trusting treatments with physical ingredients, such as herbs, or food, or therapies which involve active intervention, such as healing rituals (Kleinman 1980:95; Lee 1980).

It is interesting to note that these findings on Chinese medical practices are contradictory to a fundamental principle of Chinese medicine which emphasizes the psychological etiology of disease. A search through Chinese medical texts shows that a psychological approach is an important aspect of the health care system. This paper discusses the following four aspects of the use of psychotherapy in professional Chinese medicine.

(1) The concept of health and health care as expressed in classical Chinese texts emphasizes the relationship between the state of a person's mind and the state of his health. This relationship is especially prominent in the explanation of the effect of human emotion on pathology.

(2) There are numerous historical cases of legendary treatment through

A. J. Marsella and G. M. White (eds.), Cultural Conceptions of Mental Health and Therapy,
285–301.

psychotherapy by famed physicians. These cases can be found in scattered historical documents, local gazettes, personal diaries, and short stories. This paper reviews a number of such cases.

(3) There is the belief that formally trained Chinese physicians ought to take into consideration the patient's psychological condition and personal history in their diagnosis of illness. This concerns the method of "Four Diagnoses methods" (Ssu-chen)-*wen, wang, wen*, and *ch'ieh*, or interrogation, inspection, auscultation/olfaction, and palpation as translated by Porkert (1976:67).

(4) It is recognized among students of Chinese medicine that preventive measures rather than the curing of disease is the essence of Chinese medical care (Needham 1970; Wu 1979; and Lock 1980:44—45). Traditional Chinese hygiene stresses the importance of a balanced or disciplined life, regulation of emotions and desires, a balanced diet, and adjustment to physical changes. In other words, measures that promote, in modern terminology, mental health are regarded as more desirable in health care maintenance than remedial measures which involve medicine, treatment, or "patching up" through food (Wu 1979).

TRADITIONAL CHINESE CONCEPTIONS OF BODY AND HEALTH

To understand fully the relationship between mind and body in traditional Chinese medical theory requires a discussion of a large body of literature dealing with the place of humans in the universe, the correspondence of body and nature, and the function of mind and body in relation to health. It is beyond the scope of the present paper to undertake the task of a thorough review of this complicated philosophical and medical system. A summary of these medical theories and concepts has been provided in many published works, both in Chinese and English (Wong and Wu 1935; Chen 1937; Tseng 1973; Pa'los 1971; Kleinman et al. 1971; Leslie 1976; Bridgman 1974; Kleinman 1980; Lee 1980; Lin 1980; and Lock 1980). A review of some of the basic components in the conceptual framework of Chinese medicine will enable us to see the role of mind and emotion in medical treatment. According to the classical framework of Chinese medical systems, six components of Chinese physiology and pathology are recognized: the Yin-Yang principle, health and organism, the vital substances in the body, the *ching-lo* systems, disease etiology, and diagnosis and treatment (Jen-min 1974).

The fundamental principle of the Chinese conception of health concerns Yin-Yang and five universal elements. A sound mind will contribute to the balance of Yin and Yang, while good health depends on the equilibrium of five basic emotions and organs (Jen-min 1974:1—5).

The second component concerns the five Yin viscera and six Yang intestinal organs as the key to understanding body physiology. The five viscera comprise an interdependent system. This interdependence can be described in terms of the notion of "complementary opposition" used by anthropologists to describe social structural relationships (cf. Levi-Strauss 1963). While each of the internal organs is believed to be responsible for a particular bodily function, and each correlates with an external manifestation of the human body, the heart is considered the master of all five viscera and six intestinal organs. The heart is also believed to govern all mental activities, perceptions, and nervous activities. Malfunction of the heart in terms of symbolic imbalance may cause palpation, apprehension, memory loss, insomnia, insanity, delirium and other mental disorders.

The third essential component necessary to understand Chinese medical concepts concerns the vital substances of life, namely, ch'i, blood, semen (ching), and saliva/body liquid. The vital substances that fill the body and organs are also classified according to Yin and Yang. Ch'i and Ching (semen in a broad sense) must complement one another to maintain bodily balance, as the former is Yin and the latter Yang.

The fourth component for understanding the body in Chinese medicine concerns Ching-lo systems or "meridians". According to Chinese medical beliefs, the meridians circulate through the body; Ching-lo, which is invisible in modern anatomical terms, consists of vital points underneath the skin for acupuncture. Ching-lo connect all parts of the human body and channel ch'i — vital essence — and blood. It is believed that if ch'i becomes weak, then disease will invade the body and result in sickness.

Disease etiology is the fifth component within which emotion plays a part. Chinese categorization of the causes of disease differentiates between internal and external causes. Six evils (liu-yin), wind, cold, heat, wetness, dryness, and fire (internal), are the main external causes of disease. The internal causes are classified into three main categories; the seven emotions, irregularity of food and drink, and fatigue. The following discussion concentrates on pathology and the seven emotions: joy, anger, worry, contemplation, sorrow (grief), apprehension, and fright, which are of central interest to our discussion.

Emotion and Pathology

Excessive emotional activity (or condition) may cause imbalance of Yin and Yang, ch'i and blood, ching and lo blockage and malfunction of the organs, and thus result in illness. This theory was explained in the classical text of *Huang-ti Nei-ching Su-wen* or *The Yellow Emperor's Esoteric Canon* which, for two thousand years, has served as the bible of Chinese medicine. Even today this particular text dominates the thinking of Chinese practitioners and laypersons. Over a period of two thousand years, no less than 50 works based on this text have been written by scholars and practitioners, but they did little more than offer commentary or translation (Wong and Wu 1935:23; Porkert 1976). An examination of this original text may therefore reveal fundamental aspects of the Chinese theory of mind, body, and disease etiology (Veith 1972).[1]

On the principle of Yin—Yang and human emotion, we found entries in section five of Chapter Two entitled "The Great Treatise on the Interaction of Yin and Yang" (Veith 1972).

"Nature has four seasons and five elements. In order to grant a long life the four seasons and the five elements store up the power of creation within cold, heat, excessive dryness, moisture, and wind ...
  Man has five viscera in which these five climates are transformed to great joy, anger, sympathy (*sorrow*), grief (*worry*), and fear ...
  The emotion of joy and anger are injurious to the spirit, cold and heat are injurious to the body. Violent anger is hurtful to Yin, violent joy is hurtful to Yang ... When joy and anger are without moderation, then cold and heat exceed all measure and life is no longer secure. Yin and Yang should be respected to an equal extent" (117).

The relationship between a specific emotion and an organ is also explained in the same chapter.

"Anger is injurious to the liver, but sympathy (*sorrow*) counteracts anger" (118). "Extravagant joy is injurious to the heart, but fear counteracts happiness" (119). "Extreme grief (*worry*) is injurious to the lungs, but joy counteracts grief" (120). "Extreme sympathy is injurious to the stomach (*spleen*), but anger counteracts sympathy" (*contemplation*)" (119). "Extreme fear is injurious to the kidneys, but fear can be overcome by contemplation" (120). [Italicized words in parentheses are my translations. Contemplation should be closer in meaning to the original word, "*su*", in the text. Tseng (1973:572) translates the word into "brooding".]

  The interaction of emotion and the five viscera that cause disease is further explanation in Chapter Six, "Treatise on the Precious Mechanism of the Viscera".

Hence, when joy is felt it creates a large vacuum, and thus the force of the kidneys can ascend. The emotion of anger arises from the fullness of the liver. The emotion of sympathy arises from the fullness of the lungs. The emotion of fear releases the impulses of the spleen. The feeling of worry releases the impulses of the heart (Veith 1972:181).

  It is clear that not only may excessive emotion cause imbalance of the physical harmony of the body, but it also may damage the function of the organs and thus cause illness. The ancient text mentions disease names which denote insanity, stress, and epilepsy and attributes their cause to emotion and loss of the normal balance of Yin and Yang. On the disease of *k'uang*, hysteria or madness:

Ch'i Po said: "Yin stores up essence and prepares it to be used; Yang serves as protector against external danger and must therefore be strong". If Yin is not equal to Yang, then the pulse becomes weak and sickly and causes madness (*Treatise on the Communication of the Force of Life with Heaven*, Veith 1972:108).

On the disease of *feng-chüe*, insanity, or paralysis:

Huang Ti said: "The body is afflicted by diseases where perspiration appears and where (the patient) is troubled by fullness. This trouble of fullness does not cause the perspiration to be released; how does it affect the illness?" Ch'i Po answered: "When perspiration appears and the body is hot there will be insanity (wind). When perspiration appears and the trouble of fullness is not dispersed, there will be convulsions (*chüe*). The name of the disease indicates paralysis and convulsions (*feng-chüe*)" (Veith translated the word *feng* which literally means either wind or insanity as paralysis) (*Commentary on the Treatise on the 'Warm Illness'*, Veith 1972:248).

In this case, acupuncture and medicine are recommended as treatment. Other minor mental disorders attributed to *chüe* are *chien-chüe* and *po-chüe* which involve distress and dizziness are:

> When the force of Yang is exhausted under the pressure of overwork and weariness, then the essence (of the body) is cut short, the openings of the body are obstructed and the secretions are retained. This causes sickness in summer and *distress (chien-chüe)* . . . If the atmosphere of Yang is exposed to great anger, the force of life of the body is interrupted and the blood rushes upwards and causes *dizziness (po-chüe)* . . . The essence of the force of Yang protects the spirit, its gentleness protects the muscles (*Treatise on the Communication of the Force of Life with Heaven*, Veith 1972:106–107).

Chien-chüe, with reference to being anger prone is discussed in a later part of the text on "The Explanation of Pulse" (Jen-min 1978:269):

> There are those who are short of *ch'i* and prone to anger. This is because the force of Yang-*ch'i* is not in force. When Yang-*ch'i* is not proper the force of Yang cannot be released. Then the essence of liver which is supposed to be normal but unable to achieve makes the man become easy to get angry. A man who is prone to anger is called *chien-chüe*.

Further explanation on the etiology of *k'uang* indicates that anger is a disease symptom of insanity — *yang-chüe*. This is found in the later chapter of the text entitled *Treatise on the Function of Diseases* (for which Veith did not complete the translation).

> The Emperor said: "There are those who suffer from the sickness of violent (or insane) anger; how is the sickness originated?" Ch'i Po said: "It origines from Yang." The Emperor said: "How could Yang make a man mad (*k'uang*)?" Ch'i Po said: "The *ch'i* of Yang is due to the block of violence which makes it impossible to release. It therefore makes a man prone to anger. The name of this disease is *yang-chüe*. '

As a measure of curing, Ch'i Po suggested, "To take away his food then the disease would be cured. When the food intrudes Yin, it will nourish the *ch'i* of Yang. Thus when the food is stopped the disease will stop" (Tseng's article (1973:570) mentions this treatment of 'excited insanity').

The contemporary Chinese professional interpretation of *k'uang* and *tien* refers to the latter as the depressed type of mental disorder and to the former as the excited type (Jen-min 1974:527). When acupuncture is recommended as treatment, emphasis is placed on determination of the organs that correspond to certain emotions in order to locate particular acupunctural points. For instance,

> Too much joy causes *tien* and too much anger causes *k'uang*. Joy belongs to heart, while anger belongs to liver . . . Thus for *k'uang* needle should be placed on the point for kidney and liver. For *tien* needle should be placed on points for kidney and heart . . .

Because of these beliefs about emotions as important causes or symptoms of disease, counter emotions are used in the treatment of "mental patients". This is shown in the following discussion of clinical episodes.

EMOTION AND PSYCHOTHERAPY: CASE ILLUSTRATIONS

Since one type of emotion can counteract another type of emotion, illness caused by emotion is believed curable by inducing a counter emotion. Based on this simple principle, Chinese physicians have applied a psychological approach in the treatment of patients. Although psychotherapy is seldom discussed in medical texts, we can find examples in historical documents, popular literature and personal notes. However, this information is not readily accessible without a pain-staking search in numerous sources, an indication of the fact that psychotherapy is not a prominent part of popular medicine, but rather a special aspect of professional and scholarly views of treatment. I located some of these examples in the writings of a Chinese physician (Chen 1959) and a medical historian (Liu 1974). These examples outline sickness episodes, disease categories, and cognitive processes of therapeutic actions that support the above discussed ancient medical theory. Fifteen episodes in all are cited below. The Chinese physician (Chen 1959) classifies these clinical episodes into three categories in terms of type of treatment: (1) application of the balance theory of emotion, (2) treatment of "sickness with longing", and (3) treatment of delusion-induced illness.

Balance and Imbalance

On the treatment of "emotional diseases", a Chinese physician explained: "There is nothing special but to apply the principle of balance — to increase the positive force for the negative, and the negative for the positive" (Chen 1959: 66). In other words, from an emic, cultural conception, Chinese physicians adhere to the principle of *Nei-Ching* in correcting excessive or inadequate emotion; to balance cold emotion with heat emotion (or force), or vice versa . . . I shall comment on this explanation after examining the following six cases to exemplify the treatment of affective determined sickness:

   (1) (Famed doctor Wen Chi) The king of Ch'i had been sick. He sent for Wen Chi from Sung State (Wen was a renowned doctor of Sung State). After he had examined the king, Wen Chi explained to the prince, "I am certain the king's disease can be cured. However, as soon as the king is cured he surely will kill me." The prince asked him why. Wen Chi replied, "The king's illness cannot be cured unless he is angered; yet, when I make the king angry I will surely lose my life." The prince bowed to him and insisted that he proceed with the necessary treatment. Wen Chi approached the king, and without taking off his shoes he mounted the king's bed and put the king's clothes on himself. The king was angered and refused to speak to him. Chi then deliberately said something to offend the king further. The king jumped up in a great rage and swore at him.

Yet, the king's illness stopped" (original text in *Lü-shih Ch'un-ch'iu*, vol. II, quoted in Liu 1974:37).

(2) (Famed doctor Hua Tuo) A county mayor had been seriously ill and Tuo believed that only rage could cure him. He received many gifts from his mayor without showing any effort in giving treatment. Before long, Tuo abandoned the mayor and left a nasty letter to the mayor before escaping. The mayor, as expected, became very angry and sent some men to kill Tuo. As Tuo had gone too far to be captured, the mayor was so enraged that he vomited several liters of blood and thus became well (Liu 1974:69).[2]

(3) A woman suffered from lack of appetite although she had been without food. She frequently swore angrily. For some time she was treated by doctors without any success. When Chang Ta-jen saw her, he remarked that her illness could not be cured merely by medicine. He ordered two courtesans to be dressed and heavily made up and to perform in front of her for her entertainment. The woman was pleased. On the following day, the doctor again ordered the two courtesans to entertain her by playing a game. The woman was again pleased. The two courtesans were then asked to have a meal in front of the woman and to praise how delicious the meal was. The woman was tempted and asked for food. They gave her a small portion. A few days later, the woman lost her anger and her appetite began to increase (*Ju-men Shih-chin*, quoted in Chen 1959).

(4) A low ranking court official had just passed the highest civil examination with the highest mark and received the title of *chuang yuan*. He took a leave to visit home. When he was near the place Huai he became ill. He consulted a well-known physician and was told that his illness was beyond cure and he would die in seven days. However, if he hurried, he could still reach home. The official was depressed and hurried on the road again. After seven days he reached home, but he appeared to be in good health. A servant presented him with a letter written by the doctor who had asked him not to show it to the official until he had reached home. The official opened the letter, which said: "Since you passed the examination and acquired the highest scholarly esteem, your over-happiness has damaged your heart. The damage is beyond the remedy of medicine. I therefore dared to frighten you with death in order to cure your illness. By now you should have recovered." The official was satisfied with the explanation and had nothing but admiration for the doctor's effective treatment (*Ssu-shi I-shu*, quoted in Chen 1959).

(5) A salt vendor who was as poor as a pauper, one day was robbed of his salt and vomited several liters of blood. He crawled over to see the famous doctor Chien Tung-wen. Chien secretly enclosed half an ounce of gold in the package of the prescribed medicine. The vendor found the gold when he opened the package. He returned the gold, thinking it must belong to the doctor. Dr Chien refused to take the gold, saying to him: "How could I afford to have gold to give away." The vendor was overjoyed with this unexpected gold. He drank the medicine and was immediately cured (*Ming-yi Lie-chuan*, quoted in Chen 1959).

(6) Upon hearing the news that his father was killed by bandits, an official of the city Chi cried bitterly. He soon suffered from a heart ailment which became worse as the days went by. A month later, his heart formed a lump in the shape of an upside-down cup. He felt great pain, and medicine had no effect. Dr Chang Tsai-jen arrived. He clowned around and made a lot of jokes. The patient laughed so much that he had to turn to the wall to avoid looking at the doctor's performance. A couple of days later, the large lump beneath his heart began to disappear (*Ju-man Shih-chin*, quoted in Chen 1959).

The above stories provide some clues to the underlying hypothesis of Chinese psychotherapy in dealing with emotion and disease. From the Western point of view, the Chinese doctor in most of these cases used emotion to mediate between disease, cause and symptom. Yet, from the Chinese practitioner's point of view, disease is basically psychosomatic. Certain emotions in excess damage certain parts of the body and cause illness. Thus, a counter emotion is introduced or induced to replace the adverse emotion, and thus restore the damaged part. Rage is introduced to induce cure in the first two stories; while joy is induced to counteract anger in the third story, and to counteract grief in the sixth story. Fear is induced to cure a damaged heart due to being overjoyed. The fifth story is most interesting because it concerns the doctor's responsibility to a patient. I shall comment on this point later, after reviewing additional clinical episodes.

Sickness with Longing

The second category of sickness is *hsiang-ssu*, which in literal translation would mean "love sick". A Chinese physician's explanation (Chen 1959:67) would be that, when a person desires something which he cannot obtain, an illness will follow. This means literally "sickness with longing", and the symptom is not confined to only the unfulfilled desire for a mate of the opposite sex. From the Western viewpoint, the patient may be seen as being in a state of affective need, or melancholy, but the Chinese physician attributes the cause of *hsiang-ssu* to "desire" or *yü*. As we shall see in a later part of this paper, emotion and desire are two key concepts to the understanding of mental health in traditional Chinese medical theory. Below are four episodes of *hsiang-ssu-ping* or "sickness with longing" in Chinese medical writings:

(1) Lord Wei of Han State was sick. As it had not been raining for some time, many doctors were summoned to treat him, however, without any success. A famous doctor, Tsuo Yo-shin, arrived. After he had felt the Lord's pulse, he calculated according to the astronomical calendar and said: "It should rain on such and such a day." The Lord was anxious and thought to himself: "Is it because my illness has reached the fatal stage that the doctor would talk about the rain rather than medicine?" When the day came, rain fell in the evening. The Lord was pleased, rose from his bed and strolled in the yard. By dawn his illness seemed to have gone. He sent a servant to the doctor to inquire about his method of cure. The doctor answered: "I examined the Lord and figured out

that the cause must be over-worry. There had been a drought in the country. I figured since the Lord is loyal and kind, he must have been troubled by the drought. I believed therefore that rain will cure the Lord's illness" (source unknown, quoted in Chen 1959).

(2) A certain woman was beloved by her mother. When her mother passed away she lost her will to live, lay in bed and became seriously ill. She could not be cured with various medicines. The family sent for Han Shi-liang to treat her. Han, knowing the cause of her illness, bribed a *wu* or shaman (female spirit medium) and discussed something about the women with her. The doctor then asked the woman's husband to persuade the woman to hire the shaman. The husband said to his wife: "You have missed your mother so much, but we are not sure if your mother also missed you in the underneath land. Why not send for a *wu* to find out?" His wife was pleased with this idea and agreed to get the *wu*. After the shaman burned incense, the mother's spirit descended, for the shaman spoke and acted in the manner of the deceased mother. The sick woman cried loudly. Then her "mother" scolded her by saying: "I died of the curse of your fate. Your terrible sickness is actually my work. Although in life we were mother and child, I am now your villainous enemy." When the shaman finished talking, the sick woman changed her facial expression (from grief to anger) and began to swear. She said: "I became ill for the sake of my mother. Now that she has turned to an enemy, why should I miss her?" Her sickness was then cured (*Shan-shi I-hsüeh Tsa-chih*, quoted in Chen 1959).

(3) Chiang Tung-ming treated a young child of the Wang family. The child had suddenly refused to take mother's milk and began to lose weight. Other doctors attributed the cause to indigestion/constipation. Chiang said: "This is a symptom of longing, *hsiag-ssu-cheng*." People all laughed at him for his ridiculous diagnosis for such a young child. Chiang ordered the family to collect all the child's toys and have them displayed in front of him. The child was so pleased and laughed when he saw a wood-fish-drum. He was then cured (*Shan-shi I-hsüeh Tsa-chih*, quoted in Chen, 1959).

(4) A certain doctor named Ting was hired to treat a youth of the Ching family that suffered from emission. Many other doctors identified the youth's problem with the wet-heat which blocked the bodily function and caused the spleen to lose normal circulation. Ting entered the house and noticed an adolescent girl sewing. Ting could not tell whether the girl was a daughter or a maid. When the father saw Ting, he ordered the girl to go upstairs and then sent for the young patient. Dr Ting felt the patient's pulse and sensed the heat of his internal fire. Ting inquired about the girl. The father replied that she was an adopted daughter-in-law. Ting then requested the father to give permission to have his son formally marry the girl. The father agreed. When the young man heard about this news, he was joyful and cured (*Chung-yi Tsa-chih*, quoted in Chen 1959).

These four stories, again, provide us with some understanding of the Chinese logic in psychotherapy. Instead of active manipulation of the patient's psyche to let the patient himself realize the hidden cause of psychological problems, or to gain "insight" as Western psychotherapy attempts to do, the Chinese physician avoids verbal communication with the patient about his problems and seeks rather to change directly the internal condition of the patient believed to have caused the problem or illness. The ability to achieve "insight" is the hallmark of "psychological mindedness" and "suitability for psychotherapy" in Western psychiatry. In contrast, the Chinese approach to therapy illustrated above attempts to circumvent this need for the patient's insight and attempts to achieve a "cure" more directly. The doctor reveals the "hidden cause" only after the patient is cured, proving his correct diagnosis. Although the patient was apparently deceived by the doctor, as in the case of hiring a spirit medium to alter the patient's emotional bond with her mother, it is more important to the Chinese doctor, the patient, and the family members to obtain effective cure. For instance, it was a common belief in traditional Chinese society that arranged marriage could cure a youth of mental or physical illness (Lin and Lin 1980). More examples are presented below which illustrate the doctor's manipulation of a patient without his knowledge of the treatment process.

Delusion-Induced Illness

The third category of sickness is caused by delusion. Chinese physicians deceive the patient in their treatment as a counter measure to "Psychological problems". Five episodes illustrating this kind of sickness and treatment are given below.

(1) A woman accidentally swallowed worms at a meal and thus became ill. A famed doctor diagnosed the cause of her illness as being merely "suspicion", and prescribed emetic/laxative medicine. The doctor ordered the nurse to tell the woman that small worms were discovered in her vomit. When the patient heard this, she felt peace at heart and became well (*Pei-chuang Suo-yen*, quoted in Chen 1959).

(2) A man was drunk at a relative's house. In the middle of the night he was thirsty and drank water from the stone water tank outside of the house. When he saw the water tank the next morning, he discovered small red worms in the water. He became worried and unhappy. He could feel the worms inside his abdomen and felt sick. When he visited the famous doctor Wu Chio, the doctor realized the cause of his sickness and put small pieces of red thread into the tablets prescribed for him. The medicine caused him diarrhea. The patient saw the read thread which resembled the worms and immediately became well.

(3) A local lord suffered from diarrhea. He had to use the toilet many times and was tired. He changed several doctors but the treatments produced no results. One of his house guests recommended a certain Mr Yang from Shangtung. When Mr Yang was invited in, he started to talk about the nature of the sun, the moon, the stars, and the formation of wind, clouds, and thunder. He continued to lecture without restraint in words and gestures from morning until night and allowed no breaks. The patient was so involved with his interesting talk that he forgot to go to the toilet. Finally, Mr Yang smiled and declared that the Lord is

cured without medicine. People surrounding the Lord were surprised and pressed him for an explanation. Mr Yang said: "To treat chronic diarrhea one must first find out about the patient's hobbies. If the patient likes to play chess, then one should play chess with him. If the patient enjoys fun, then one should have fun with the patient. It will induce the patient to pay full attention to what attracts him and forget about his suffering" (*Ju-men Shih-chin*, quoted in Chen 1959).

(4) A woman suffered from a sickness which caused her to bend forward, unable to raise her head. Men Shun asked the woman to sit on a chair, then he produced a long needle as if he was about to attack her with it. When the woman attempt to avoid the needle she gradually raised her head (*Wu-chin Hsien-chih*, quoted in Chen 1959).

(5) Once upon a time, a certain official's daughter, who was 16, when picking flowers from a tree, felt a sudden numbness and could not lower her arms. Many doctors failed to help her. The family called a famous doctor whose name was Tseng to examine her. After determining the cause of illness, the doctor had a discussion with the official. He recommended that he and the girl be confined to a room, with all the windows and doors locked, and both should strip naked. The girl would not agree to such a treatment. She finally yielded to her parents after lengthy persuasion. The doctor told the official that nobody should be allowed to enter the room until they hear the daughter scream. Inside the room Dr Tseng stared at the naked girl, making her so ashamed and angry. Tseng suddenly jumped at the girl as if he was about to launch an assault. The girl screamed and tried to cover her body with her hands without realizing that she had lowered her arms. By the time the official entered the room, the girl already could move her arms freely (*Ch'uan-chie Jiu-lu*, quoted in Chen 1959).

The professional conception in Chinese medicine makes no distinction between the modern concept of disease and illness (cf. Kleinman 1980; Loudon 1976), the former being biomedical and the latter personal. Some Chinese physicians believe that many diseases are in some way related to psychological and especially emotional disorder which, like any other kind of bodily disorder, can be "cured". The above stories show that traditional Chinese psychotherapy seeks to manage or relieve symptoms of psychiatric disorder. However, the doctors do not trace the internal origin of psychological problems, or share it with their patients as seen in the treatment process in Western psychiatry. Deception, therefore, is perfectly acceptable as long as desirable results are produced and illness is cured. The Chinese physician omits part of the treatment necessary in Western psychotherapy, namely, "talk therapy", and attempts to alleviate directly the patient's problem by changing both internal as well as external causes, or environments.

Furthermore, the Chinese doctor deals with not only the patient's illness but also with the patient's *social reality*, which in most of our stories turned out to involve the "true" causes of sickness. To achieve an effective cure a good Chinese doctor plays the additional roles of matchmaker, entertainer, and philanthropist. In contrast, direct intervention in the patient's life or social relations is not part of the cultural tradition of Western medicine or psycho-therapy. Chinese patients' avoidance of Western psychiatrists may be due not so much to their distrust of "talk-therapy" as to a number of factors associated with the practitioner-client relationship and interaction. Contemporary, formally trained Chinese physicians are supposed to incorporate in thier diagnoses discus-sions with patients about their psychosocial problems which are regarded as one of the prime sources of disorder. This is why the above-mentioned method of "four means of diagnosis" is deemed to be an integral part of Chinese medicine.

Research I conducted in Singapore among Chinese physicians revealed that they recognized that patients of particular socio-economic backgrounds who seek treatment in traditional medicine, may share certain psychological problems and stresses. As a result, the physicians usually take the individual patient's socio-economic background into consideration in their diagnoses (Wu n.d.). A Chinese physician may start his clinical notes (like a medical chart in Western medicine) with a statement about the patient's current psychological and social condition. These conditions are then related to the nature of the illness, which is explained in terms of emotive-somatic disease etiology. For instance, a physician wrote the following note about a patient who complained of diarrhea: "A few days ago this woman quarreled with a friend of hers and her agony still stays with her (lingered on) . . . " And a Chinese physician wrote of a patient who suffered pain and swelling underneath his arm pits (and who had been diagnosed previously in a Western hospital as suffering from no disease at all and had been dismissed without treatment), that:

The patient is young and physically strong. He has recently been troubled by problems at work and he is worried about his business . . . It leads to congestion of *ch'i* and depression (*yü*) of liver . . . (Hsieh 1979:58).

Discussion of the above cases has been aimed at illustrating that Chinese practi-tioners' models of etiology and treatment may resemble psychotherapeutic procedures, although the Chinese doctors seldom label their treatments as such.

DISEASE PREVENTION AND MENTAL HEALTH

Disease prevention in modern medical research may be perceived as a core function of the health care system (Dunn 1976), although some may perceive this function as meaningful in terms of a much broader "health system" (see Kleinman 1980:71–83). As mentioned before, a key concept in traditional Chinese medical theory is that preventive measures outweigh remedial measures in health maintenance. This concept has become an integral part of the Chinese philosophy of maintaining harmony with nature, in the social value of managing appropriate interpersonal relationships, and in the cultural value of self control (Kleinman and Lin 1980, *passim*). Proper management of one's emotions and desires is believed to be the secret to health and wisdom. *Huang ti Nei ching* describes sages as persons who have,

Attained harmony with Heaven and Earth and followed closely the laws of the eight winds. They were able to adjust their desires to worldly affairs, and within their hearts there was neither hatred nor anger. They did not wish to separate their activities from the world; they could not be indifferent to custom. They did not over-exert their bodies at physical labour and they did not over-exert their minds by strenuous meditation. They were not concerned about anything, they regarded inner happiness and peace as fundamental, and contentment as the highest achievement. Their bodies could never be harmed and their mental faculties never be dissipated. Thus they could reach the age of one hundred years or more (Veith 1972:11).

The teaching of seeking inner happiness through contentment is popular in Chinese folklore and in contemporary writings. A study of Chinese proverbs on health and hygiene reveals that folk beliefs in many parts of traditional China conform to this classical medical teaching (Chu 1970). Chinese individuals are all familiar with the following sayings; *Shen an pu ju shin an* — A peaceful mind is more important than a healthy body; *chi chu chang lo* — contentment ensures happiness; and *sui yu erh an* — one should feel at ease whatever the circumstance. Consistent interpretation of medical theory, philosophy of life, and personal attitude has enabled traditional Chinese medicine to deal with psychological and psychosocial disorders (cf. Dunn 1976:147). In Taiwan, Singapore (Wu 1979) and Hong Kong, I have observed Chinese paying more attention to preventive medicine and self medication than to seeking professional help, which usually is the last resort after long "endurance". Although studies have revealed how Chinese improve their health through medical tonics, broth, and nutritious food, little is known ethnographically about how individuals deal with psychological problems — stress or distress — in a traditional way, before deciding to approach professional help, be it a doctor, spirit medium, or fortune teller.

According to cultural beliefs, what is most important to an individual to protect his health is the avoidance of stress, which is often equated with the repression of emotion (Hsu 1949; Kleinman and Lin 1980). Some of the cases presented above exemplify the principle of Chinese medicine that proper "release" or channeling of emotion is beneficial to the mind and body. However, in normal situations in Chinese society a moderate display of emotion is more desirable than full expression. In the Confucian tradition, stress avoidance is associated with a person's ability in achieving *shiu-yang* ("self-discipline" is a close but not synonymous translation. *Shiu-yang* is an abbreviated expression of *Shiu-shin yang-shing*; correct the mind and training the temperament.) Lin (1980) makes a similar point in noting that the Chinese cultural emphasis on social harmony makes equanimity and the suppression of emotion a psycho-cultural coping mechanism.

At the level of external, social interaction, *shiu-yang* means individual ability to control outbursts of adverse emotion in displays of bad temper. In terms of a person's mental state, *shiu-yang* indicates that a person is not easily disturbed. While equanimity or even-mindedness is a cultural ideal, these qualities are regarded as difficult to achieve. *Shiu-yang* is particularly expected, but not necessarily achieved, among learned persons with higher education and higher social standing. It is believed that persons who follow the ideal norm of *shiu-yang* will be able to dilute social conflicts and psychological stress. The inter-relation of levels of education, achievement of *shiu-yang*, the art of emotional disguise, and the inner ability to cope with stress in Chinese society are topics worth pursuing in future research.

Psychiatrists have observed (Tseng 1975; Kleinman 1980:135–136; Lin and Lin 1980) that Chinese have difficulty in expressing emotional and psychological problems in clinical situations. However, in ordinary life, Chinese have rich and subtle ways to display emotion and inner feelings, even though full expression is thought to be inappropriate under certain circumstances. In fact, the entire area of emotional control – repression or suppression – in Chinese culture has not been carefully examined. What is lacking in the literature on Chinese psychotherapy are observations about (1) the difference between unconstrained expression of emotion and culturally determined rules of emotional display; and, more importantly, (2) the difference between controlled display of emotion and possibly unconscious behavioral cues which could still be recognized by others as signs of emotion. Ekman and Friesen's (1969, 1974) studies of American psychiatric patients' facial expression and body movement shows that ordinary people may detect emotion through "deception clues" and nonverbal "leakage". Boucher (1979:175) summarizes emotion research to date and remarks that there are few studies of the socially learned aspects of affective behavior, calling for further research on culturally based "display rules". More research on "deception clues" and nonverbal "leakage" in Chinese social interaction, may provide a better understanding of the cultural and behavioral significance of "somatization" among Chinese patients.

It is logical to assume that the more a culture emphasizes formal, ritualized, display rules, the more the members of that culture are likely to recognize nonverbal cues which reveal emotional dispositions. While Chinese are socialized to restrain the expression of emotion, especially those considered negative, parents will often press a child to reveal possible psychological problems or *hsin-shin* ('heart-business'). They also learn the skill of *ch'a-yen kuan-se* to examine constantly the other party's intentions, emotions, and true feelings duing social interaction. The ability of ordinary Chinese to observe "deception clues" and nonverbal "leakage" enable them to rely less on verbal complaints in communicating with others, especially kin, close friends, and superiors about their feelings. In the same manner, a Chinese patient expects an authoritative doctor to detect physical or psychological disorders without elaborate com-plaints. The stories cited above are examples of how "famed doctors" – those who had mastered the "true art" of Chinese medicine – would treat patients through balancing or manipulating emotion to achieve effective cures, though none of them used "insight"-oriented methods characteristic of Western psycho-therapy. When stress is detected in another person, close friends and relatives do not hesitate to offer advice. The cases given in this paper illustrate a kind of psycho-somatic explanation for illness which is evident in advice commonly given among Chinese that one must not allow oneself to be governed by emotions lest one damage oneself physically. This type of reasoning contrasts with the more common somato-psychic mode of explanation which has been described by other scholars of Asian medicine (Obeyesekere 1977; Lock 1980; Kleinman 1980).

CONCLUSION

Chinese medicine has demonstrated positive adaptive advantages (Dunn 1976: 147). It is not accidental that China has applied both Western and Chinese health care systems in practice, while traditional medicine still plays a prominent role in many overseas Chinese societies.

Awareness (by self) and recognition (by others) of disease symptoms are culturally patterned, as is the expression of emotion and psychological problems. If indeed the conception of body, emotion, and health in modern Chinese societies still conforms to the traditional medical paradigm of balance, mental health services should take account of this conception before appropriate and effective programs can be developed. It is important for cross-cultural researchers to study Chinese interpersonal problems and coping strategies in contributing to the field of mental health. We need to know, for instance, how Chinese in day to day life manage their interpersonal problems, how they cope with stress and the frustration of goals (desires). At what point is imbalance of emotion and physical state recognized and either "self medication" or professional help considered? Are there distinctions between physical illness and psychosocial adjustment problems? How are they connected? Ethnomedical research on these topics will benefit not only medical science in Chinese societies, but also the cross-cultural study of medicine and psychiatry (cf. Kleinman 1980:385).

In this paper I have attempted to call attention to the emphasis of mind and body in Chinese classical texts as well as in popular folklore. A better understanding of this indigenous Chinese health care system may strengthen the ethnomedical study of psychiatry and counseling and contribute to the development of culturally appropriate mental health programs.

ACKNOWLEDGMENTS

I am grateful to Geoffrey White, Arthur Kleinman and Mary Brandt for useful comments on this paper, although they may not agree with everything I have said. I alone am responsible for the views expressed here.

NOTES

1. For the Chinese text, I used a 1974 version published in China (Jen-min 1974). Veith's (1972) English translation provided a convenient reference for our discussion, although I may not completely agree with the translation.
2. According to historical studies, Hua Tuo was born in A.D. 190 (Wong and Wu 1932:605).

REFERENCES

Boucher, J. D.
    1979 Culture and Emotion. *In* Perspectives on Cross-Cultural Psychology. A. Marsella
          et al. (eds.), pp. 159–178. New York: Academic Press.
Bridgman, R.
    1974 Traditional Chinese Medicine. *In* Medicine and Society in China. J. Z. Bowers and
          E. F. Purcell (eds.), pp. 1–21. New York: Josiah Macy, Jr. Foundation.
Chen, Pang-Shien
    1937 Chung-kuo I-shüe-shih (History of Chinese Medicine). Taipei: Shang-wu (1977
          edition).
Chen, Ts'un-jen
    1959 Chung-kuo Hsin-li-ping Liau-fa Shih (History of Chinese Psychotherapy). *In* Spe-
          cial Issue of Thong Chai Hospital 92nd Anniversary. pp. Shing 65–67. Singapore.
Chu, Chieh-fan
    1970 A Study of Chinese Proverbs on Health and Hygiene. Bulletin of the Institute of
          Ethnology, Academia Sinica, No. 30:165–237.
Croizier, R.
    1968 Traditional Medicine in Modern China. Cambridge: Harvard University Press.
Dunn, F.
    1976 Traditional Asian Medicine and Cosmopolitan Medicine as Adaptive Systems. *In*
          Asian Medical Systems. C. Leslie (ed.), pp. 133–158. Berkeley, University of
          California Press.
Ekman, P. and W. V. Friesen
    1969 Nonverbal Leakage and Clues to Deception. Psychiatry 32(1):88–105.
    1974 Nonverbal Behavior and Psychopathology. *In* Psychology of Depression: Contem-
          porary Theory and Research. R. J. Friedman and M. M. Katz (eds.), pp. 203–232.
          Washington, D.C.: Winston and Sons.
Hsieh, Ta-fu
    1979 Five Case Records. *In* the Fourth Graduation Souvenir Magazine of Chinese Medi-
          cal Studies. p. 58. Singapore: The Association for promoting Chinese Medicine.
Hsu, F. L. K.
    1949 Suppression Versus Repression. *Psychiatry* 12(3):223–243.
Jen-min, Wei-sheng Chu-pan She
    1973 Huang-ti Nei-ching Su-wen. Peking: People's Health Press.
    1974 Hsin-pien Chung-i-hsüe Kai-yau (New Guidelines of Chinese Medicine). Peking:
          People's Health Press.
Kleinman, A.
    1977 Depression, Somatization and the "New Cross-Cultural Psychiatry". Social
          Science and Medicine 11:3–10.
    1980 Patients and Healers in the Context of Culture. Berkeley: University of California
          Press.
Kleinman, A. and T. Y. Lin (eds.)
    1980 Normal and Abnormal Behavior in Chinese Culture. Dordrecht, Holland, and
          Boston: D. Reidel.
Kleinman, A. et al.
    1975 Medicine in Chinese Cultures. Washington: U.S. Government Printing Office.
Lee, Rance P. L.
    1980 Perceptions and Uses of Chinese Medicine Among the Chinese in Hong Kong.
          Culture, Medicine and Psychiatry 4:345–375.
Leslie, C.
    1976 Asian Medical Systems: a Comparative Study. Berkeley: University of California
          Press.

Levi-Strauss, C.
    1963   Structural Anthropology. New York: Doubleday.
Lin, K. M.
    1980   Traditional Chinese Medical Beliefs and Their Relevance for Mental Illness and
           Psychiatry. *In* Normal and Abnormal Behavior in Chinese Culture. A. Kleinman
           and T. Y. Lin (eds.), pp. 95–111. Dordrecht, Holland, and Boston: D. Reidel.
Lin, T. Y. and M. C. Lin
    1980   Love, Denial and Rejection: Responses of Chinese Families to Mental Illness. *In*
           Normal and Abnormal Behavior in Chinese Culture. A. Kleinman and T. Y. Lin
           (eds.), pp. 387–401. Dordrecht, Holland, and Boston: D. Reidel.
Liu, Pei-chi
    1974   History of Chinese Medical Studies.
Lock, M. M.
    1980   East Asian Medicine in Urban Japan. Berkeley: University of California Press.
Loudon, J. B.
    1976   Social Anthropology and Medicine. London: Academic Press.
Needham, J.
    1970   Hygiene and Preventive Medicine in Ancient China. *In* Clerks and Craftsmen in
           China and the West. J. Needham (ed.), pp. 340–378. Cambridge: Cambridge
           University Press.
Obeyesekere, G.
    1977   "The Theory and Practice of Psychological Medicine in the Ayurvedic Tradition".
           Culture, Medicine and Psychiatry. 1:155–181.
Pa'los, S.
    1971   The Chinese Art of Healing. New York: Herder and Herder.
Porkert, M.
    1976   The Intellectual and Social Impulses Behind the Evolution of Traditional Chinese
           Medicine. *In* Asian Medical Systems. C. Leslie (ed.), pp. 63–76. Berkeley: Univer-
           sity of California Press.
Tseng, Wen-shing
    1973   The Development of Psychiatric Concepts in Traditional Chinese Medicine.
           Archives of General Psychiatry 29:569–575.
    1975   The Nature of Somatic Complaints Among Psychiatric Patients: the Chinese Case.
           Comprehensive Psychiatry 16:237–245.
Veith, I.
    1972   Huang ti Nei ching Su wen [The Yellow Emperor's Classic of Internal Medicine].
           Berkeley: University of California Press.
Wong, K. Chimin and L. T. Wu
    1932   History of Chinese Medicine. Tientsin: Tientsin Press.
Wu, D. Y. H.
    1979   Traditional Concepts of Food and Medicine in Singapore. Singapore: Institute of
           Southeast Asian Studies, Occasional Paper, No. 35.
    n.d.   Adaptation and Professionalization of Traditional Chinese Medicine in Singapore.
           Unpublished manuscript.

13. SHAMAN-CLIENT INTERCHANGE IN OKINAWA: PERFORMATIVE STAGES IN SHAMANIC THERAPY

INTRODUCTION

From the early years of this century, the leading Okinawan newspapers have denounced the persistence of shamanism, placing the responsibility principally upon uneducated females over 40 years of age (Ryukyu Government 1969). Even earlier, during the last 150 years of the Okinawan Kingdom, when Confucian values dominated in official circles, there had been periodic, though presumably ineffective, efforts to proscribe the practice (Uezu 1977). With the exile of King Sho Tai and formal assumption of Japanese control in 1879, even more restrictive laws and measures came to apply, for among the progressive enactments of the new Restoration Government were laws not only abolishing shamanism, but banning spirit possession as well. Thus, until the conclusion of World War II the shaman practiced with caution, more or less *sub rosa*. With the advent of a more democratic climate in the postwar era, religious toleration obtained, allowing the shaman to surface and proliferate. In today's affluent society they are very much a part of the scene, despite the fact that universal education has been a reality for more than 65 years.

Although I am unable to provide any firm proof, I suspect that their numbers are greater than ever. In 1960 the Central Police Headquarters estimated about one shaman for every 500 of population, and my limited survey of that year in a district reputed to be shaman-prone, suggested one per 600 as somewhat more accurate. In any case, they significantly outnumber(ed) the medical doctors, who have been long aware of their impinging activities. Apparently improved communications have served to enlarge their sphere of influence, for accoding to a colleague presently engaged in a study of Okinawan fishing operations in the Solomon Islands, it is a common practice when the catch declines to radio back requesting shamanic inspiration and divine guidance.

I have attributed the persistence of shamanism in Okinawa primarily to the weak development of a concept of impersonal causation in traditional thinking and to the practice of ascribing the ultimate cause of misfortune to the spirit world (Lebra 1964, 1966, 1969). The shaman alone with socially recognized supernatural powers of seeing and hearing, predominates as the final authority in determining the cause of misfortune and, in generally, prescribing remedial action.

While the cause of adversity may be attributed to an angry offended god, to a malevolent spirit, to cursing (or, very rarely, to sorcery), largely trouble with the spirit world seems to derive from the ancestors as a consequence of their past actions and/or present interactions(s) with living relatives. There is an

303

A. J. Marsella and G. M. White (eds.), Cultural Conceptions of Mental Health and Therapy, 303–315.

elaborate complex of beliefs and rituals comprising the ancestral cult, and virtually all households are organized on a principle of patrilineality into lineages and clans. Tombs generally appear to be properly maintained, and the annual tomb cleaning rites well attended. Visits to homes reveal carefully tended altars, not uncommonly somewhat ostentatious in comparison with other evidences of material wealth. Attendance at a clan meeting can bring exposure to expressions of pride in the ancestors and their accomplishments. But all of this may go hand in hand with a substantial amount of ambivalence, for ancestors also can be inconveniencing and even make you ill!

Overwhelmingly the clients of the shaman are females, and superficially this may appear to be the result of most males being better educated, as they will readily tell you. But in truth the spiritual burdens of Okinawan society seemingly always have been carried by women, far back in time, before history into the protohistoric and mythological past. In the Kingdom there was a political hierarchy of males, headed by King, paralleled by a religious hierarchy of females extending down from the Chief Priestess — eldest daughter, eldest sister, or aunt of the ruler — through the regional, district, and villages priestesses. Ritual within the patri-clans was (is) dominated by female priestesses, and the bulk of the shaman were (are) females, about 95% presently.

Within the family-household the senior female — mother or wife of the male household head — functioned, and continues to function, as principal ritualist on behalf of her family. Should illness, misfortune, or anything untoward or unexpected occur in the family, she will likely consult a shaman. It is also her duty in the early months of the lunar year, to obtain from the shaman the prospective fortunes for the family and each individual member. Thus, every family should seek a spiritual checkup (*hachi unchi* or *suu unchi*) at least yearly, and this is regarded as virtually mandatory by those who carry this responsibility. Yet, much like the annual physical checkup, people often procrastinate, and perhaps for the very same reasons — vague, apprehensive fears that something serious might be uncovered. Not uncommonly the client will state that the visit is for the first fortune, but what comes out in the ensuing interchange is that someone is at home sick. Some shamans are well aware of this and, after rendering a fortune, may ask directly, "Now, what brings you here today?"

The shaman-client encounter ordinarily takes place in the home of the former (house calls are relatively infrequent and cost dearly), usually in a living room much like that of others. *Tatami* mats cover the floor, and the room is largely bare of furniture, save for a low table which the shaman sits behind facing her clients. At her back is a small shrine which she may often turn to in the process of consulting the spirits. Clients may gather in front of her in a semi-circle seated on the tatami or thin cushions. On two sides of the room the outer walls are made up of sliding wooden panels which permit opening the room to the outside in good weather. Overflow from this room and latecomers may gather outside on the *engawa*, a narrow porch-like extension of the floor covered by the eaves.

Clients are given audience in the order of their arrival; some arriving even before the shaman has completed breakfast to await their turn. Depending on the reputation, a popular shaman may manage as many as 30 or more clients per day; those less popular may see only one or two, sometimes fewer. Each client addresses the shaman in front of the others waiting in the room, and if something highly interesting or entertaining should develop, even those outside the room, but within hearing distance, may stretch their necks or attempt to put their heads inside. The shaman-client encounter with audience has some similarities with group therapy, but here the others are not expected to interrupt or to intrude in the interchange, rather they are limited to join in laughing, crying, murmuring and similar passive, empathetic involvement.

In comparison with shamanic performances which I have observed in Taiwan and Korea and with some of the literature which I have read, the Okinawan is rather tame, if not subdued. I can scarcely imagine their reaction to seeing the head of a live chicken bitten off; such a shaman would be regarded as deserving to be caged, the common mode of treatment for violent mental cases until recently. Save for her shrine, incense, and minor offerings (usually rice, wine, money, or food), there are no props. The shaman wears an ordinary street dress (if an older woman, she may be more informal during the hot summer months and reduce her garb to a slip), little different from that of her clients. Only one of my informants was inclined toward the bizarre in her dress, and this was taken by some as evidence of her lack of stability. Their ritual interaction with clients does not involve massage, laying on of hands, etc.; in fact, I have rarely seen a shaman touch a client. They tend, in fact, to be physically distanced from one another.

Music, drumming, and dancing are notably absent from the Okinawan shamanic performance. Some may follow a rhythmical, monotonously intoned, chant in rendering a fortune; many others dispense with this altogether. The shaman is expected to enter a trance-like state which would facilitate seeing and hearing and/or induce possession trance enabling an ancestral spirit to speak directly to living kin.[1] There are a number of terms to denote the various kinds of trance and possession trance — to see, hear, possess, be carried, be ridden, be leaned upon, etc. (Lebra 1964) — which applied to the ordinary shaman-client interchange infer not so much a loss of control as a heightening of faculties. While I am convinced that most of my shaman informants had experienced altered states of consciousness, in the ordinary routine handling of clients on a day to day basis trance or possession trance were obviously simulated, and not too impressively in most cases, I might add. Nonetheless, I am equally persuaded that the performance had emic validity for the majority of watching clients.

Essentially, the shaman-client encounter is a verbal exchange, primarily involving persuasion, whereby the shaman establishes the client's confidence in her powers. It is not that the client commences resistant to the shamanic message in general, rather the client, engaging a new shaman for the first time, retains a skeptical attitude toward this particular shaman until proven to the contrary. It is well known that some, posing as servants of the gods, do this for money or personal gain, and, as a consequence, lie to and otherwise deceive their clients. The shaman, of course, is well aware of this and strives to overcome the client's resistance by rendering a credible performance which confirms the client's personal and cultural expectations, in other words, making sense in terms of the individual client's cognitive structure.

Although there are some variations in routine from shaman to shaman, what I have observed struck me as following a fairly conventional pattern (the work of Ohashi (1978) and others confirms this). From my perspective, the process includes three principal steps or stages which might be termed (1) negotiating shamanic reality, (2) determining spiritual cause, and (3) prescribing remedial action. In addition, there are some minor or subsidiary phases, occurring from time to time, fashioned or inserted by the shaman; three of these also will be described.

PERFORMATIVE STAGES IN SHAMANIC THERAPY

Negotiating Shamanic Reality

This first stage is by far the most important aspect of the transaction for the shaman, for here the shaman establishes dominance through providing proof of her credibility. The clues as to what the shaman "sees" or "hears" must be skillfully elicited from the client at this time (assuming no previous knowledge). It is essential for the shaman to manifest clearly that she has some mastery over the spirits, being able to control seeing, hearing, or even possession by them.

Ordinarily, the shaman-client session (we are here describing a new client or an infrequent one) commences with the client identifying herself in terms of place of residence and husband's or family's occupation. The family name may or may not be given; more often, where there is one, the house name is preferably presented instead. Members of the family-household are then specified in terms of their kin status, birth order, and animal birth year (according to the Chinese lunar-solar calendar); thus, for example: husband dog man, first son monkey, second son pig person, first daughter horse, etc. For greater clarification, approximate age or the number of cycles passed may be added; hence a fourth cycle person would indicate someone over 48 and less than 60 years of age. Given the present animal year, people can rather easily calculate the age.

When the purpose of the visit is the first fortune of the year, that may be so stated at the outset. But as noted before, the spiritual checkup is often postponed until a crisis occurs, usually sickness, and the shaman are aware that a request for a general fortune for an entire family may conceal the fact that a serious problem exists. Aside from this indication of a first fortune, however, a (new) client does not initially reveal "I have a back ache" or "My husband is at home sick today." Instead they appear to hold back, hedging somewhat, in expectation that some demonstration of shamanic power is warranted first. "Show me that you are privy to my world!" seems to be the implicit challenge. Thus, a transaction ensues with the features of a verbal skirmish or game with the shaman actively attempting to elicit some clues or hints as to what might be seen or heard in the trance state. One is reminded of Twenty Questions and the like. With a satisfactory response from the shaman, the client can reciprocate with further clues and encouragement.

Shaman (in trance): I see a house with a corrugated iron roof.
Client: Our neighbor's.

or

Shaman (in trance): Kamii? Who is Kamii?
Client: Kamee?
Shaman: Yes, Kamee!

or

Shaman (in trance): Shotoku? Who is Shotoku?
Client: Seitoku?
Shaman: Yes, Seitoku!

Among the oldest generation of Okinawans there are a limited number of personal names; so, oftentimes the shaman strikes the name of some relative on the first round.

There are other clues inadvertently provided by the client which a clever shaman can piece together and construct a realistic characterization of the family. A house containing a grandmother or grandfather suggests a first son line with patrilocal residence, whereas a young couple living alone or with a small child intimates the branch house of a younger son with neolocal residence (a first son inherits the parental house, and brothers do not co-reside after marriage; so, younger brothers establish new houses).

Shaman (in trance): I can see two houses.
Client: One is my father's.
Shaman: Why don't you live with your father? You are a first son aren't you?

House names, formerly universal in Okinawa, and still common in the rural areas and among the old gentry and nobility in Shuri (the former capital) also provide clues to class rank (in the Kingdom), antiquity within a lineage and/or within a village, and sometimes to occupation. Thus, for example, the house name Ufu Irii (Great West) would imply a strong likelihood of considerable antiquity within a kin group and community, whereas Sannan Naka Ufu Irii (Third Son Middle Great West) indicates a newer house and more derived status. The shaman, of course, can employ these clues to construct a reasonable approximation of the client's family-household, which will be taken as convincing evidence of the shaman's powers and will bring forth further clues from the client.

As the negotiations progress, the client gaining confidence in the shaman tends to provide the clues more quickly and/or to overlook more readily an inaccuracy or blunder on the part of the shaman.

Shaman (in trance): I see a well in your house lot.
Client: Yes, there is.
Shaman: It is near the gate.
Client: No, it is rather (far) inside.
Shaman: Yes, but it can be seen from the gate?
Client: Yes.

In negotiating shamanic reality the shaman at times seems to be imposing her interpretations on the client, but more often it appears that between them they are jointly constructing a scenario. Occasionally, a client is obdurate, or plainly obtuse, in playing negotiations. The transaction then flounders, and the shaman becomes frustrated, because not enough information is coming across.

Shaman (clearly exasperated): I cannot see! By the way, did you pray at the (ancestral) altar before coming here?
Client: No.
Shaman: Go home and do so! You should always pray at the (ancestral) altar before visiting here; then if there is any problem, your ancestors will come with you and speak to me.

Most clients, however, usually know how to perform, and once sufficient rapport has been created and the shaman has established herself as in command, the exchange can move on to the next stage.

Determining Spiritual Cause

The second stage of the interchange is the most crucial from the client's point of view, for here there should be obtained an explanation for the illness, misfortune, or other problem which occasioned the visit. Many types of problems are brought to the shamans or are skillfully elicited from their clients. Among these, health clearly outstripped all others combined running as high as 80% of the subjects discussed with the shaman by our count. This included not only those problems raised by the client, but also those which were anticipated through the shaman's seeing, hearing, or being possessed. So not infrequently, some people, who assumed themeselves and their families to be well, found themselves with a health problem, or rather the threat of a health problem as a result of having asked for the spiritual checkup.

When the shamans came to ascribe cause, purportedly by means of seeing and hearing or by possession-trance, we found that in seven out of ten cases the ancestors were held to be accountable. Most commonly this appeared to result from one of three possibilities:

(1)   the ancestor(s) displeased by insufficiency of prayer, ritual neglect, or ritual oversight had withdrawn support.

(2) atavism: a behavior trait, unwelcome or socially disruptive, of an ancestor(s) is recurring in descendants, because they failed to undertake proper ritual remedy.
(3) the unhappiness and/or envy of a female relative who died unmarried or may have married, but died without male heir. Also included here would be the woman who was unable to marry a man for whom she had great passion.

Not only do the ancestors appear to be the most common cause for illness and misfortune, but among them female spirits are indicated more often than male. Thus, in our sampling female spirits showed up with a frequency two to three times greater than that of male ancestral spirits as the precipitating agent for illness or misfortune. For example, a woman who had lost her first son to tuberculosis and thereafter suffered from chronic headaches:

Shaman (in trance): I see a woman who married into your family and was unable to bear a child. She is giving you and your family these notifications.

Another woman had experienced severe back pain for more than half a year, and the medical doctors were said to be unable to bring relief:

Shaman (in trance): Your younger sister who died away from home during the war is making these requests.

In ascribing spiritual cause the shaman is often obviously guided by information obtained during the first stage of negotiations. For older houses (of several or more generations) ancestral entanglements are likely to be suggested, whereas for a new house the offending spirit may be an angry Earth God. Not infrequently, the new branch house is accused of neglecting to maintain ritual ties with the parent or origin house, a not unlikely possibility for a young couple just establishing themselves. In the following example a young housewife, clearly from a new branch house, was a bit distraught because her small son was unaccountably ill.

Shaman (in trance): Your child has spirit loss ("has dropped his spirit").
Client (with obvious relief): Oh, yes! His swing broke the other day. It must have happened at that time.

A new house is without ancestors; so, for the shaman to have mentioned an ancestral spirit in this case would not have made much sense. An angry Earth God might have sufficed, but then everyone knows that small children are susceptible to startle and subsequent spirit loss.

Those who seek out the shaman for resolution of serious problems of health and other misfortune are usually, needless to say, highly frustrated. Frequently, they claim not to have found solution through medical treatment, often contending, rightly or wrongly, the medical doctors could not give a name to their disorder. Moreover, at least for the older generation, a medical cure might be viewed as only a partial solution or settlement lacking final ascription of spirit cause. More than once we were told, "A medical doctor may cure, but that would not explain why you were sick!"

Prescribing Remedial Action

Assuming that the client has been persuaded to accept the shaman's definition of the situation, there remain the final steps of prescribing a remedial course of action. Usually, however, these guidelines are phrased in very general terms. "Pray to clear this matter up", is a not uncommon injunction. This means that the client carries the burden of praying, investigating (going around and questioning older relatives, if an ancestral problem), and awaiting some signs, perhaps an hallucinatory experience (*imi-gukuchi* = dream-like experience). Some more bold clients may not tolerate this and demand more, but even should the shaman provide more specific instructions, the burden rests primarily with the client. When a frustrated and disappointed client returns, this can transpire:

Shaman: Tell me how you did your praying.
Client: First at A, then B, next C, etc.
Shaman: No, no! You should have started with C, then B, and last A!

Not infrequently the prescribed course of action combines a ritual solution with a good measure of common sense. For instance, a child's hare lip was attributed to the fact that the father had been orphaned quite young and was unsure of his ancestry (his mother had died when he was young, his father was unknown, and, therefore, he had never prayed to his ancestors). The recommendation was to make a strenuous effort to clear up the matter of his background, identify his patri-line, pray to his ancestors, and meanwhile take the child to a hospital for surgery.

An 85-year-old man was described as having degenerated into a severe state of mental incapacity, probably senile psychosis. His 76-year-old wife was told that the cause was a lack of worship by the young people in the clan. She was advised to get together with other old people and educate the young regarding clan history and ritual. Not curative certainly, but the activity at least would have served to deflect her frustration over her husband's debilitation which was likely beyond cure. Moreover, I suspect that the shaman was steering her toward consideration of the prospect of becoming a clan priestess, a role which commonly falls to widows and older women.

There was relatively little attention devoted to helping a client develop self-insight. Similar observations have been made for shamans in Taiwan (Tseng 1976) and in Korea (Harvey 1976). Of course, some exceptions may occur. When a mother proposed the notion of setting aside her first son, because of his drinking problem, in favor of the second son as heir, the shaman snapped, "Perhaps you did not give him enough love!" But usually impaired human relationships, and especially beyond the immediate members of the family, tend to be transferred into the supernatural realm for explanation. Thus, when a young woman reported her husband injured in a knife fight at work, no attempt was made to analyze the motives or social relationships of the principals. In another case, a group of townpeople were infuriated by the mayor's proposed highway widening plan which would substantially decrease the size of all front-ing property; yet, his anxious wife was simply told by the shaman, "His only problem is that he doesn't pray enough to his ancestors."

In this respect the Okinawans share resemblance with the Ifaluk (Spiro 1952); both in their traditional culture placed high value on communalism and coopera-tion, and strongly disvalued interpersonal aggression. Both also projected the cause(s) for problems of health and misfortune into the supernatural, but in place of the alien, malevolent *alus* the Okinawans employed their otherwise benevolent ancestors.

Miscellaneous Contingencies

The three stages in the shaman-client transactions described in the above appear with regularity, but in addition there may occur from time to time additional phases or stages which might be termed contingencies serving to alter the typical routines. In some instances the shaman may initiate the new course of action, and in other instances respond to the action initiated by the client or by some wholly unexpected turn of events. In any case the manner in which these con-tingencies are handled, often marks the difference between a master and a hack, between a popular performer and a mundane player of the shamanic role. Three of these contingencies will be described − (1) challenge and confrontation, (2) the fortuitous event, and (3) comic interlude.

Challenge and Confrontation should not be an unexpected event for any Okina-wan shaman, for the new client approaches the shaman, as I have indicated, with skepticism about the valdity of performance which is retained until the shaman proves herself. When confronted with obvious error, a skillful shaman can often recover the situation in a dramatic fashion as in the following. The shaman was clearly near exhaustion after having put on an impressive hour-long performance for the previous client, who was said to be in an early stage of shaman-sickness. The event had been marred by the interference of the shaman's mother who accused the client of lacking initiative and being too dependent upon the shaman. This had angered the shaman to the point of unsettling poise and composure. The next client approach the table.

Shaman (after preliminary negotiations): How many days ago did your husband die?
Client: Days? He died during World War II! This is 1960!
Shaman slumps to the floor, stretches out full length, closes eyes.
Client: Please continue my fortune!
Shaman (still reclining): You moved some bones in the tomb which were laid out like me. That is why I was made to lie down by the spirit.
Client (impressed): Oh!

You can't win them all, however, and occasionally even a seasoned profes-sional is trapped. In this case the shaman had forgotten what had transpired with the client on a previous occasion. After the preliminary negotiations, the shaman appeared to be possessed by a male spirit who wanted to talk with the client, but the client did not respond (to the spirit), remained silent for a few minutes, and looked very displeased.

Client: With my last *hanji* (shaman) I spoke to my daughter (deceased); so, today I am here for *hichi-ati* (comparison)!
Shaman (scoffingly): What? Who said that? Where?
Client (disputatiously): It was you! Right here!
Shaman (incredulous and angry): What! Get out! You never make comparisons with the same shaman! *Hichi-ati* must be done with different shaman; not the same one! That is all for you today! Go to another shaman!

The Fortuitous Event permits a resourceful shaman to take advantage of an unexpected opportunity, sometimes to convert disadvantage into asset. For example, a client reported that a medical doctor had recommended an operation for goiter. Two other shaman had separately declared the doctor wrong, asserting the matter was wholly spiritual; so, now the client was seeking comparison with a third shaman. Our shaman, who had served as a nurses' aide in the Japanese Army during World War II, supported the doctor and was silently pondering what to say in order to discount the pronouncements of the other two. At that moment a large rat ran through the room causing the client to scream.

Shaman: That was a sign from the gods! This is rat year, and the gods sent a rat to tell me that you should go to the hospital and have that operation!

Sufficiently impressed, the client did enter the hospital, and later credited this shaman with having saved her life (the doctor was not mentioned).

Comic Interludes occurred in a number of client-shaman transactions which we observed. A majority of the shaman whom I knew possessed a sense of humor, or rather they were good performers who employed humor to their advantage. Most assuredly they were not above grandstanding, playing to the audience sometimes at the expense of a client, when it served their purpose. While a comic interlude might arise spontaneously, it was my impression that these were often staged. This seemed to take place particularly after a long and emotionally laden session. There would be a rather abrupt switch over to joking and heavy laughter. In the following example, the shaman was obviously privy to some aspects of the client's more private life. The client, a 35-year-old farmer, stated that he had come on behalf of his mother who was unable to come (though not ill) for a general family fortune; after that he added somewhat hesitantly that his cow was not eating.

Shaman (in trance): Your mother should be careful of fire throughout all of this year. Except for that, all of your family will be good, nothing wrong. (The shaman moved as to indicate that the session was at an end.)

Client (somewhat indignant): Is that all?
Shaman: Yes!
Client: You must have something more to say!
Shaman: Yes, but do you really want to find out?
Client: Of course! You should know better than that!
Shaman: I know, but I cannot say it.
Client: Why?
Shaman: I do not want to make you ashamed here in front of everyone.
Client: That's all right! Speak up!
Shaman: All right then! Who is it that I see coming into your house?
Client: A woman?
Shaman: Yes.
Client: At night?
Shaman: Yes.
Client: *Akisamiyoo* (Oh, my God!). You can see that too (incredulous)? (Shaman and room full of people convulsed with laughter).
Shaman: Yes.
Client (all composure gone): And that is why I have trouble?
Shaman: Of course! You know it doesn't work since you already have a wife in your house.
Client: Yes, but what shall I do then?
Shaman (feigning indifference): I don't know. That is a problem which you alone should enjoy since you created it. (Audience broken up with laughter.)
Shaman (relenting): Do prayers for this fate (*innen*) to go away from you. Talk this matter over with that woman, so that she will understand. But do not talk to your wife about it; otherwise you will make a bigger problem for your family!
Client (subdued): Then will my cow eat?
Shaman: Yes, your cow does not eat because of sharing your fate. The cow is having sickness because of you.

I believe that a similar technique is employed in the Okinawan theater, especially in tragedy when emotions reach a high pitch. A curtain drops suddenly, and there emerge two comedians, a straight man and a fall guy, who rapidly proceed to reduce the audience into helpless laughter. Frankly, I found the interruption disconcerting, and particularly so when the tension-laden previous scene set in a fifteenth-century castle was now replaced by a bus stop and two comics arguing over a space on the waiting bench. Perhaps limitations of language and cultural bias kept me over-distanced (Scheff 1979) from participating in the generally shared catharsis. In watching the shaman lead the clients through a comic interlude, I was reminded of grade school days when after a strenuous drill in arithmetic or the like, we were asked to stand, stretch, wave our arms, and stamp our feet before resuming lessons.

CONCLUSION

Okinawan shamanic therapy must be labelled as a 'putative' psychotherapy, for there is lacking any hard scientific evidence of its efficacy. There were numerous informants, however, who were quite willing to affirm their conviction, and the numbers attending the popular shamans were positive expression of sustaining belief with action. It would appear, therefore, that shamanic therapy for a goodly segment of contemporary Okinawan society has emic validity. Beyond that I can only speculate as to the possible underlying processes contributing to an actual reduction of stress.

It should be noted, first of all, that the shamans are readily accessible and relatively inexpensive for the bulk of the population. Some accept clients shortly after breakfast and work into the evening. Not a few of them follow a work pattern of 14 days followed by one day off (the first and the fifteenth of the lunar month). It is not difficult task then to see a shaman, even a popular one, without much delay of time. Their fees are low enough so that most people resort to comparing, consulting two or more, and then pragmatically following prevailing opinion. Redundancy, of course, serves to provide assurance of certainty.

The social-physical setting for the client would seem to be a congenial one. The shaman's living room is much like that in other homes, and usually tea is readily available and sometimes inexpensive hard candy to suck on. Most clients may spend their waiting time listening, smoking, and sipping tea. The talking out of a problem in the presence of receptive, even sympathetic, listeners surely has cathartic benefit for the individual concerned as well as for other clients who can perceive the common nature of many problems.

Additionally catharsis may be provided through the discharge of emotion. The comic interlude, described previously, provides one instance of this, as does occasional banter, in stimulating laughter. Frequently clients in describing their problems may commence weeping, and in resonance most of the listening females will have their eyes brimming with tears. Empathetic crying provides further release.

Nearly always the shaman prescribes a course of action, usually general ritual action directed toward the ancestors, which may serve to replace some of the frustration of inaction with new hope for more positive outcomes through activity. Moreover, as noted earlier, a prescribed course of action may deflect the individual, or family group, from being obsessively absorbed with their problem.

A recurring complaint among those consulting the shaman is that the doctors or hospitals were not only unable to effect a cure, they also failed to provide a diagnosis or name for the illness. In mental health the labeling theorists have contended that the mere fact of labeling a transitory behavior deviance as mental disorder may result in a patient acting out a social role on a long term basis. But labeling might also work positively when a believing client is advised by the shaman that her (his) problems are not those of a medical nature but of an impaired spiritual relationship. The sick role is thereby eliminated, and the client may (or may not) measure up to the demands of the new role and social situation. Happily, each of us is restricted to but one fatality per lifetime, and as Alland (1970) and others have pointed out, most illness are of limited duration, and people recover, more or less, more often than not.

ACKNOWLEDGMENTS

Support for this research was provided by the National Institute of Mental Health, Grants M–3084 and MH09243, which is gratefully acknowledged. Principal periods of field research were 1960, 1961, and 1974.

NOTE

1. Usage of trance and possession trance follows that of Bourguignon (1973).

REFERENCES

Alland, A.
  1970 Adaptation in Cultural Evolution: An Approach of Medical Anthropology. New York: Columbia University Press.
Bourguigon, E.
  1973 Religion, Altered States of Consciousness, and Social Change. Columbus: Ohio State University Press.
Harvey, Y. K.
  1976 The Korean *mudang* as a Household Therapist. *In* Culture-Bound Syndromes, Ethnopsychiatry, and Alternate Therapies. W. P. Lebra (ed.), Honolulu: University Press of Hawaii.
Lebra, W. P.
  1964 The Okinawan Shaman. *In* Ryukyuan Culture and Society: A Survey. A. H. Smith (ed.). Honolulu: University of Hawaii Press.
  1966 Okinawan Religion: Belief, Ritual, and Social Structure. Honolulu: University of Hawaii Press.
  1968 Ancestral Beliefs and Illness in Okinawa. *In* Proceedings of the VIIIth International Congress of Anthropological and Ethnological Sciences, Volume III. Tokyo: Science Council of Japan.
  1969 Shaman and Client in Okinawa. *In* Mental Health Research in Asia and the Pacific. W. Caudil and T. Y. Lin (eds.). Honolulu: East-West Center Press.
Ohashi, H.
  1978 Okinawa ni okeru shaman (*yuta*) no seitai to kino (Function and mode of life of the shaman (yuta) in Okinawa). Tohoku Daigaku Bungakubu Kenkyu Nempo (Annual Research Bulletin, Faculty of Letters, Tohoku University) 28:1–46.
Ryukyu Government
  1969 Okinawa-ken shi (Okinawa Prefecture History). Volume 19 Naha.
Scheff, T. J.
  1979 Catharsis in Healing, Ritual and Drama. Berkeley: University of California Press.
Spiro, M. E.
  1952 Ghosts, Ifaluk and Teleological Functionalism. American Anthropologist 54: 497–503.
Tseng, W. S.
  1976 Folk Psychotherapy in Taiwan. *In* Culture-Bound Syndromes, Ethnopsychiatry, and Alternate Therapies. W. P. Lebra (ed.). Honolulu: University Press of Hawaii.
Uezu, T.
  1977 Yuta no rekishi to shakai-teki yakuwari (Social and historical role of the *yuta* (shaman). Aoi Umi 67:121–131.

14. *SUNAO*: A CENTRAL VALUE IN JAPANESE PSYCHOTHERAPY

INTRODUCTION

Any psychotherapy which is accepted by a society must embody — either implicitly or explicitly — the values of that society. In the early history of psychoanalysis, the new innovative therapy drew from and reinforced new emerging values associated with modernization. In the case of Japanese psychotherapies, *Naikan* and Morita, we find the reverse pattern. The methods used are essentially revivalistic, and oriented towards a rediscovery of the core values of Japanese society.

What are these values? How are they related to Japanese culture? How do they contrast with Western values? This paper examines these questions by discussing *Naikan* and Morita therapies and their relation to the central Japanese value of *Sunao*.

A BRIEF OUTLINE OF *NAIKAN*

Goals

Naikan (*Nai* meaning "inside" or "within" and *Kan*, "looking" or "observing oneself") is a particular kind of introspection based on a fixed method of recollection and of self-reflection. The procedure aims to achieve two parallel and interwoven goals: (1) the discovery of personal, *authentic* guilt for having been ungrateful and troublesome to others in the past, and (2) the discovery of a positive gratitude towards individuals who have extended themselves on behalf of the client at some time in the past. In short, guilt and gratitude. When these goals are attained, a profound change in self-image and interpersonal attitude occurs.

Procedure

The *Naikan* client sits in a quiet place surrounded by a folding partition and walls so that he is cut off from outside distractions. He is therefore free to concentrate exclusively on his inner world. For seven successive days he starts his *Naikan* examination at 5:30 in the morning and continues until 9:00 in the evening. He is visited briefly by an interviewer every 90 minutes.

The client is asked to look at himself *vis-à-vis* his relationships with others from the following three perspectives:

(1) Care received. The first instruction is to "recollect and examine your

A. J. Marsella and G. M. White (eds.), Cultural Conceptions of Mental Health and Therapy,
317–329.

memories on the care and kindness that you have received from a particular person during a particular time in your life". The client usually begins with an examination of his relationship to his mother, proceeds to talk about relationships with other family members, and then moves on to close persons, always following a progression from childhood to the present. For example, in the first day he may remember how his mother cared for him when he was sick in grammar school.

(2) Repayment. During that particular period "recollect what you have done for that person in return".

(3) Troubles caused. "Recollect what troubles and worries you have caused that person in that same period."

This examination is conducted in a boldly moralistic manner, placing the burden of blame on the client rather than "on others". Only in the earlier meetings when the interviewer is more lenient and tends to listen to what the client describes to him, are excuses, rationalizations or aggressions toward others permitted.

The role of the *Naikan* interviewer is quite different from that of the ordinary professional counselor or therapist. His primary function is to directly supervise the client in a very specific routine of concentration on his past. His main concern is that the client follows instructions and reflect successfully on the topics assigned for self-examination.

Process

It usually takes two to three days for clients to adjust to the new situation. Occasionally forgotten memories may come unexpectedly to the surface, bringing sporadic or diffuse feelings of guilt and gratitude. As the process goes on, the client becomes more and more meaningfully connected with his past. Insights into the guilty aspects of his present and past life emerge. He also gains insights into other people's love for him and into his dependence upon them for that love. Toward the end of the therapy, he accepts the *newly* recognized guilt along with the feeling of actual self-criticism. He also feels truly grateful for the love he has received from others and begins to empathize with them for the pain and suffering that they must have experienced.

There are three basic themes which flow from this process: (1) authentic guilt, (2) gratitude and (3) differentiation of self from others. Let us examine the underlying meaning of each.

(1) Authentic guilt. In contrast to the prevalent Western concept of guilt as more or less negative or even pathological, "authentic guilt" in *Naikan* has a profound, positive effect. Guilt in *Naikan* is coupled with the client's empathy for others, making empathy a prerequisite for the guilt. The client who confronts his own guilt accuses himself in a strict manner. This strong self-recrimination counters any narcissistic or egotistic orientations which he might have. It must be noted, however, that this painful experience can only be endured and

overcome by the experience of gratitude towards others which will be discussed in detail later.

In addition, the authentic guilt breaks down some of the rationalizations for past and present behavior. Most of us tend to take what we receive from others for granted and are often even unaware that we have received anything to begin with. Yet once we realize that we have done so little for all the trouble we have caused "others", this "authentic guilt" begins to develop. Therefore, our entire outlook on the world starts to change. One of the clients put it this way: "All of a sudden I was struck by a profound gratitude towards my parents and others for all their caring and kindness, despite the fact that I've been so egotistic." At the same time, resistance against changing oneself or accepting others fades rapidly. Clients who regarded themselves as victims to justify their hostility and distrust, now acknowledge that it is *they* — not the world — who are the real aggressors. They then become deeply sorry for the harm they have caused others. They become humble, open-minded and free from defenses. They feel that they can no longer take others for granted.

Another outcome of the authentic guilt experience is a clearer consciousness of one's social ties. Since guilt is related to a sense of indebtedness to the society one belongs to, it intensifies one's feelings of responsibility, first to the people around us, and then to the society in general.

(2) Gratitude. The experience of gratitude comes from the discovery of what the client has received from the people related to him. As described by Fromm (1956), there is a "basic love" acquired from birth which changes with time. During *Naikan*, one has the opportunity to relive this "basic feeling" connected with mother-child love and crucial to one's infancy. This extremely positive experience is similar to "creative regression" described by Kris (1952), and to *Amae*, the sweet feeling of dependency described extensively by T. Doi (1963, 1973). Because the sense of being accepted by others has its roots in this basic mother-child love, the client regains his trusting relationship with the world.

(3) Differentiation of self from others. Unlike Westerners, Japanese children are not encouraged from an early age to emphasize individual independence or autonomy. They are brought up in a more or less 'interdependent' or *amae* culture, where differentiation of self from others is a necessary task to be accomplished by socialization. In other words, one must resolve his not yet socialized *amae* to live as a mature and psychologically healthy person. The instruction requires that the client examine himself in his relationships with several significant others in his life, while directing and encouraging this differentiation.

For the first time in their lives, *Naikan* clients come to see their parents as individuals distinct and separate from themselves. They then realize that they do not have the right to expect so much from their parents, or to cause them so much harm. This differentiation of self from others is the prerequisite for becoming aware of one's responsibility to others.

Outcome

How might one describe the total picture of the final state of mind brought about by the *Naikan* experiences described above? The most striking and common feature found among successful *Naikan* clients is the deep realization that they actually exist for the sake of others. Another important discovery is their awareness of the extensive love and care they have received, in spite of the immeasurable harm they have caused. In *Naikan*, this combination of gratitude and guilt often causes crying spells and, in the Japanese language, is expressed in the common phrase *sumimasen* or "I'm sorry".

One more important characteristic in *Naikan* is the minimization of self and the maximization of others – a shift from an 'ego-centered' way of thinking and living to a relationship-oriented outlook. A strong emphasis is put on acceptance and harmony rather than assertiveness and competitiveness. Usually the Japanese *Naikan* clients experience satisfaction in establishing a relationship-oriented outlook. Although this may sound paradoxical, individuals who have successfully done *Naikan* feel they have encountered their authentic selves in this newly experienced relationship-oriented outlook. It can be said that self-realization in Japanese traditional culture is achieved only by the minimization of self. From this point of view, the special positive meaning that honesty and openmindedness has for the Japanese may be well understood, while facade, defence, and strategy have in contrast been valued negatively (Nakamura 1964).

Let me now turn to the new state of mind described by *Naikan* clients themselves at the end of their therapy. The most clear-cut features are found in the remarks they make concerning their past behaviors, attitudes and personality, which are consistently valued negatively after therapy. Clients' views of their psychological state of mind are expressed frequently with words such as the following: *Gohjoh*: Literally, strong emotion – actually meaning stubborn or obstinate; *Wagamama*: Selfish or capricious and wayward; *Ga*: Literally means ego but the implication is basically very negative. Thus, if someone's *Ga* is strong, it implies the same meaning as that of *Wagamama* or selfish mentioned above; *Ga o tohosu*: Have one's way, stick to one's own opinion, assert oneself; *Ga o haru*: Do as one pleases, almost the same meaning as that of *Ga o tohosu*; *Go o dasu*: Show the negative aspects of the self; *Jibun-katte* or *Migatte*: Selfish; *Gashuu*: Egotistic attachment; *Namaiki and Unobore*: Self-conceit, impertinence, forwardness; *Omoiagatta*: Boastful, conceited; *Iji-waru*: Ill-natured or unkind; *Higamu*: To become jaundiced, jealous; *Ekoji*: Obstinate, stubborn; *Teikoh-suru*: Resist against someone.

All of these expressions describe rigid, onesided and other negative aspects of the ego which are viewed as hampering smooth communication and harmony with others. *Naikan* attempts first to change or overcome these negative aspects of the ego, and then to achieve the reverse state of mind. In contrast to this wide range of negative expressions, there are very few expressions describing the positive aspects of the ego. In fact, the antithesis of all these qualities can, and is, expressed in a single word: *sunao*.

DEFINITION OF *SUNAO*

Many of the successful *Naikan* clients report that they became *sunao* as the result of their *Naikan* therapy. Indeed, Mr Yoshimoto, the founder of *Naikan*, states that becoming *sunao* is the main goal of the therapy. *Sunao* is such a popular term in Japanese that its meaning has broadened to the point where a literal translation is practically impossible. Therefore, both psychological and popular definitions are discussed below.

The word *sunao* consists of two parts; '*su*' and '*nao*'. '*Su*' means things in their original state without any transformation. The etymology of the word is said to be plain white silk cloth. '*Nao*', which literally means 'straight' or undistorted, implies being 'upright at heart', 'right-minded', 'authentic or genuine', or 'having no falsehood'. Since *sunao* has such broad, diffused meaning, its actual usage generally appears in a variety of terms which give it specificity. For example, *sunao de otonashii* (*sunao* and obedient), *sunao de shojiki* (*sunao* and honest), *sunao ni ayamaru* (apologizing with *sunao*).

As an adjective, *sunao* has several different psychologically interrelated meanings in both the interpersonal and intrapersonal realms.

In the interpersonal realm, someone who is *sunao* is: (1) obedient or docile (without the negative connotation of English); (2) more acceptance-prone and obedient rather than self-assertive or aggressive; (3) more passive and dependent rather than autonomous; (4) free from egotism, self-centeredness and therefore in harmony with one's social environment; (5) open-minded, disclosing, candid, honest, and truthful to oneself; (6) free from resistance, opposition, antagonism, rivalry.

In the intrapersonal realm, the meanings of *sunao* include: (1) smooth, relaxed and flexible; (2) gentle, soft, mild and tender; (3) free from conflict, struggle, frustration and suppression; (4) without preconceptions, bias or distortions; and (5) in tune with joy and gratitude.

Sunao has an essentially positive implication in Japanese culture, such that to say someone is *not sunao* is to make a decisively negative judgment of character or attitude. Possible psychological states of mind which consist of "not being *sunao*" are: (1) a state where some forms of resistance, conflict and suppression are found both among oneself and in one's relation to the environment, and (2) somewhere in one's mind and behavior, a '*muri*' or 'quirk' which prompts one to behave unnaturally in certain situations; (3) a somewhat tense or anxious state of mind; (4) a state which is often onesided, one-way communication; (5) a state where one's perspective is very limited, narrow, and one cannot get a whole picture.

These descriptive meanings of the word *sunao* may be clarified through consideration of several different contextual usages of this word.

Example 1. An adolescent girl, who previously resented her parents is now thinking with a more *sunao* mind. She looks back at her childhood and suddenly she feels sorry for her parents because she has not fulfilled their expectations. In this context, *sunao* is used to describe her newly-found attitude approximating obedience.

Example 2. An excerpt from the Asahi newspaper: "His way of living is amazingly *sunao* and 'free' without being annoyed by any constraints of shame, convention, or criticism by others." In this case, a genuine and authentic attitude toward oneself and toward the world at large is emphasized.

Example 3. She behaves like a delinquent but if you get to know her better, you will realize she is both *sunao* and smart. In this case, *sunao* conveys the nuance of not being "an antisocial" girl at heart.

Example 4. "Looking with *sunao* eyes, it is obvious that the evidence provided by the prosecutor is inadequate." In this example, *sunao* means unprejudiced, objective.

SUNAO AND MORITA THERAPY

As we have seen, *sunao* is a key concept underlying *Naikan* therapy. Our next question is: Does this also hold true for another major Japanese psychotherapy, namely Morita therapy? Since a number of excellent summaries of this method are now available in English (Murase and Johnson 1974; Reynolds 1976), I shall confine my comments to its relation with *sunao*.

A very significant feature of Morita therapy is that it has a definite limit in terms of the kinds of patients who can be successfully treated. The Morita method is applicable only to a specific personality type called "Morita nervosity" or "Morita *shinkeishitsu*", which can easily lead to a pathological state. Those falling into this category tend to be sensitive and introverted with a perfectionistic attitude and a high need for achievement. They tend to become extremely subjective.

Thus, when they become anxious they readily resort to defensive intellectualization, which prevents them from seeing themselves through the eyes of others. They tend to be overly sensitive to mild disturbances such as stray thoughts or fear of eye-to-eye contact and prone to uncontrollable blushing, compulsive ideas, and so on. Therefore, they plunge into a variety of unrealistic attempts to consciously suppress or overcompensate for these problems.

Before coming to Morita therapy for help, *shinkeishitsu* people often resort to various kinds of coping devices. But in their very effort to reduce their troubles, they often wind up mobilizing their intellect in an essentially rigid and arbitrary way, exacerbating their problems and creating a vicious circle. For example, one male patient with a chronic fear of blushing in front of girls tried to count to 100 in a vain effort to get his mind off his problem. In another case, patients sought absolute concentration while studying, or tried to maintain a totally relaxed and confident attitude during an oral examination.

One patient suffering from fear of eye-to-eye contact tried to cope with his fear by starting fixed at others. The outcome was quite inevitable his fear incresed all the more. Morita describes these clients as "egocentric" in the sense that, for the purpose of resolving their anxieties triggered by external stimuli, they focus too much attention on themselves and pay insufficient attention to what others are really saying, thinking or feeling.

According to Morita, the cause of this is quite simple: the clients do not face and accept their *natural* psychological reality. They do not recognize that it is natural to feel uncomfortable with direct eye contact; that it is common to lose one's power of concentration on a task in which one has little interest; and that anyone can get tense during an oral examination. In short, they do not see their reality as it is. However, if they had a *sunao* mind it would be obvious to them that they have been trying to achieve the impossible. With a *sunao* mind they would be able to endure their anxiety and dissatisfaction. Accepting oneself means admitting one's weaknesses, demerits, discomforts, and undesirable feelings as they are.

In typical Morita therapy, overcoming this psychological state is achieved by two entirely different steps: first, 'absolute bed-resting'; and, secondly, gradual adaptation to one's outer reality by means of everyday physical work in groups.

In the first step, the individual is isolated from the outside. Books, TV, music and conversation are not allowed. Therefore, the patient is forced to confront himself and attempt to give up his old ways of coping with his sufferings. Translated literally, the Japanese expressions for this process are "throwing away one's (negative) self or "breaking one's *ga*". This is the same kind of change that takes place in *Naikan* when the patient "faces his guilt".

In the next step, as the patient does various minor daily tasks such as cleaning the house, taking care of the plants and so on, he learns to see things as they are. The need to work effectively gradually shakes him loose from his anxieties and again his obstinate, self-centered orientation diminishes. He accepts things as they are (*arugamama*), which is one of the basic goals of Morita therapy. Morita's "accepting things as they are" is almost the same as Naikan's *sunao*. In fact, Morita therapists often use the term *sunao* in describing their goal. The difference between the two regarding this goal is more a matter of tone and emphasis than actual content. Morita tends to be more philosophical and objective; whereas *Naikan* tends to be more moralistic and emotional, using the term *sunao* in an interpersonal context.

SUNAO AND JAPANESE CULTURE

Two Levels of Sunao

A naive, trusting and empathic relationship with others — and even with the non-human world — is a precondition for the *sunao* mind. In short, as indicated by the popular expression 'he is *sunao* like a child', the prototype of *sunao* is found in the mind of early childhood, when one's ego is not yet fully developed. How can we reconcile this ideal with the therapeutic goal of helping individuals to adjust to an adult world? One possible solution is to differentiate two levels of *sunao* — (1) original or pristine and (2) socialized or developed.

(1) Original or pristine. The "original *sunao*" in *Naikan* is typically associated with the baby's trusting attitude toward his mother and is somewhat similar to what Balint (1970), an English psychoanalyst, classified as the "good type of regression". It is in this oral stage of life that we can find the most naive, submissive and nondefensive state of mind. Any baby in a trusting relationship is by definition *sunao*.

Through *Naikan* a state approaching "original *sunao*" can be experienced — but only temporally. Despite its limited duration and intensity, however, the therapeutic significance of this experience should not be overlooked. Re-experiencing the mother-child union and love seems to play a decisive role for reconfirming one's feelings of trust towards the world. The client then feels a profound security that appears to reach the innermost core of his identity.

(2) Socialized or developed. With the original *sunao* as a foundation, *Naikan* clients proceed to differentiate their individuality by becoming more objective and critical about themselves. This *Naikan* process is parallel to the psycho-analytic developmental theory. Thus, the original *sunao* is transformed along the same line as the socialization process, in that it is imbued with a clearer sense of responsibility and a greater empathic ability — in short a better integration of past, future and present. Unconditional trusting of others, rather than self gain, becomes the ideal sought by the client. Naturally, his empathy is far more differentiated than that in original *sunao*. Both this *sunao* and the ego described by Western psychoanalytic theory can be viewed as agents of socialization. The contrastive nature of these two socialization processes are described below in a brief comparison of *Naikan* and Western psychotherapies and the social ideals upon which they are based.

Sunao and Japanese Religious Traditions

The plain, natural and honest states of mind associated with *sunao* are also the central values of the ancient Shinto religion which centers around respect for the pristine and unembellished state of man or nature.

This leads us to a conclusion that may be startling to many in the practice: since *sunao* is in turn closely linked to Shintoism, it follows that Shintoism plays a significant role in both therapies. Although it has been recognized that *Naikan* was influenced by both the Buddhistic and Confucianistic traditions, and that Morita therapy was developed under the *indirect* influence of Zen, we must now go one step beyond this observation and realize that beneath the influence of these relatively recent religious traditions, the ancient Shinto tradition of *sunao* has survived and thrived. In fact, the role of Shinto may be the most fundamental.

On the other hand, this conclusion should not come as a surprise at all to students of Japanese culture and history. If we look back at the long history of Japanese culture, we soon notice a pattern wherein strong undercurrents of this ancient value reassert themselves repeatedly in reaction to hasty introduction of imported values from China, Korea, and the West.

The two Japanese psychotherapies do essentially the same thing; they periodically restore and maintain the oldest of traditional values.

Many key-words have been proposed as representing the essential nature of Japanese culture. To cite some of them: *"amae"* (Doi 1962, 1973), "empathy culture" (Minamoto 1969), "maternal principle" (Kawai 1976), "egg without eggshell" (Mori 1977), "self-negation" (Araki 1976), and "between man and man" (Kimura 1972). All these key-words are very closely related to *sunao* value and, like *sunao*, symbolize a merging of the relationship between mother and child. The key point is that the relationship *per se* is far more important than the individuals themselves. *Sunao* value reinforces trustful relationships which in turn provide the appropriate climate for *sunao* attitudes such as openness and dependence.

'Sunao Culture' and 'Ego Culture'

In short, Japan is a *'sunao* culture' whereas most of the Western world is an 'ego culture'. In a *'sunao'* culture, there is a tendency to view the ego as a negative force such that the ideal of socialization becomes the negation of this ego. At first glance, it might appear that this is a paradox because one has to repress oneself in order to *realize* oneself. However, Japanese in general and the Japanese therapies in particular, distinguish between two kinds of ego as in the expression "throw away your lesser ego (*shohga*) so that you may achieve a greater ego (*taiga*)". The latter is on an entirely different plane than the ordinary ego, and is considered to be harmonious with one's outer world. The negation of *shoga* (lesser ego) and the aspiration to reach *taiga* (greater ego) may be a tendency common to most Japanese. As I proposed earlier, the original *sunao* develops into socialized *sunao*. But this *sunao* can develop even higher ideal levels which one might call "universal *sunao*" (in Japanese *taiga sunao*). This universal *sunao* contains the quality of original *sunao* more clearly than does the ordinary socialized *sunao*.

In contrast to this *sunao* culture, ego culture is primarily concerned with the strengthening of the ego. It is expected that the negative aspect of the ego can be overcome not by the denial of ego itself but by allowing the positive aspects of the ego to gain control over it. In this sense ego culture seems to be fundamentally realistic and progression-prone; where *sunao* culture is idealistic and regression-prone. It is possible to list a series of related oppositions which contrast the social ideals and socialization patterns of *'sunao* culture' with those typical of the Western 'ego culture'. These are shown in Table I.

TABLE I

Two patterns of socialization

Sunao culture	"Ego" culture
1. Relationship-oriented	Individual centered
2. Unconditional relationship	Contractual relationship
3. Self-realization through union with the group	Self-realization through interaction within the group
4. Non-defensive, disclosing	Healthy defense
5. Feelings are dominant	Intellect and will are dominant
6. Simple, plain, and less structured	Complex, sophisticated and more structured
7. Mild and tender	Harsh and solid
8. Passive, obedient, and non-aggressive	Active, assertive, and aggressive
9. Humble, self-limiting	Self-expanding
10. Dependent	Autonomous
11. Intrapunitive	Extrapunitive
12. Harmonious	Competitive
13. Flexible and adaptable	Strong
14. Maternal principle	Paternal principle

How does this relate to psychotherapy, our primary concern? The negation of oneself, becoming free from *shohga*, is seen as an elevation of the individual. These are the prevalent ideals of *sunao* culture which appear to permeate various activities, including psychotherapy and even some of the traditional sports. Thus, *Naikan* may be one of the most direct and effective ways of attaining this goal; while Morita is a more indirect, but equally effective method.

Since Western ego culture has a different view regarding socialization (See Table I), the person and especially individualism (see Shweder and Bourne, this volume), its therapeutic strategies also reflect differences from those of *sunao* culture. Western psychotherapies, especially psychoanalysis, rely heavily on the individual intellect, and attempt to lead the client on a somewhat unstructured path to self-improvement by probing the past for the causes of disorder in infantile conflicts or traumata. As Reynolds and Kiefer (1977) note, this type of verbal analysis, aimed at increasing self-awareness, tends to separate the individual from the here-and-now of his environment. This orientation contrasts with Morita's "accepting things as they are". In the Morita view, the intellectual examination of past experience would be regarded as a continuation of mentalistic self-absorption. The Japanese therapies are aimed more at achieving adaptation through accommodation, rather than resolving internal conflicts, strengthening the individual ego, and gaining mastery over the social environment (Murase and Johnson 1974). The "insight" in *Naikan* therapy involves the discovery of relations of responsibility, obligation and dependency which structure Japanese social reality. Social ideals and personal objectives are thus brought into alignment. Conformity, or the merging of self and other is consistent with self-actualization, as defined by the premises of *sunao* culture.

CONCLUSION

The goal of *Naikan* can be summarized by a single Japanese word – *sunao*, a uniquely Japanese term and value system. Generally speaking, *sunao* implies the harmonious and natural state of mind *vis-à-vis* oneself and others. It is directly associated with honesty, humility, docility and simplicity. Although these qualities are not necessarily valued positively in Western culture, in Japanese culture *sunao* is an extremely important positive value. In this model, value orientations in *sunao* culture are essentially passive, relationship-oriented and regression-prone; whereas ego culture is active, individual-centered and progression-prone.

Since *sunao* culture has been changing under the strong influence of the Western ego culture, a major question which remains unanswered is what influence it will have in the future. *Sunao* may be a useful concept for understanding the primary nature of Japanese culture as a *sunao* culture, in contrast to Western societies as ego cultures.

It can be differentiated into at least two levels, the original, prototypical *sunao* found among infants who experience a trusting relationship with their mothers, and the socialized *sunao* of the more mature adult. Both levels of *sunao* play a significant role in *Naikan* therapy.

Morita, another Japanese therapy, has essentially the same goal, in spite of considerable differences in methodology and terminology. Usually *Naikan* and Morita are considered to have been influenced – directly or indirectly – by Buddhism and other imported cultures. *Sunao* does not, however, belong to these 'imported' religions but is essentially derived from ancient Shintoism – a value system which remains a strong undercurrent of Japanese culture. Both of the Japanese therapies embody the same latent system, but at the same time neither has made the origin of these values explicit. *Sunao*, an essentially Japanese concept with no English equivalent, is an important link between Japan's distant past and the practical therapies being used successfully today.

ACKNOWLEDGMENTS

The author wishes to express his appreciation to Mr and Mrs Weiss for their help in improving the English expression of ideas in this paper.

REFERENCES

Araki, H.
  1976 Nihonjin No Shinjoh-Ronri (Feelings and Logics of the Japanese). Tokyo: Kohdansha.

Balint, M.
    1968 The Basic Fault: Therapeutic Aspects of Regression. London: Tavistock.
DeVos, G.
    1960 The Relation of Guilt toward Parents to Achievement and Arranged Marriage
          among the Japanese. Psychiatry 23:287–301.
Doi, L. T.
    1962 "Amae: A Key Concept for Understanding Japanese Personality Structure." In
          Japanese Culture, its Development and Characteristics. R. J. Smith and R. K.
          Beardsley (eds.). Chicago: Aldine.
    1973 The Anatomy of Dependence. Tokyo: Kohdansha International Ltd.
Fromm, E.
    1956 The Art of Loving. New York: Harper.
Kimura, B.
    1972 Hito To Hito To No Aida (Between Person and Person). Tokyo: Kohbundoh.
Kawai, H.
    1976 Bosei Shakai Nihon No Byori (Psychopathology of the contemporary Japan as
          the maternal society). Tokyo: Chuo Koronsha.
Kris, E.
    1952 Psychoanalytic Explorations in Art. New York: International University Press.
Lebra, T. S. and W. P. Lebra, eds.
    1974 Japanese Culture and Behavior: Selected Readings. Honolulu: The University
          Press of Hawaii.
Lebra, T. S.
    1976 Japanese Patterns of Behavior. Honolulu: The University Press of Hawaii.
Minamoto, R.
    1969 Giri To Ninjo (Obligation and Human Feelings). Tokyo: Chuo Koronsha.
Mori, J.
    1977 Nihonjin: 'Kara-Nashi-Tamago' No Jigazoh. (The Japanese: His Self-Image as an
          'Egg without its Eggshell') Tokyo: Kohdansha.
Murase, T.
    1974 Naikan Therapy. In Japanese Culture and Behavior: Selected Readings. T. S.
          Lebra and W. P. Lebra (eds.). Honolulu: The University Press of Hawaii.
Murase, T. and F. Johnson
    1974 Naikan, Morita and Western Psychotherapy: A Comparison. Archives of General
          Psychiatry 31:121–130.
Murase, T.
    1977 Naikan Ryoho to Morita Ryoho (Naikan Therapy and Morita Therapy). In Gendai
          No Morita Ryoho. K. Ohara (ed.). Tokyo: Hakuyosha.
Nakamura, H.
    1964 Ways of Thinking of Eastern People: India, China, Tibet, Japan. Philip Wiener, ed.
          Honolulu: The University Press of Hawaii.
Nakane, C.
    1970 Japanese Society. Berkeley: University of California Press.
Pattison, E. M.
    1969 Morality, Guilt and Forgiveness in Psychotherapy. In Clinical Psychiatry and
          Religion. E. M. Pattison (ed.). Boston: Little Brown.
Reynolds, D. K.
    1976 Morita Therapy. Berkeley: University of California Press.
    1977 Naikan Therapy – An Experiential View. The International Journal of Social
          Psychiatry 23:256–267.
    1980 The Quiet Therapies. Honolulu: The University Press of Hawaii.
Reynolds, D. K. and C. W. Kiefer
    1977 Cultural Adaptability as an Attribute of Therapies: The Case of Morita Psycho-
          therapy. Culture, Medicine and Psychiatry 1:395–412.

Tahara, T.
  1968 Motoori Noringa. Tokyo: Kohdansha.
Tanaka-Matsumi, J.
  1979 Cultural factors and Social Influence Technique in Naikan Therapy: A Japanese
        Self-Observation Method. Psychotherapy: Theory, Research and Practice 16:
        385–390.

SECTION IV

ISSUES AND DIRECTIONS

PAUL PEDERSEN

15. THE INTERCULTURAL CONTEXT OF COUNSELING AND THERAPY

INTRODUCTION

By viewing counseling and therapy in their intercultural context, several points will become apparent: (1) That these functions have spread rapidly to a complex social industry on a world-wide basis; (2) That counseling and therapy as we know them are labels for one of the many alternatives for intervention to influence a person's mental health; (3) That counseling and therapy as the *preferred* alternatives are based on assumptions generic to a very small portion of the world's people; (4) That an interculturally appropriate application in counseling and therapy is necessarily responsive to the social context.

The historical spread of counseling and therapy has been documented in a wide range of cultures. While mental health problems and solutions are continuous, the labels have changed from one culture to another over time. Support services and problems have been around for a long time. What has changed has been the complex classification of the environments where counseling and therapy is being applied, and the categories of problems, illness, difficulty, or crisis. A specialized therapeutic industry has developed to meet this defined configuration of need with numbers of consumers as well as numbers of providers increasing in proportion to the increasingly liberal definition of "appropriate" criteria for entering counseling and therapy.

The ambiguities of intercultural therapy might be diminished by identifying the range of contextual situations in which it might occur. Wohl (1981) describes seven different operational contexts for intercultural therapy. First, representatives of one culture study the therapeutic modes of another culture. This most obvious example emphasizes an anthropological or research interest, including studies of culture-bound disorders, traditional healers, folk treatment procedures and topics of psychological anthropology (Lebra 1976).

A second category includes problems related to culturally-different "minorities" within the larger cultural context, which have been enlarged to include special populations of age, life style, sex role and socio-economic status as well as ethnic and nationality groups. Culturally differentiated groups have special and unique needs; overemphasizing those demographic variables will result in cultural stereotyping just as under-emphasizing them will result in cultural insensitivity.

A third category includes a therapist working with culturally different clients through culturally-different approaches. Work with immigrants, foreign students or sojourners, or a foreign medical resident coming to practice in the United States would be examples of this category.

A. J. Marsella and G. M. White (eds.), Cultural Conceptions of Mental Health and Therapy,
333–358.

A fourth category would include therapists applying their "back home" methods of therapy in a culturally foreign society, whether through research or service delivery. The visitor is usually temporarily working in the host culture and is less likely to have a permanent influence, unless the foreign therapy is somehow adapted to the local context.

A fifth category would include the exploration of a system of therapy independent of the person or persons transporting it. The basic premise of intercultural therapy is that a particular system of ideas and theories can be adapted to many culturally-different societies.

A sixth category would include a therapist from one culture and a client from a second culture working in the context of a third culture. Wohl suggests the even more complicated possibility of their using a system of therapy developed in a fourth culture!

The seventh category Wohl outlines, occurs when members of one culture have lived for a long time in another culture, borrowing elements from both their home and host culture. As a consequence a "third culture" is developed (Useem and Useem 1967) to suit the special needs of these "bi-cultural" persons.

Each of these categories has been described as examples of cross-cultural counseling and therapy within the other papers of this book. It will be important to keep these categories in mind as we consider the domestic and international development of this field. I will discuss the field of intercultural therapy from five perspectives.

THE MINORITY PERSPECTIVE

The "contact hypothesis" tests the assumption that just bringing people from different groups together will result in more positive intergroup relations. Amir (1969) reviewed the literature from social psychology in a classic article on the contact hypothesis that drew three basic conclusions. First, when groups come together under favourable conditions, the intergroup contact does indeed result in more positive relationships. Second, when groups come together under unfavorable conditions, the intergroup contact results in more negative relationships and disharmony. Third, the spontaneous intergroup contact is more likely to occur under unfavorable conditions than favorable conditions. These unfavorable conditions are most easily illustrated in the relationships between dominant and minority groups. Atkinson et al. (1979) include the *condition of being oppressed* as an important defining characteristic of any minority group. This might be the case even when the group is not a numerical "minority" as in the literature about women as a minority group. The literature on minority relations is therefore characterized by the struggle of each minority against a dominant majority group and, more recently, of some minority groups against other minority groups competing for limited resources.

With increased publications on minority group counseling in the late 1960s and 1970s, a great deal of confusion has occurred in the use of terms like race, ethnicity, culture and minority (Atkinson et al. 1979). The term "race" technically refers to biological differences, while ethnicity rightly refers to group classifications where members share a cultural heritage from one generation to another. People of the same ethnic group within the same race, might still be culturally different. Other terms such as "culturally deprived" or "culturally disadvantaged" and even the more modern "culturally different" and "culturally distinct" were created to explain why a "minority" group is out of step with the "majority" population. Minorities, then, are people singled out for unequal and different treatment and who regard themselves as objects of discrimination (Atkinson et al. 1979).

Intercultural counseling and therapy in the domestic context has been characterized by the political and economic interaction of special interest and minority groups throughout the country. The domestic context of intercultural relations has been characterized by political influence and socio-economic impact. The basis of dissatisfaction, ironically, was written into the practically unfulfilled idealistic promises of the Declaration of Independence. As a nation, we have experienced a social revolution that has idealized a state of equality among races, sexes, generations and peoples. We have been taught that only those who make use of their opportunities and develop special skills can be assured of their fair share. The concept of equality is thereby diluted to a doctrine of equal opportunity, granting us the equal right to become unequal, as perceived by the minorities, through competing with one another (Dreikurs 1972). Bryne (1977) has pointed out how the perception of equality has politicized the delivery of mental health services in our domestic social context. Aubrey (1977) likewise pointed out the trend in mental health to emphasize normal developmental concerns of individuals to the exclusion of special group's concerns, in the name of "equality".

With the Civil Rights movement of the 1950s, the militancy of minorities for change gained momentum. With the growth of the community mental health movement of the 1960s, mental health care was now the right of all citizens and not just the wealthy or middle-class dominant majority (LeVine and Padilla 1980; Atkinson et al. 1979). The issues of feminism and popular dissent nurtured by the anti-Vietnam war movement fostered a climate of discontent where protest was accepted and in some cases even demanded. The stigma of discrimination became synonymous with any attempt to treat groups differently. Sue (1981) suggested that minority groups may not be asking for equal treatment as much as equal access and opportunity. Differential treatment is not necessarily discriminatory or preferential. One of the conclusions of cross-cultural counseling is that interculturally skilled counseling is almost necessarily and inevitably differential across cultures in providing an appropriate mental health service. In response to the same problem, a therapist may help one client be more dependent and another be less dependent, depending on the context.

There is abundant evidence that came to light in the 1970s that mental health services were being underutilized by minority groups and that behavior described as pathological in a minority culture such as individualistic assertiveness may be viewed as adaptive in a majority culture client (Wilson and Calhoun 1974; Grier and Cobbs 1968). Asian-Americans, Blacks, Chicanos, American Indians and other minority groups terminate counseling significantly earlier than Anglo clients (Sue 1977; Atkinson et al. 1979). In most of the literature, these examples of differentiation are credited to cultural barriers that hinder the formation of good counseling relationships, language barriers, class-bound values and culture-bound attitudes. To some extent these conditions certainly do exist and do result in a minority group's disillusionment with the professional field of mental health as a solution for social and individual coping. Dinges et al. (1981) offer a contrasting view which is not frequently mentioned but which may also account for underutilization based on cultural boundary maintenance functions. This viewpoint suggests that mental health services perceived as alien by the minority group may be avoided in a desire to avoid the erosion of personal identity-sustaining forces in the minority culture. From this point point of view, more attractive and effective mental health services might result in *increased* acculturative stress among those being served.

There have been numerous efforts to compensate for inequitable practices in providing mental health services to minorities in culturally sensitive ways. One example of such an effort is in the area of testing. There have been extensive studies of problems in the use of psychological tests with American minority clients and particularly in mental tests of intelligence of ability across cultures. Most of these research efforts are cited by Brislin et al. (1973) and more recently by Lonner (1981). The development of "culture free" and more recently "culture-fair" intelligence tests are, included in the several attempts to measure intelligence across cultures (Brislin et al. 1973). Frijda and Jahoda (1966) pointed out that a culture-fair test would need to be either equally familiar or equally unfamiliar to persons from responding cultures, which would be an impossible pre-condition. Tests are more widely accepted as inevitably biased, and in the more recent intercultrual research, the emphasis has been placed on accounting for cultural differences in the interpretation of test results that are sensitive to these inherent biases.

A second area of activity that recognizes the reality of cultural bias is in public policy statements that acknowledge the importance of mental health consumer's cultural environment. The National Institute of Mental Health (Fields 1979), The American Psychological Association (Korman 1974), the American Psychological Association Council of Representatives (APA 1979), the American Psychiatric Association's Task Force on Ethnocentricity among Psychiatrists (Wintrob and Harvey 1981), and the recent President's Commission on Mental Health (Fields 1979) have all emphasized the ethical responsibility of counselors and therapists to know their clients' cultural values, and public responsibility of professional organizations to meet the culturally-different mental health needs within a pluralistic society.

This has resulted in culturally-sensitive guidelines for accreditation of mental health training programs, special funding for research on cultural differences in mental health services and the development of resources for collective pressure to make mental health services more responsive to cultural differences. The adjustment has not been trouble-free however. Atkinson, Staso and Hosford (1978) describe problems in meeting federal standards for admitting minority applicants to counseling while maintaining a single admission standard on test scores and selection following the Bakke decision in California. Jaslow (1978) describes some of the problems in the desegregation of schools and the difficulty in retraining school personnel, students, counselor educators and communities in the skills for working in a racially mixed school.

Although these visible efforts have increased, the field of mental health is still a long way from providing diverse services that are culturally responsive. That situation is likely to change as the numbers and influence of various minority groups increase, through acculturation by both minority and majority group members and perhaps through the weakening of the ethnic family of community support systems as the defenders of traditional values. Hopefully there will also be a development of more knowledgable and relevant mental health services, more adequate and comprehensive cross-cultural training for mental health professionals, and more power in the laws and professional licensing criteria related to the delivery of culturally appropriate mental health services. Allen Ivey (1980, 1981) speaks for the field of counseling in forecasting the importance of the cultural dimension.

In short, a broadly-based counseling psychology which seeks to foster human development in a person-environment perspective, of necessity, must consider cultural factors of primary importance in any treatment plan, community intervention or multi-faceted program of assistance. (Ivey 1980:6).

THE INTERNATIONAL PERSPECTIVE

Although culture as a concept is ancient, the systematic study of culture and psychopathology is a phenomenon of the twentieth century. Initially the fields of psychoanalysis and anthropology were the focus of interest in studying culture and mental health, later expanding to include epidemiology and sociology and more recently the sub-specialty of social psychiatry. The focus of study has shifted from the anthropological study of remote cultures to the cultural variations in modern pluralistic and complex societies (Marsella 1979).

Through the work of men like Kiev (1972); Prince (1976) and Kleinman (1979) the indigenous approaches to mental health in non-Western cultures began to be taken more seriously, replacing the "crazy shaman" notion of curiousity and fascination with indigenous healers' techniques and even sometimes integrating them with other modern mental health services. Major cross-cultural studies of psychiatric evaluation and diagnosis (WHO 1979) have resulted in a more careful assessment of culture beyond the exotic, dramatic, and more conspicuous manifestations (Draguns 1980) as a "near-to-home" phenomenon of everyday life as well. Torrey (1972) went so far as drawing direct parallels between the techniques of "witchdoctors" and "psychiatrists" in naming their treatment, identifying a cause, establishing rapport, developing client expectation for improvement, and demonstrating legitimacy. Kleinman (1979) among others however, opposes any conclusion that would imply shamans and psychiatrists do the same thing and considers this identification an over-simplication that does "a profound disservice to both psychiatry and anthropology" (99).

Draguns (1977) describes research by Collomb (1973) on additional "pitfalls" of adapting mental health services including attitudes of "*pseudouniversalism*" that populations vary but services are immutable, "*idealization* of the host culture" with a corresponding denigration of one's home culture, and "*denial* of any validity" for outside mental health services in the host culture. Dubreuil (1975) reviews Collomb's (1973) book about work in Senegal that suggests problems in adapting mental health services modeled on Western values to non-Western cultures. The system must be matched with the cultural context. Explorational, open-ended, insight-oriented therapy is less successful in cultures favoring authoritarian-totalitarian political régimes (Draguns 1981).

There is likewise more emphasis on what developed-cultures can learn about providing mental health services from less-developed cultures. Prince (1976, 1980) demonstrates how the activity of all healers and healing institutions depends on endogenous self-righting mechanisms for healing to occur, rather than on exogenous experts. In non-Western cultures with fewer formal healing institutions, there is more dependence on these endogenous self-righting mechanisms such as dreams, sleep or rest, altered states of consciousness, religious experience, or even psychotic reaction as a healing resource. Some of the renewed interest in learning how these self-righting mechanisms work is because of their proven effectiveness in managing psychiatric disorders, the shortage and expense of modern psychiatric facilties, the high prestige of some endogenous approaches in their home cultures and the evidence that "modern" treatment methods tend to be culture-bound (Prince 1980; Marsella and Higginbotham, in press).

Kleinman has developed ethnomedical models from his work in China and other non-Western cultures that contrast with the biomedical models of modern medical treatment. Kleinman (1978b) attacks the "discipline-bound compartmentalization" of medical research through ethnography, ethnoscience, epidemiology and cultural systems analysis.

The cultural context does not merely tell us about the social and cultural environment within which a particular local system of medicine is situated, but also tells about the specific cognitive, behavioral and institutional structure of that system and the cultural constructional principles (values and symbolic meanings) underlying and determining that structure. (Kleinman 1978b:415).

David Reynolds (1980) has adapted *Naikan*, Morita and several other systems of traditional Japanese therapy to Western cultures as uniquely appropriate to mental illness in Western as well as Asian society. While Reynolds is careful to acknowledge the unrealistic claims in much of the popular literature about meditation, Zen-related therapies and other non-Western approaches, he also demonstrates the value and adaptability of these therapies when appropriately presented. Many other non-Western derived therapies have gained popularity, but frequently without documentation and careful standards of delivery. (Pedersen 1977).

As a consequence of being culturally relevant, phenomena are inevitably culturally perceived, so that even in psychobiological processes such as the perception of space and cognition, there are cultural differences (Diaz-Guerrero 1977; Marsella and Golden 1980). These culturally-specific characteristics challenge the universality of psychology, not its scientific character. There are alternative cultural assumptions which are not related to the "American ideal" (Sampson 1977) or to the premises of the Protestant Ethic (Rotenberg 1974; Draguns 1974) and pervasive assumptions of individualism (Hsu 1972; Pedersen 1979). It is increasingly clear that Western-style mental health services are inappropriate, too expensive, too dependent on technology and are frequently destructive to the non-Western host setting. There are numerous assumptions, beginning with individualistic biases, that require us to look to non-Western alternatives (Pedersen 1979).

There appears to be a contrast between Western and non-Western approaches to counseling and therapy that has to do with the importance of "psychological balance" (Pedersen 1977). In the non-Westernized systems there is less emphasis on *"solving"* problems or *"curing"* illness where the therapy separates the person or persons from the presenting problem or source of difficulty. There is less tendency to locate the difficulty inside the isolated individuals, but rather to relate that individual's difficulty to other persons or even the cosmology. Health describes a condition of order and predictability in a context where all elements (even problems and pain) serve a useful and necessary function. The emphasis is more holistic in acknowledging the interaction of person and environment in *both* their positive and negative aspects. This insight may be one of the most significant contributions of ethnoscience to mental health. Therapy is integrated with cultural context in every application, suggesting generalized universal similarities across cultures. The *restoration of "balance"* is likely to replace the medical model's more individualized goals of *"cure"* in the definition of good mental health across cultures. In a context of balance, therapy is perceived as continuous and not episodic, a process and not a conclusive event. The contrasting assumptions of a balanced, as against an "unbalanced" approach to mental health might account for the contradictory conclusions of therapy-outcome studies in different cultures.

THE THEORETICAL PERSPECTIVE

There is no agreement on a theoretical or conceptual framework for matching therapy interventions with culturally complex personal problems to facilitate intercultural adjustment. In the most comprehensive recent reviews of the literature, Marsella (1979), and Strauss (1979) comment that there is no paradigm to focus the increasing research studies or to test the consistency of contradictory theories that are offered to explain the relationship of personality and culture. LeVine (1972) provides a useful classification for organizing the theories of culture and personality. First, *anticulture and personality* states that culture determines personality and that the individual has little influence on the cultures. Second, *psychological reductionism* states that all human activity can be explained by studying individuals. Third, *personality as culture* equates personality dynamics with culture. Fourth, *personality mediation* assumes a chain reaction where culture creates an individual personality who in turn changes the culture. Fifth, the *"two systems" approach* avoids the question of whether culture or personality is more basic, but assumes a continuous and parallel interaction and compromise between the two. Study of personality and culture has increased in the 1970s (Tapp 1980).

Culture and mental health research has failed to develop grounded theory based on empirical data for several reasons. First, the emphasis has been on abnormal behavior across cultures isolated from the study of normal behavior across cultures (Katz and Sanborn 1976). Second, it is only in the 1970s that a pancultural core has emerged for the more serious categories of disturbance such as schizophrenia and affective psychoses, so that they are recognizable according to uniform symptoms across cultures even though tremendous cultural variations continue to exist (Draguns 1980). Third, the complexity of research on therapy across cultural lines is difficult to manage beyond pre-quantificated stages (Draguns 1981). Fourth, the research which is available has lacked an applied emphasis related to practical concerns of program development, service delivery, and techniques of treatment (Draguns 1980). Fifth, there has been insufficient interdisciplinary collaboration from psychology, psychiatry, and anthropology among the more directly related disciplines, each approaching culture and mental health from different perspectives (Favazza and Oman 1977). Sixth, the emphasis of research foci has been on the symptom as a basic variable, to the neglect of the interaction of person, professional, institution and community (Ivey 1980). Cultural differences introduce barriers to understanding in those very areas of interaction that are most crucial to the outcome of therapy, through discrepancies between counselor and client, experiences, beliefs, values, expectations and goals. Cross-cultural counseling describes conditions that are most unfavorable for successful therapy (Lambert 1981). It is no wonder therefore that there is disagreement concerning the theoretical criteria of interculturally skilled counseling.

THE THERAPIST PERSPECTIVE

Wrenn (1962) defined the "culturally encapsulated counselor" as one who had substituted symbiotic modal stereotypes for the real world, disregarded cultural variations among clients, and dogmatized technique-oriented definitions of counseling and therapy. Counselors can become "addicted" to one system of cultural values, resulting in the same disorientation and dependency as with any other addiction by analogy (Morrow 1972). Pluralistic therapy then recognizes a client's culturally-based beliefs, values and behaviors; is sensitive to the cultural environment and the network of interacting influences. Sue (1978) suggests that culturally-effective counselors have at least five characteristics: First, they recognize their own values and assumptions in contrast with alternative assumptions, with the ability to translate those values and assumptions into action. Second, they are aware of generic characteristics of counseling that cut across schools and classes and cultures and any other contextual variables that influence the counseling process. Third, they understand the socio-political forces that influence the attitudes of culturally-different minorities or otherwise oppressed groups. Fourth, they can share a client's world view without negating its legitimacy and without cultural oppression of their client's viewpoint. Fifth, they are truly eclectic in their own counseling style, generating a variety of skills from a wide range of theroretical orientations.

Tseng and Hsu (1980) have discussed how therapy might compensate for culturally-different features so that highly controlled and overregulated cultures might encourage therapies that provide a safety-valve release for feelings and emotions, while underregulated or anomic cultures would encourage therapies with externalized social control at the expense of self-expression. There is a constant re-adjustment of the balance between interacting therapeutic and cultural variables. It is as though the individual is participating in a social game based on conventional rules that define boundaries between the individual and the cultural context. Watts (1961) defines the duty of the therapist to involve participants in a "counter game" that restores a unifying perspective of ego and environment so that the person can be liberated in a balanced context. To the extent that the therapist is distanced from the client, culture becomes a more significant barrier. Kleinman (1979) describes the problems which result when the explanations of the clinician and the patient are in conflict. Kleinman characterizes most clinicians as schooled in the biomedical paradigm to recognize and treat *disease* as the malfunction or maladaptative biological and or psychological process. By contrast, the patient is more likely to experience *illness* as interruptions in the social and cultural network created through the experience. Patients evaluate treatment as a "healing process" more than as a "cure outcome", recognizing that there are no clear beginnings or endings in the complex interaction of variables. The best a clinician can hope for is restoration of balance.

Draguns (1977) suggests several guidelines for adjusting therapy modes to fit the culture. The more complex the social and cognitive structure, the more a society will prefer hierarchy and ritual characterized by elaborate techniques for countering psychological distress. The stronger a society believes in changeability of human nature and plasticity of social roles, the more they will favor therapy techniques as vehicles of change. Where attitudes toward psychological disturbance reflect deep-seated prejudices about human nature, the less tolerant and accepting they will be of the mentally ill. The emphasis is rightly on dynamic rather than static variables across cultures.

The therapist needs to form a facilitative relationship with culturally different clients so that, ideally, the client will experience being warmly received, deeply accepted and fully understood (Lambert (1981). To establish that relationship, the client needs to perceive the counselor as a crediable expert (well informed, capable, and intelligent) and trustworthy (Sue 1981). The counselor needs to accommodate a wide range of therapist and client roles, integrating them with the client's world view without at the same time losing the counselor's own integrity as a culturally integrated person (Sue 1977). These prerequisites incorporate a blend of the goals of helping through insight, self-actualization, behavior change and immediacy, with the appropriate process. A client may be exposed to appropriate process and appropriate goals, appropriate process and inappropriate goals, inappropriate process and appropriate goals or inappropriate process and inappropriate goals (Ivey 1981).

Ultimately these counselor characteristics result in rapport, empathy, interest and appreciation of the client's culture, understanding the special terms, knowing the language, knowing the community and the problems of living in a bicultural world (Sundberg 1981a, 1982b). Given that therapists experience the same rates of stereotyping and ethnocentrism as the general public (Bloombaum et al. 1968), our expectations for the cross-cultural therapist seem somewhat unrealistic. Cross-cultural counselors ask for special techniques, assuming it is better for minorities to counsel other minorities, since these cultural barriers are so formidable. Vontress (1981) suggests that few counselors really want to change themselves. Most are products of a racist socialization, and this condition is not likely to change as a result of a few courses, without the impact of affective confrontation as through cultural immersion. Sometimes it would seem that the advancement of cross-cultural counseling implies the abandonment of counseling theory, therapy techniques and our traditional understanding of a client's psychological processes, when counseling techniques we have learned don't seem to work. Wohl (1981) is critical of the "super-flexibility" of counselors and "elastic modifications" of sound principle as dominant values in the conventional wisdom of cross-cultural counseling. Even before students acquire the fundamentals of counseling and therapy they are urged to abandon them in favor of some unorthodox method that is presumed to be cross-cultural. Patterson (1974, 1978) argues also that the proper approach is not to be "flexible" in modifying the method to fit the client's expectations and wishes, even though this is the most popular attitude among cross-cultural counselors because it subverts the counseling goals of self actualization.

THE CLIENT'S PERSPECTIVE

There is considerable controversy on the issue of whether counselors and clients should ideally be culturally similar. Carkhuff and Pierce (1967) are frequently cited as evidence that counselors who are most different from their clients in ethnicity and social class or who are not of the same sex have the greatest difficulty effecting constructive changes. LeVine and Campbell (1972) likewise are cited with evidence that groups who perceive themselves similarly are more likely to relate harmoniously. Mitchel (1970) suggested that most White counselors can't help Black clients because they are part of the problem. Stanges and Riccio (1970) demonstrated that counselor trainees preferred same-race and culture clients while Harrison (1975) and Berman (1979) demonstrated that black counselors preferred black clients. However there are other factors which have tended to exaggerate the apparent importance of racial similarity and have resulted in contradictory research findings. Parloff et al. (1978) conclude that cultural matching of counselors and clients is not clearly preferred. Not all research supports the preference for clients and counselors from the same culture, and some research (Gamboa et al. 1976) has demonstrated special conditions where the clients actually preferred culturally-different counselors.

Several issues are involved. First, as Peoples and Dell (1975) demonstrated, the preference for counseling style may be more important than racial match among black and white clients, among Asian-Americans (Atkinson et al. 1978) and among lower class people as compared with middle class people (Aronson and Overall 1966). Blacks also used more active expression skills and fewer attending skills than White counselors. Muliozzi (1972) indicated that Whites felt more genuine and empathic with Whites, although Blacks didn't see them as less genuine or understanding, and in other research (Ewing 1974) Black students reacted more favorably to Black and to White counselors than White students. Bryson and Cody (1973) indicated that Black counselors understood Black clients best, but White counselors were more acceptable than Black counselors for *both* Black and White. Part of this apparent contradiction might be accounted for in Acosta and Sheehan's (1976) finding that Mexican Americans and Anglos attributed more skill, understanding and trust to Anglo professionals or to Mexican American non-professionals. It appears that variables such as more active intervention styles for positive change through counseling are more important than racial similarity in building rapport (Atkinson, Maruyama and Matsui 1978; Peoples and Dell 1975). Tseng and Hsu (1980) point out how styles of therapy are closely related to the sociocultural system.

For example, in a highly organized sociocultural system in which regulation and control is overemphasized, institutionalized 'catharsis' is needed; whereas, in a poorly organized society, where lack of goal regulation and guidance is characteristic, 'control' is the therapeutic approach used (Tseng and Hsu 1980:337).

Second, Korchin (1980) is critical of the tendency to decide on an *a priori* basis that membership in one particular ethnic or cultural group, class or culture relegates a client to less-qualified therapists for shorter periods of time. Warheit et al. (1975) and Ambrowitz and Dokecki (1977) identify socio-economic status as the most powerful predictor of poor mental health conditions, Fierman (1965) and Korchin (1980) and Gomes-Schwartz et al. (1978) have attacked the assumption that therapy cannot be successful with lower socio-economic groups. Lorion (1974) provides a comprehensive review of other literature in the relationship between therapy and low status or poverty as a predictor of mental health. Lower-income persons are less likely to be in therapy, or are in therapy for shorter periods of time with similar symptoms, even though those similar symptoms are typically described as being more severe among lower-class clients. Lower-class clients are treated by less experienced staff and through less-sophisticated modes of therapy.

Third, minority clients may even respond with anger when confronted by a minority counselor (Jackson 1973), either because they perceive that minority person to be associated with a majority-controlled institution, because they perceive majority counselors as more competent, or out of jealously toward the minority counselor who has "made it" (Atkinson et al. 1978). The minority counselor may also not prefer a minority client out of a tendency to deny identification with, or overidentify with minority client problems, or because he or she views counseling other minority clients as lower status work (Gardner 1971; Sattler 1970; Calnek 1970).

Fourth, a compromise solution might introduce two counselors, one similar to the client's culture and one dissimilar. Bolman (1968) advocates the approach of using two professionals, one from each culture, collaborating in cross-cultural counseling with traditional healers as co-counselors. Weidman (1975) introduced the notion of a "culture broker" as an intermediary for working with culturally different clients. Slack and Slack (1976) suggest bringing in a co-client who has already effectively solved similar problems in working with chemically-dependent clients. Mediators have been applied to family therapy in problems of pathogenic coalitions (Satir 1964) with the therapist mediating to change pathogenic relating styles. Zuk (1971) describes counseling itself as a "go-between" process where the therapist mediates between parties. In these various examples, the use of a third person provides an additional "cultural punch" (Opler 1959) that might be uniquely suitable for working with some cultures. Trimble (1981) recommends bringing in a third person as frequently suitable for working with American Indian clients as a means of helping the American Indian client become more comfortable in therapy.

Fifth, when the counselor is indeed bi-lingual or bi-cultural, then the process of counseling might itself become a process of mediation. Meadows (1968) goes back to the early Greek notion of the counselor as a mediator between the client and a "superordinate world of powers and values". Mediation is not without its own unique problems. Miles (1976) points out how these "boundary-spanning activities" of counselors can result in role ambiguity and role diffusion for either the counselor or the client expected to coordinate the conflicting demands of multiple membership. To some extent Stonequist's (1937) 'marginal person' describes the role of a mediating person. Mediation also presents opportunities. Ruiz and Casas (1981) describe a bi-cultural counseling model for helping counselors become both more bi-lingual and bi-cultural appropriate to their client's needs, in the transition between majority and minority cultural affiliations. Berry (1975) suggests that bi-cultural individuals have higher potential to function with cognitive flexibility and are more creatively adaptive to either culture. Szapocznik and Kurtines (1980) further suggest that bi-lingual and bi-cultural individuals are better adjusted and perform at a higher level in either of their two cultures. As a mediator, the counselor serves to interpret either culture, and it is therefore important for the counselor to be accepted by both cultures in a well-defined role to be effective (MacKinnon and Michels 1971).

Given the complications in understanding and communicating with culturally different clients, and given that few therapy variables other than relationship correlate with outcome, Lambert (1981) suggests the possibility that cross-cultural therapy is not only difficult but even contra-indicated in most circumstances.

DEVELOPING A CONCEPTUAL FRAMEWORK

Once a paradigm or frame of reference has become accepted by science, it functions as a screening device for selecting and defining problems which, coincidentally, can fit into the paradigm's framework. Other problems which do not fit are rejected as irrelevant, belonging to another discipline-paradigm, or too chaotic to consider. As a consequence, only those problems which can be stated in the conceptual and instrumental tools of the paradigm are allowed (Kuhn 1962). The paradigm becomes the criteria for selecting data which in turn confirm and validate the paradigm. Disconfirming data are likely to be labeled invalid or non-scientific. To the extent that the paradigm does not describe reality, society is insulated from real contact by the fixed form of the paradigm. In a parallel observation Bateson (1979) cites Gresham's "Law of Cultural Evolution", according to which the oversimplified ideas will always displace the sophisticated and the vulgar or hateful will always displace the beautiful. And yet, as Bateson points out, the beautiful persists. The greatest danger facing cultural conceptions of human behavior are in the *reductionist* oversimplifications of those interactions in terms of paradigms and models.

In an attempt to understand the complexity of intercultural contact we tend to make simplified models, which can more easily be understood, but which fail to reflect aspects of complex reality with any authenticity. The imbedded rationality of our perspective requires us to construct simplified models of the complex real situation in order to deal with it. We behave rationally with respect to this model and such behavior is generalized to the real world. To predict behavior, therefore, we must understand *both* the complex interaction of the real world *and* perceptions of that world through simplified models, that is, both the real world and the labels we use to describe it. Inevitably confusion results when we confuse the labels with reality. We have little tolerance for the entropy of aggregate, mixed up, unsorted, undifferentiated, unpredictable and random data and quickly move to sort, order and predict emerging patterns.

The contribution of culture to mental health has been to guarantee that interacting complexities will not be overlooked. Categories are derived to reduce limitless variation and uncertainty to manageable proportions. Rosch (1975: 197) stated

In informational terms, a category is most useful when, by knowing the category to which a thing belongs, the organism thereby knows as many attributes of the thing as possible. Segmentation of the same domain would be progressively less useful the fewer the properties of things predictable from knowing the category.

Weaknesses of the "digital" model of sorting categories in logical conjunctions of discrete criterial attributes, becomes obvious in dealing with natural data. The alternative "analog" or "family resemblance" model describes natural categories characterized by internal structure and prototypes (the clearest cases or best examples) of the category where members of the category are described on a continuum of increasing or decreasing similarity and "degrees of membership" (Rosch 1975). The clearest example of this phenomenon is in color category membership where each color is represented by a prototype surrounded by colors of decreasing similarity (Kay and McDaniel 1978). The analog model reflects the "fuzzy" nature of category membership. The family resemblance model applied to social relations permits category content variation across age and cultural groups without viewing such differences in value laden terms as correct and incorrect (Brandt 1980).

Considerable attention to differentiation in the area of cognition and culture seems to provide insights to culture and mental health as well. The concept of differentiation refers to the complexity of a system's structure, with less differentiated systems having a more homogeneous structure and more differentiated systems a more heterogeneous structure (Witkin and Goodenough 1981). With increased differentiation there is also increased specialization and integration of data into new systems (Berry 1975). Triandis (1975) points out how cognitive complexity is used by different writers to refer to at least four phenomena in addition to the literature on differentiation; (1) complexity as a perceptual variable influencing other psychological functions; (2) complexity as an interpersonal cognitive variable; (3) complexity as a personality variable; (4) and complexity as a general cognitive variable applied to different cognitive domains (Triandis 1975:62–63). Triandis elsewhere suggests that groups share the same "subjective culture" in proportion to their isomorphic attributions suggesting a similar pattern of differentiation and discrimination between two individuals (Triandis et al. 1972).

This overview of culture and counseling therapy is a history of our attempts to sort out or differentiate the influences of cultural categories or "families" interacting with cognitive variables in overlapping patterns of influence. The complexity of that interaction involves interaction between group affiliation variables and cognitive patterns of behavior, expectation and values – interactions best represented in an *open-ended* paradigm (Hines and Pedersen 1980).

Cultural labels can be selected to fit any particular situation where different labels will vary in importance and definition relative to each label's "prototype". The complexity of meanings, feelings and thought will probably prevent the creation of any deterministic science of human behavior analyzing human events into limited categories. The alternative is what Reynolds (1980) calls "phenomenological operationalism".

If limited categorical definitions of human experience are all science can use, then perhaps no accurate understanding of human experience is possible. But if we allow empathy, introspection and operational approaches to experience entry into respectable scientific circles, we might begin to map out a fuller predictive science of the mind. (Reynolds 1980: 2)

The history of cross-cultural counseling and therapy from a Western perspective has consistently constrained data into linear progressions toward an illusion of causality in analytic methodologies. By contrast, non-Western descriptions have developed a more syncretic, visual-spatial rather than verbal-sequential mode of thought (DeVos 1980). Consequently, the new and perhaps more promising direction is toward non-Western descriptions of how culture is related to human behavior. This will require a radical shift in the research and perhaps in therapy modes as well, even though the supporting data for such a shift are already published and implicit in the conclusions of interactional psychology.

INTEGRATION OF CROSS CULTURAL THERAPIES

The future will require us to advance the field of culture and mental health in four areas. First, we will need to advance the conceptual and theoretical approaches to the interaction between culture and mental health beyond the diffuse and incomplete theoretical alternatives now available. Second, we will need to sharpen our research efforts to identify those primary variables which will allow us to explain what has happened, interpret what is happening and perhaps predict what is going to happen in the migration of persons and ideas across cultures. Third, we will need to identify criteria of expertise for the education and training of professionals to work interculturally, adequately prepared to deal with the problems of a pluralistic society. Fourth, we will need to revolutionize our mode of providing services based on the new theory, new research, and new training so that mental health care is equitably and appropriately provided to members of a pluralistic society.

Developing a *conceptual framework* for cross-cultural therapy is perhaps the most difficult and the most basic of these four tasks. Western culture is dependent on individualistic priorities and rationalistic methods. Much of the data we do have lends illusory support to the mistaken belief that individual differences can be described in a language consisting of context-free global traits, factors or dimensions (Shweder 1979). We will require a convergence of disciplines and fields and sources of information that have thus far been classified as disparate or unrelated, in a redefinition of the basic questions from a variety of cultural perspectives. We will need theories linking biological, behavioral and social phenomena, with the emphasis centered on relatively small social units rather than the pan-societal mega-units which have been favored by the "social philosophers" among us (Westermeyer 1976b:5). We will need to include workers beyond the academics and researchers trained in anthropology, psychiatry, psychology and sociology who have focused on *ex-post-facto* explanations of phenomena rather than *a priori* pragmatic concerns that anticipate applied usefulness. We may look to analogies and metaphors from other fields for alternative models. Stewart (1981) compares cultures to a hologram, where each cultural event contains cues for understanding a client if appropriately illuminated by insight, in a multi-dimensional depiction of cultural complexity.

Our *research focus* needs to focus on more holistic frames of reference, recognizing the reductionistic fallacy of "atomistic" exclusivism based on the illusion that we can control and isolate cultural phenomena. We will need to focus on the complexity of the whole person or whole organism interacting with a complex and ever-changing environment. This shift of assumptions will require a radical revolution in cross-cultural research methodology. The dangers of continuing to depend on personality measuring instruments and single method research are that they tell us more about the methodological artifact than the subject and remain more stable across cultures than the people measured (Shweder 1979:259). One such holistic model has already been tried.

Hologeistic methods which (1) draw on a worldwide data base (2) examine a sample of societies or cultures (3) test hypotheses about whole societies or cultures and (4) test those hypotheses by statistical correlations (Shafer 1976) have attempted to look at the *holos* (whole) *ge* (earth) through cross-cultural, cross-polity, cross-historical and cross-archeological surveys. The weaknesses of this approach have been in the precise definition of sample societies (unit definition); failure to control for cultural diffusion to explain correlations (Galton's problem); failure to control for representativeness in the sample (sample bias); failure to present documentation of codings and sources (data documentation); and failure to deal with the systematic bias among coders, ethnographers, and informants (demand function) (Shafer 1976).

A second research direction with a holistic emphasis is the search for cultural universals. Triandis (1977) has emphasized the importance of identifying those universals that apply across cultures as the primary task of modern psychological research. Westermeyer (1976b) has commented on the convergence of research interests and data to bridge the etic/emic, universalistic/particularistic categories as a documented trend. He cites the examples of (1) increasing sophistication, rigor and power of mathematically-derived methodologies, (2) overlap of accruing psychopathological data and case studies from different cultures, fields and disciplines, (3) the effects of reflective anthropology through informant-interviewer feedback loops, (4) the accumulating data from altered states of perception and consciousness, (5) increasing convergence of information on states and classifications of mental illness and deviant behavior, (6) increasing use of individualistic sources for many general statements to include the exception, (7) payoffs from applied areas or neo-utilitarian theory, (8) emergence of non-typological non-modular experiments to explain thinking with epistomological flexibility, (9) the use of systems theory and process in epistomology, and (10) the increasingly vast information field. The difficulty with this position is the danger of creating "pseudo-etic" phenomena that result in mistaking the particularistic perspective of one group for a universal truth (Triandis 1977).

Sundberg (1981) cites a wide range of 15 research hypotheses needed to advance the field of culture and therapy which attends to complexity relating to mutuality of purposes and expectations, counselor's intercultural understanding, client's intercultural attitudes, cultural consideration of the client's options and aspects of group commonality. In a similar mode, Draguns (1981) suggests that four areas of information are needed, including: first, intercultural data on the effects of indigenous therapy techniques; second, comparisons of effectiveness of techniques in various cultures; three, comparisons of indigenous and extraneous therapies within the same culture; and fourth, the effect of using indigenous mental health specialists on therapy outcomes. In each case the emphasis of future research is on applied rather than theoretical problems based on direct contact with clients, in locus.

In developing a more relevant and appropriate *educational and training mode* we are assuming that persons who have learned to relate to others in the host culture will function more effectively and intentionally. Furthermore, people who have learned to relate in one social environment will have difficulty relating in other social environments unless they have been trained to make appropriate differentiations. Triandis (1975) suggests that culture training should (1) familiarize students of one culture with dimensions that make a difference in the other cultures, (2) that the transfer of learning or new information to new situations can be improved through training, (3) that increased isomorphic attributions between persons from different cultures is a measure of successful training and (4) that training will familiarize the learner with typologies of culture and differentiated exchange. Triandis further suggests that culture training involves increased cognitive complexity with stimulus generalization decreasing as stimulus differentiation increases.

A variety of training models have been developed to prepare counselors to work with culturally-different clients. Atkinson et al. (1979) review the most popular models of Bryson et al. (1974), Lewis and Lewis (1970), Mitchell (1970) and Pedersen (1981). Arrendondo-Dowd and Gonslaves (1980) describe a rationale for the developing of cross-cultural counselor training programs to prepare culturally effective counselors. Ivey (1980) likewise describes a variety of active training approaches being used in preparing counselors. The difficulty in each of these approaches has been characterized by a lack of uniformity, systematic development of method, comparisons of training outcomes and definition of agreed-upon outcome criteria.

Ivey (1980) integrates the educational and training variables more adequately than any of the other publications on counseling with his notion of "intentionality". Cultural expertise and intentionality imply (1) the ability to generate a maximum number of verbal and nonverbal sentences to communicate with self and others, (2) the ability to communicate with diverse groups within the culture and (3) the ability to formulate plans and possibilities in a cultural context (Ivey 1980). Intentionality can be modified to become the central outcome measure of cross-culturally skilled counselors *both* in their cultural self-awareness and control over their own basic cultural biases, prejudices or predispositions *and* in their cultural other-awareness of the alternative systems of client-needs and therapy-responses to those needs that are alive and healthy in a pluralistic society and global village. The fact that we have not yet defined the criteria of interculturally skilled counseling enormously complicates the evaluation of existing education and training for cross-cultural skills.

A variety of training approaches have been modified to fit the needs of cross-cultural training and education (Pedersen 1981a). Human relations training focuses on increasing counselor empathy, warmth and genuineness. The problem is, these are defined differently in each culture and reflect a bias toward middle class values. Microtraining emphasizes a single skill at a time with expert modeling, rehearsal and operationalizing of the counseling process, one skill at a time. The difficulty is that the same skill has a different effect in each culturally defined context and microtraining could be misinterpreted as an oversimplified solution. Life development training emphasizes increased understanding of yourself, knowledge of helping skills and experience. The difficulty is in the assumption that we already know how to train counselors to work in cross-cultural situations that present an infinite variety of combinations. Structured learning and behavioral approaches emphasize modeling, role playing and social reinforcement. However some cultures resist the intervention of the outside stranger and it is difficult in any case to identify appropriate reinforcing rewards for each culturally different context. Interpersonal process recall emphasizes training from responses modes, self confrontation and mutual recall through feedback. However, it requires a high tolerance for self-disclosure and considerable resources of time and money to complete the training. Other skill training methods generally are isolated from the interview context itself as abstractions and presume a hierarchical role for the counselor as the "help giver" which introduces its own cultural bias.

CONCLUSION

In the *application* of intercultural counseling services we have the ultimate criteria and judge of effectiveness. Although the ultimate delivery of services should no doubt be foremost in our examination of the field, most emphasis has, in fact, been on basic research questions "unwittingly, yet effectively separated from the practical concerns of program development, service delivery and techniques of treatment" (Draguns 1980:64). We need to draw out practical implications from the available information. This may include re-defining the role of counselors to include outreach workers, consultants, ombudsmen, change agents, and facilitators of indigenous support systems (Atkinson et al. 1979).

The constraints of cross-cultural counseling include elements from theory, research and training as well. We need more attention to cultural variables to increase a counselors measured accuracy and effectiveness, to accommodate ethical imperatives of culturally different consumers, and to measure counselor competency in communicating with culturally different clients. We need increased understanding of the intercultural dimension within all counseling contacts. We need to integrate cross-cultural variables into the core curricula of counselor-education programs rather than as a sub-specialty. We need to get more cross-cultural materials into the research literature of main-line professional journals of counseling and therapy. We need to develop alternatives to counseling from other cultures. We need more accuracy in matching counseling intervention skills to different cultures, and we need to translate counseling and mental health into the language of other disciplines, fields and professions of social management. Psychology plays an important role as the new popular ideology and religion to justify social programs (Sampson 1977). That role can isolate and atomize, individualize and alienate counselors from their clients, or it can nurture fundamental interdependencies within a pluralistic society.

ACKNOWLEDGMENTS

Support for completing this paper was received through a grant from the NIMH (#IT24-MH15552). The author also acknowledges helpful comments from Anne Hines and Norman Sundberg on early drafts of this paper.

REFERENCES

Acosta, F. and J. Sheehan
    1976 Preferences Toward Mexican American and Anglo-American Psychotherapies. Journal of Consulting and Clinical Psychology 44:272–279.
Ambrowitz, D., and P. Dokecki
    1977 The Politicals of Clinical Judgment: Early Empirical Returns. Psychological Bulletin 84:460–476.

American Psychological Association (APA)
    1979 Council of Representatives Minutes From the Meeting of January 19–20, 1979.
Amir, Y.
    1979 Contact Hypothesis in Ethnic Relations. Psychological Bulletin 71(5):319–342.
Aronson, H. and B. Overall
    1966 Treatment Expectancies in Patients in Two Social Classes. Social Work 11:35–
          41.
Arrendondo-Dowd, P. and J. Gonslaves
    1980 Preparing Culturally Effective Counselors. Personnel and Guidance Journal, June.
Atkinson, D. R., M. Maruyama, and S. Matsui
    1978 Effects of Counselor Race and Counseling Approach on Asian American's Percep-
          tions of Counselor Credibility and Utility. Journal of Counseling Psychology 25:
          76–83.
Atkinson, D. R., G. Morton, and D. W. Sue
    1979 Counseling American Minorities: A Cross-Cultural Perspective. Dubuque, Iowa:
          William C. Brown Company.
Atkinson, D. R., D. Staso, and R. Hosford
    1978 Selecting Counselor Trainees With Multicultural Strengths: A Solution to the
          Bakke Decision Crisis. Personnel and Guidance Journal 56(9):546–549.
Aubrey, R. F.
    1977 Historical Development of Guidance and Counseling and Implications for the
          Future. Personnel and Guidance Journal 55:288–295.
Bateson, G.
    1979 Mind and Nature. New York: Dutton.
Berman, J.
    1979 Individual Versus Societal Focus in Problem Diagnosis of Black and White Male
          and Female Counselors. Journal of Cross-Cultural Psychology 10(4):497–507.
Berry, J. W.
    1975 Ecology, Cultural Adaptation and Psychological Differentiation: Traditional
          Patterning and Acculturative Stress. In Cross-Cultural Perspective on Learning.
          R. Brislin, S. Bochner, and W. Lonner (eds.). New York: John Wiley and Sons.
Bloombaum, M., J. Yamamoto, and Q. James
    1968 Cultural Stereotyping Among Psychotherapiests. Journal of Consulting and
          Clinical Psychology 32(1):99.
Bolman, W.
    1968 Cross-Cultural Psychotherapy. American Journal of Psychiatry 124:1237–1244.
Brandt, E.
    1980 Effects of Typicality on Recall and Clustering in a Free Recall Task: A Develop-
          mental Study. Ph.D. Dissertation. Department of Psychology, University of
          Hawaii.
Brislin, R. W., W. J. Lonner, and R. M. Thorndike
    1973 Cross-Cultural Research Methods. New York: John Wiley and Sons.
Bryne, R. H.
    1977 Guidance: A Behavioral Approach. Englewood Cliffs, New Jersey: Prentice-Hall.
Bryson, L. and J. Cody
    1973 Relationship of Race and Level of Understanding Between Counselor and Client.
          Journal of Counseling Psychology 20:495–498.
Bryson, S., G. A. Renzaglia, and S. Danish
    1974 Training Counselors Through Simulated Racial Encounters. Journal of Non-
          White Concerns in Personnel and Guidance 3:218–223.
Calneck, M.
    1970 Racial Factors in the Countertransference: The Black Therapist and the Black
          Client. American Journal of Orthopsychiatry 40:39–46.

Carkhuff, R. R. and R. Pierce
  1967 Differential Effects of Therapist Race and Social Class Upon Patient Depth of
        Self-Exploration in the Initial Clinical Interview. Journal of Consulting Psychology
        31(6):632–634.
Collomb, H.
  1973 L'avenir De La Psychiatrie En Afrique. Psychopathologie Africaine 9:343–370.
DeVos, G.
  1980 Afterward. In The Quiet Therapies: Japanese Pathways to Personal Growth. D.
        Reynolds (ed.). Honolulu: The University Press of Hawaii.
Diaz-Guerrero, R.
  1977 A Mexican Psychology. American Psychologist 32:934–944.
Dinges, N., J. E. Trimble, S. M. Manson, and F. L. Pasquale
  1981 The Social Ecology of Counseling and Psychotherapy with American Indians and
        Alaskan Natives. In Cross-Cultural Counseling and Psychotherapy. A. Marsella and
        P. Pedersen, (eds.). Elmsford, N. Y.: Pergamon.
Draguns, J. G.
  1974 Values Reflected in Psychopathology: The Case of the Protestant Ethic. Ethos
        2:115–136.
  1977 Mental Health and Culture. In Overview of Intercultural Education, Training and
        Research, Volume 1, Theory. P. B. Pedersen and G. Renwick (eds.). Chicago:
        Intercultural Network.
  1980 Psychological Disorders of Clinical Severity. In Handbook of Cross-Cultural
        Psychology, Volume VI, Psychopathology. H. C. Triandis and J. G. Draguns
        (eds.). Boston: Allyn and Bacon.
  1981a Counseling Cultures: Common Themes and Distinct Approaches. In Counseling
        Across Cultures, Second Edition. P. Pedersen, J. Draguns, W. Lonner and J.
        Trimble (eds.). Honolulu: University Press of Hawaii.
  1981b Cross-Cultural Counseling and Psychotherapy: History, Issues and Current Status.
        In Cross-Cultural Counseling and Psychotherapy. A. Marsella and P. Pedersen
        (eds.). Elmsford, New York: Pergamon.
Dreikurs, R.
  1972 Equality: The Life-Style of Tomorrow. The Futurist, August.
Dubreuil, G.
  1975 Review of L'avenir De La Psychiatric En Afrique, by H. Collomb. Psychopatho-
        logic Africaine 9:343–370. In Transcultural Psychiatric Research Review 12:
        171–174.
Ewing, T. N.
  1974 Racial Similarity of Client and Counselor and Client Satisfaction With Counseling.
        Journal of Counseling Psychology 21:446–449.
Favazza, A. F. and M. Oman
  1977 Anthropological and Cross-Cultural Themes in Mental Health: An Annotated
        Bibliography 1925–1974. Columbia and London: University of Missouri Press.
Fields, S.
  1979 Mental Health and the Melting Pot. Innovations 6(2):2–3.
Fierman, T. B.
  1965 Myths in the Practice of Psychotherapy. Archives of General Psychiatry 12:
        408–414.
Frijda, N. and G. Jahoda
  1966 On the Scope and Methods of Cross-Cultural Research. International Journal of
        Psychology 1:109–127.
Gamboa, A. M., D. J. Tosi, and A. C. Riccio
  1976 Race and Counselor Climate in the Counselor Preference of Delinquent Girls.
        Journal of Counseling Psychology 23:160–162.

Gardner, L. H.
    1971 The Therapeutic Relationship Under Varying Conditions of Race. Psychotherapy:
          Theory, Research and Practice 8(1):78—87.
Gomes-Schwartz, B., S. W. Hadley, and H. H. Strupp
    1978 Individual Psychotherapy and Behavior Therapy. Annual Review of Psychology
          29:435—472.
Grier, W. H. and P. M. Cobbs
    1968 Black Rage. New York: Bantam Books, Inc.
Harrison, D. K.
    1975 Race as a Counselor-Client Variable in Counseling and Psychotherapy: A Review
          of the Research. The Counseling Psychologist 5(1):124—133.
Hines, A. and P. Pedersen
    1980 The Cultural Grid: Matching Social System Variables and Cultural Perspectives.
          Asian Pacific Training Development Journal 1.
Hsu, F. L. K., ed.
    1972 Psychological Anthropology. Cambridge: Massachusetts: Schenkman.
Ivey, A.
    1981 A Person-Environment View of Counseling and Psychotherapy: Implications for
          Social Policy. In Cross-Cultural Counseling and Psychotherapy. A. Marsella and
          P. Pedersen (eds.). New York: Pergamon Press.
Jackson, A. M.
    1973 Psychotherapy: Factors Associated with the Race of the Therapist. Psycho-
          therapy: Theory, Research and Practice 10(3):273—277.
Jaslow, C.
    1978 Exemplary Programs, Practices and Policies. In Transcultural Counseling: Needs,
          Programs and Techniques. G. Walz and L. Benjamin (eds.). New York: Human
          Sciences Press.
Katchadourian, Herant
    1977 Culture and Psychopathology. In Psychological Dimensions of Near Eastern
          Studies. L. C. Brown and N. Itzkowitz (eds.). Princeton: The Darwin Press.
Katz, M. and K. Sanborn
    1976 Multiethnic Studies of Psychopathology and Normality in Hawaii. In Anthropology
          and Mental Health. J. Westermeyer, (ed.). The Hague: Mouton.
Kay, P. and C. McDaniel
    1978 The Linguistic Significance of the Meanings of Basic Color Terms. Language
          54:426—437.
Kiev, A.
    1972 Transcultural Psychiatry. New York: The Free Press.
Kinloch, G.
    1979 The Sociology of Minority Group Relations. Englewood Cliffs, New Jersey:
          Prentice-Hall, Inc.
Kleinman, A.
    1978 Problems and Prospects in Comparative Cross-Cultural Medical and Psychiatric
          Studies, 407—440. In Culture and Healing in Asian Societies. A. Kleinman, P.
          Kunstadter, E. B. Alexander and J. L. Gate (eds.). Cambridge, Massachusetts:
          Schenkman Publishing Company.
Korchin, S. J.
    1980 Clinical Psychology and Minority Problems. American Psychologist 35:263—269.
Korman, M.
    1974 National Conference on Levels and Patterns of Professional Training in Psychol-
          ogy: Major Themes. American Psychologist 29:441—449.
Kuhn, T.
    1962 The Structure of Scientific Revolutions. Chicago: University of Chicago Press.

Lambert, M. J.
  1981 The Implications of Psychotherapy Outcome Research on Cross-Cultural Psychotherapy. *In* Cross-Cultural Counseling and Psychotherapy. A. Marsella and P. Pedersen (eds.). New York: Pergamon Press.
Lebra, W. P., ed.
  1976 Culture-Bound Syndromes, Ethnopsychiatry, and Alternative Therapies. Honolulu: The University Press of Hawaii.
LeVine, D.
  1972 A Cross-Cultural Study of Attitudes Toward Mental Illness. Journal of Abnormal Psychology 80:111–112.
LeVine, R. and D. Campbell
  1972 Ethnocentrism: Theories of Conflict, Ethnic Attitudes and Group Behavior. New York: Wiley.
LeVine, R. and A. Padilla
  1980 Crossing Cultures in Therapy: Pluralistic Counseling for the Hispanic. Monterey, Calif.: Brooks/Cole.
Lewis, M. D. and J. A. Lewis
  1970 Relevant Training for Relevant Roles: A Model for Educating Inner-City Counselors. Counselor Education and Supervision 10(1):31–38.
Lonner, W.
  1981 Psychological Tests and Intercultural Counseling. *In* Counseling Across Cultures, Second edition. P. Pedersen, J. Draguns, W. Lonner and J. Trimble (eds.). Honolulu: University Press of Hawaii.
Lorion, R. P.
  1978 Research on Psychotherapy and Behavior Change with the Disadvantaged. *In* Handbook of Psychotherapy and Behavior Change: An Empricial Analysis, Second edition. S. L. Garfield and A. E. Bergin (eds.). New York: Wiley.
MacKinnon, R. A. and R. Michels
  1971 The Psychiatric Interview in Clinical Practice. Philadelphia: W. B. Saunders.
Marsella, A. J.
  1979 Culture and Mental Disorders. *In* Perspectives on Cross-Cultural Psychology. A. J. Marsella, R. Tharp and T. Ciborowski (eds.). New York: Academic Press.
Marsella, A. and C. Golden
  1980 The Structure of Cognitive Abilities in Americans of Japanese and of European Ancestry in Hawaii. The Journal of Social Psychology 112:19–30.
Marsella, A. J. and H. N. Higginbotham
  1980 Applications of Traditional Asian Medicine to Psychiatric Services in Developing Nations. WHO/NIMH Schizophrenia Research Center, The Queen's Medical Center, Honolulu, Hawaii.
Meadows, P.
  1968 The Cure of Souls and the Winds of Change. Psychoanalytic Review 55:491–504.
Miles, R. H.
  1976 Role Requirements as Sources of Organization Stress. Journal of Applied Psychology 61:172–179.
Mitchell, H.
  1970 The Black Experience in Higher Education. The Counseling Psychologist 2:30–36.
Morrow, D. L.
  1972 Cultural Addiction. Journal of Rehabilitation 38(3):30–32.
Muliozzi, A. D.
  1972 Inter-racial Counseling: Does It Work? Paper presented at the American Personnel and Guidance Association Meeting, Chicago.

Opler, M. K.
  1959 The Cultural Backgrounds of Mental Health. *In* Culture and Mental Health. M. K. Opler (ed.). New York: Macmillan Co.
Parloff, M. B., I. E. Waskow, and B. E. Wolfe
  1978 Research on Therapist Variables in Relation to Process and Outcome. *In* Handbook of Psychotherapy and Behavior Change, Revised edition. S. Garfield and A. Bergin (eds.). New York: John Wiley and Sons.
Patterson, C. H.
  1974 Relationship Counseling and Psychotherapy. New York: Harper and Row, 1974.
  1978 Cross-Cultural or Intercultural Psychotherapy. International Journal for the Advancement of Counseling 1:231–248.
Pedersen, P.
  1977a Asian Theories of Personality. *In* Contemporary Theories of Personality. R. Corsini (ed.). Itasca: Peacock.
  1977b The Triad Model of Cross-Cultural Counselor Training. Personnel and Guidance Journal 56:94–100.
  1979 Non-Western Psychologies: The Search for Alternatives. *In* Perspectives in Cross-Cultural Psychology. A. Marsella, R. Tharpe, and T. Ciborowski (eds.). New York: Academic Press.
  1981 The Cultural Inclusiveness of Counseling. *In* Counseling Across Cultures, Second edition. P. Pedersen, J. Draguns, W. Lonner, and J. Trimble (eds.). Honolulu: University Press of Hawaii.
Peoples, V. Y. and D. M. Dell
  1975 Black and White Student Preferences for Counselor Roles. Journal of Counseling Psychology 22:529–534.
Prince, R.
  1976 Psychotherapy As the Manipulation of Endogenous Healing Mechanism: A Transcultural Survey. Transcultural Psychiatric Research Review: 13:155–233.
Reynolds, D. K.
  1980 The Quiet Therapies: Japanese Pathways to Personal Growth. Honolulu: The University Press of Hawaii.
Rosch, E.
  1975 Universals and Cultural Specifics in Human Categorization. *In* Cross-Cultural Perspectives on Learning. R. Brislin, S. Bochner, and W. Lonner (eds.). New York: John Wiley and Sons.
Rotenberg, M.
  1974 The Protestant Ethic Versus Western People-Changing Sciences. *In* Readings in Cross-Cultural Psychology. J. Dawson and W. Lonner (eds.). Hong Kong: University of Hond Kong Press.
Ruiz, R. A. and J. M. Casas
  1981 Culturally Relevant and Behavioristic Counseling for Chicano College Students. *In* Counseling Across Cultures, Second edition. P. Pedersen, J. Draguns, W. Lonner and J. Trimble (eds.). Honolulu: University Press of Hawaii.
Sampson, E.
  1977 Psychology and the American Ideal. Journal of Personality and Social Psychology 11:767–782.
Satir, V.
  1964 Conjoint Family Therapy. Palo Alto, CA: Science and Behavior Books.
Sattler, J. M.
  1970 Racial "Experimenter Effects" in Experimentation, Testing, Interviewing and Psychotherapy. Psychological Bulletin 73:137–160.

Shafer, J.
 1976 A Review of Methods in Holocultural Studies in Mental Health/Illness. *In* Anthropology and Mental Health. J. Westermeyer (ed.). The Hague: Mouton.
Shweder, R.
 1979 Rethinking Culture and Personality Theory. Ethos 7:255–287, 9:60–94.
Slack, C. W. and E. N. Slack
 1976 It Takes Three to Break a Habit. Psychology Today, pp. 46–50. February.
Stanges, B. and A. Riccio
 1970 A Counselee Preference for Counselors: Some Implications for Counselor Education. Counselor Education and Supervision 10: 39–46.
Stewart, E.
 1981 Cultural Sensitivities in Counseling. *In* Counseling Across Cultures. P. Pedersen, J. Draguns, W. Lonner and J. Trimble (eds.). Honolulu: University Press of Hawaii.
Stonequist, F. V.
 1937 The Marginal Man: A Study in Personality and Culture Conflict. New York: Russell and Russell, Inc.
Strauss, J. S.
 1979 Social and Cultural Influences on Psychopathology. Annual Review of Psychology 30:397–416.
Sue, D. W.
 1977 Barriers to Effective Cross-Cultural Counseling. Journal of Counseling Psychology 24:420–429.
 1978 Editorial: Counseling Across Cultures. Personnel and Guidance Journal 56:451.
 1981 Cross-Cultural Counseling. New York: Wiley and Sons.
Sundberg, N. D.
 1981a How Best to Counsel a Stranger: Overview and Hypotheses for Research on Effectiveness of Cross-Cultural Counseling and Psychotherapy. *In* Cross-Cultural Counseling and Psychotherapy. A. Marsella and P. Pedersen (eds.). Elmsford, N. Y.: Pergamon Press.
 1981b Overview of Research and Research Hypotheses About Effectiveness in Intercultural Counseling. *In* Counseling Across Cultures, Revised and Expanded Edited. P. Pedersen, J. Draguns, W. Lonner and J. Trimble (eds.). Honolulu: University Press of Hawaii.
Szapocznik, J. and W. Kurtines
 1980 Acculturation, Biculturalism and Adjustment Among Cuban Americans. *In* Acculturation: Theory, Models and Some New Findings. A. Padilla (ed.). Boulder, Colorado: Westwood Press.
Tapp, J. L.
 1980 Studying Personality Development. *In* Handbook of Cross-Cultural Psychology, Volume IV, Development Psychology. H. C. Triandis and A. Heron (eds.). Boston, Massachussetts: Allyn and Bacon.
Torrey, E. F.
 1972 The Mind Game: Witchdoctors and Psychiatrists. New York: Emmerson Hall.
Triandis, H. C.
 1975 Culture Training, Cognitive Complexity and Interpersonal Attitudes. *In* Cross-Cultural Perspectives on Learning. R. Brislin, S. Bochner and W. Lonner (eds.). New York: John Wiley and Sons.
 1977 Interpersonal Behavior. Monterey, CA: Brooks/Cole.
Triandis, H. C., V. et al.
 1972 The Analysis of Subjective Culture. New York: John Wiley and Sons.
Trimble, J.
 1981 Value Differentials and Their Importance in Counseling American Indians. *In* Counseling Across Cultures, Second Edition. P. Pedersen, J. Draguns, W. Lonner and J. Trimble (eds.). Honolulu: University Press of Hawaii.

Tseng, W. S. and J. Hsu
   1980 Minor Psychological Disturbances of Everyday Life. *In* Handbook of Cross-Cultural Psychology, Volume VI, Psychopathology. H. C. Triandis and J. G. Draguns (eds.). Boston: Allyn and Bacon.
Useem, J. and R. Useem
   1967 The Interfaces of a Binational Third Culture: A Study of the American Community in India. Journal of Social Issues 23:130–143.
Vontress, C. E.
   1981 Racial and Ethnic Barriers in Counseling. *In* Counseling Across Cultures, Second Edition. P. Pedersen, J. Draguns, W. Lonner, and J. Trimble (eds.). Honolulu: University Press of Hawaii.
Warheit, G. J., C. E. Holzer, and S. A. Areye
   1975 Race and Mental Illness: An Epidemiological Update. Journal of Health and Social Behavior 16:243–256.
Watts, A. W.
   1961 Psychotherapy East and West. New York: Mentir Press.
Weidman, H.
   1975 Concepts as Strategies for Change. Psychiatric Annals 5:312–314.
Westermeyer, J.
   1976 Clinical Guidelines for the Cross-Cultural Treatment of Chemical Dependency. American Journal of Drug and Alcohol Abuse 3(2):315–322.
Westermeyer, J., ed.
   1976b Anthropology and Mental Health. The Hague: Mouton.
Wilson, W. and J. F. Calhoun
   1974 Behavior Therapy and the Minority Client. Psychotherapy: Theory, Research and Practice 11(4):317–325.
Wintrob, R. M. and Y. K. Harvey
   1981 The Self-Awareness Factor in Intercultural Psychotherapy: Some Personal Reflections. *In* Counseling Across Cultures, Second edition. P. Pedersen, J. Draguns, W. Lonner and J. Trimble (eds.). Honolulu: The University Press of Hawaii.
Witkin, H. A. and D. R. Goodenough
   1981 Cognitive Styles: Essence and Origins. New York: International Universities Press.
Wohl, J.
   1981 Intercultural Psychotherapy: Issues, Questions and Reflections. *In* Counseling Across Cultures, Second edition. P. Pedersen, J. Draguns, W. Lonner, and J. Trimble (eds.). Honolulu: University Press of Hawaii.
Wohl, J.
   1980 Some Observations on Counseling and Psychotherapy Theory in Cross-Cultural Counseling and Psychotherapy. Unpublished manuscript.
World Health Organization (WHO)
   1979 Schizophrenia: An International Follow-Up Study. New York: John Wiley and Sons.
Wrenn, G. C.
   1962 The Culturally Encapsulated Counselor. Harvard Educational Review 32(4): 444–449.
Zuk, G.
   1971 Family Therapy: A Triadic Based Approach. New York: Behavioral Publications.

ANTHONY J. MARSELLA

16. CULTURE AND MENTAL HEALTH: AN OVERVIEW

INTRODUCTION

Recent decades have witnessed an increased interest in the cross-cultural study of mental disorders. This interest has manifested itself across a variety of disciplines and has served as an impetus for the development of a number of subdisciplinary specialities which have been variously termed *vergleichende psychiatrie* or comparative psychiatry (Kraepelin 1904), primitive psychiatry (Devereux 1940), culture and psychopathology (Slotkin 1955), ethnopsychiatry (Devereux 1961), transcultural psychiatry (Wittkower and Rin 1965), cross-cultural psychiatry (Murphy and Leighton 1965), psychiatric sociology (Weinberg 1967), cultural psychiatry (Kennedy 1973), and the "new" transcultural psychiatry (Kleinman 1977).

Regardless of the different names which have been applied, the central concern of all of these specialities has been to illuminate the role of cultural factors in the etiology, expression, course, and outcome of mental disorders. From their success in achieving these purposes, it is clear that the cross-cultural study of mental disorders has contributed greatly to our understanding of the role of cultural factors in mental disorders. The purpose of the present paper is to discuss some of these contributions and, in the process, to call attention to the fact that all aspects of mental disorders are inextricably linked to the sociocultural milieu in which they are generated.

A number of literature reviews on cross-cultural studies of mental disorders have appeared. The first of these was published by Benedict and Jacks (1954). Following a brief hiatus, many other reviews of the literature appeared including publications by Opler (1967), Al-Issa (1970), Draguns and Phillips (1971), Kiev (1972), German (1972), Draguns (1973), Pfeiffer (1974), Kennedy (1973), King (1977), Strauss (1979) Sartorius (1979), Marsella (1979), and Draguns (1980). In addition to these general reviews, a number of reviews were also published on cross-cultural studies of specific disorders such as schizophrenia (e.g., Sanua 1969, 1980; Mishler and Scotch 1965; Odegard 1975; Jablensky and Sartorius 1975; Sartorius and Jablensky in press) and depression (e.g., Prince 1968; Fabrega 1974, 1975; Singer 1975; Marsella 1980; Marsella et al. n.d.).

The sheer number of review papers which have been published lend credence to the fact that cross-cultural studies of mental disorders have now achieved the critical mass necessary to exercise an effect upon our traditional approaches to the problem of mental disorder. No longer can the role of cultural factors in mental disorders be ignored or cast aside as being unfounded or spurious. It is time for the community of mental health researchers and practitioners around

A. J. Marsella and G. M. White (eds.), Cultural Conceptions of Mental Health and Therapy,
359–388.

the world to re-examine their assumptions and practices and to introduce cultural factors into their efforts to understand and treat mental disorders.

Although the contributions of the cross-cultural study of mental disorders have been numerous, the present paper will address itself to only a few of the areas in which these contributions have occurred. Their areas include the following: Culture, Self, and Mental Disorder; Defining Normality and Abnormality; the Concept of Mental Health; the Epidemiology of Mental Disorders; the classification of Mental Disorders; the Etiology of Mental Disorders; and Psychotherapy and Healing. The areas will be discussed in order. Prior to the discussion, however, it would be useful to provide a historical perspective on the development of cross-cultural studies of mental disorders.

HISTORICAL PERSPECTIVES

The history of the study of culture and mental health relationships is relatively new, but is nevertheless very complex. This is because it reflects many of the ideological trends of the nineteenth and twentieth centuries. In the author's opinion, the history of culture and mental health can be divided into four different periods (see Marsella 1979).

In the pre-1900 era, mental health professionals revealed an extensive concern for the role of civilization in producing madness. Indeed, a number of psychiatrists and public health specialists like Jarvis remarked that "Insanity is then a part of the price we pay for civilization. The causes of the one increase with the developments and results of the other" (Jarvis 1851; quoted in Rosen 1969:21). The idea that culture is related to mental disorders was part of the legacy of Jean-Jacques Rousseau, whose thoughts were largely responsible for the entire romanticist movement, which stresses the evils of civilization and the beauty of the primitive. When Rousseau stated, "Man is by nature good and only our institutions have made him bad!" (Durant and Durant 1967:19), he launched an ideological revolution which focused Western thought on the role of the sociocultural environment. It was this turn of events which represents the earliest recognition of the culture and mental health relationships we currently pursue.

By the turn of the century, a growing number of psychiatric researchers began exploring mental disorders in non-Western cultures. For example, Kraepelin, the father of modern psychiatry, journeyed to Southeast Asia and there registered his bewilderment regarding the absence of depression among various Asian populations. In addition, many investigators began to study the so-called "culture specific" or "exotic" syndromes among non-Western people. These included disorders like "latah" (Van Brero 1895), "myriachit" (Czapligka 1914), "amok" (Van Loon 1927), and "pibloktoq" (Brill 1913). Further, some investigators initiated studies of Western diagnostic disorders in non-Western countries. By the 1940s, there were numerous epidemiological studies of mental disorders under way in Japan, Germany, and the United States. But, in spite of the cultural variations that emerged in the rates of disorders across cultures (e.g., Akimoto et al. 1942; Uchimura et al. 1942), and also the differences which were revealed in the studies of the "culture specific" disorders, there was considerable resistance against incorporating cultural variables into causal theories of mental disorder.

The period between 1950–1970 can be considered the third major era for the study of culture and mental health, because it was during this time that there was a proliferation of publications regarding culture and mental health. Numerous books were published detailing the findings of cross-cultural studies of mental disorder (e.g., *Transcultural Psychiatric Research Review*; *International Journal of Social Psychiatry*). In addition, the National Institute of Mental Health started a training program in cross-cultural studies of mental health at the University of Hawaii under the direction of William Lebra, an anthropologist. This training program produced many books and scientific papers which helped define the field.

The time from 1970 to the present constitutes the last major period in the development of culture and mental health relationships. In many respects, our proximity to this period makes it difficult to appraise the current trends. In the opinion of the author, however, there are some recognizable directions which are emerging.

First, it is clear that more and more mental health scholars and practitioners are invoking sociocultural factors in their conceptions of causality and treatment of mental disorders. Indeed, the entire community mental health movement as well as the growing concern with minority mental health needs, reflects this increased interest in the sociocultural aspects of mental disorders. This is likely to continue in spite of the continuing popularity of biological models.

Second, There will probably be an increase in the number of multi-national psychiatric research studies of various mental disorders (e.g., the WHO Collaborative Projects on schizophrenia, depressive disorders, etc.). These efforts will serve to highlight the ethnocentricity of many Western concepts of mental health and therapy.

Third, it is likely that there will be an increased respect for and broader utilization of indigenous healers and natural support networks in the development of mental health services in non-Western countries. As a correlate of this, there will probably also be greater sensitivity to cultural factors in the delivery of mental health services in Western countries (e.g., Marsella and Pedersen 1981a; Reynolds 1981; Higginbotham 1980; Marsella and Higginbotham 1981).

Fourth, it would not be surprising if Western psychiatry begins to alter its diagnostic systems to conform with the many findings emerging from cross-cultural research. For example, in many non-Western cultures, psychotic disorders often have rapid onset, and brief durations, and good prognoses (e.g., Sartorius et al. 1978). One possible reason for this is that these psychoses are, in fact, not schizophrenic disorders but rather different types of psychoses which can be considered hysterical or benign in nature. If this turns out to be the case through careful study (i.e., the WHO Benign Psychosis Project), it will mean that a new psychotic pattern will have to be added to DSM-III and ICD-9.

The 1970s witnessed an explosion of interest in cross-cultural studies of mental disorder. These studies explored virtually every aspect of mental disorder from etiological agents to epidemiology to therapy. As a result, a critical mass of information was developed which will make it exceedingly difficult to ignore cultural factors in our understanding of mental disorder. The 1980s promises to continue that trend.

CULTURE, SELF, AND MENTAL DISORDER

One of the major avenues by which culture and mental disorder are related is the concept of self or "personhood" that a culture codifies (Marsella 1981). It is clear that mental disorders cannot be understood apart from the concept of self, because it is the nature of the self which serves to identify "reality" for a given cultural group and which dictates the definition of what constitutes a symptom. In addition, the experience of "disorder" is ultimately mediated by the self, since it is the context in which the patient interprets the meaning of what is occurring. Self as object and self as process constitute two different modes of experiencing reality which have profound effects for all aspects of mental disorder. For example, in a factor analytic study of psychiatric symptomology across three different ethnic groups, Marsella and his co-workers found that different groups expressed depressive disorders in different dimensions which were related to their concept of self. Marsella (1973:448—449) stated,

... what emerges is the possibility of interpreting complaints ... as reflections of the self perceived as somatic functioning, as interaction, as cognitive process, and as an ... existential process ... One value of considering complaints within this framework is that the concept of self provides a rather interesting and heuristic metapsychological bridge for examining the influence of culture and individual differences on behavior ... Different cultures may condition their members to develop particular dimensions of self over others.

Thus, since cultures condition different concepts of self, and since self is inextricably linked to the definition, experience, and expression of mental disorder, it is clear that cultural factors are closely related to mental disorders. Self is the bridge for mediating these relationships. Efforts to understand mental disorder, apart from self are ultimately doomed to failure because they ignore the organism as a total being. It is the total person that experiences mental disorder and not a neurosynapse or an isolated psychological conflict. Most of the papers in the present book as well as a forthcoming book on culture and self (Marsella et al. n.d.) take up the issue of self and its relationships to culture and to mental health. In the future, it is likely that more anthropological studies of self will be implicated in cross-cultural studies of mental disorder, because of their logical relationships to one another. These studies will add to the growing number of reports which point out that mental disorders are not universal but rather are "culture specific". The discussion by Shweder and Bourne in this volume reveals some of the assumptions which guide "universalist" and "relativist" perspectives in cross-cultural research. Marsella (1981:29) stated,

We cannot separate our experience of an event from our sensory and linguistic mediation of it. If these differ, so must the experience differ across cultures. If we define who we are in different ways (i.e., self as object), if we process reality in different ways (i.e., self as process), if we define the very nature of what is real, and what is acceptable, and even what is right and what is wrong, how can we then expect similarities in something as complex as madness?

The present book addresses the interdependency among cultural conceptions of person, mental disorder, and therapy in recognition of the important relationships of these three variables. Shweder and Bourne (Paper 4), Gaines (Paper 6), and White (Paper 3) provide persuasive scholarly and empirical accounts of these relationships in their analyses of the concept of person across cultures. The future will bring many more efforts which link culture, self, and mental disorder.

DEFINING "NORMALITY" AND "ABNORMALITY"

The first challenges to the assumption about the universality of "normal" and "abnormal" behavior emerged in the early 1930s with the writings of such famous cultural anthropologists as Sapir, Hallowell and Benedict. Sapir (1932: 230) wrote,

Cultural anthropology has the healthiest of skepticisms about the validity of the concept of "normal behavior" .... It (cultural anthropology) is valuable because it is constantly rediscovering the normal. For the psychiatrist and the student of personality in general, this is of the greatest importance, for personalities are not conditioned by a generalized process of adjustment to the "normal" but by the necessity of adjustment to the greatest possible variety of idea and action patterns according to the accidents of birth and biography.

A few years later, Benedict (1934) and Hallowell (1934) published strong statements on the relativity of normal behavior based on the growing number of culture and personality studies. Hallowell's words are as meaningful today as when he wrote them 45 years ago. He stated that the cross-cultural investigator must,

... have an intimate knowledge of the culture as a whole, he must also be aware of the normal range of individual behavior within the cultural pattern and likewise understand what the people themselves consider to be extreme deviations from this norm. In short, he must develop a standard of normality with reference to the culture itself, as a means of controlling an uncritical application of the criteria that he brings with him from our civilization (Hallowell 1934:2).

One of the first medical people to respond to the growing ideas about the relativity of normality was Ackerknecht (1942). He suggested that behavior could be divided into four categories: *autopathological* (behavior abnormal in the culture in which it is found but normal in other cultures), *autonormal* (behavior normal in the culture which it is found but abnormal in other cultures), *heteropathological* (behavior which is abnormal in all cultures), and *heteronormal* (behavior which is normal in all cultures). Obviously Ackerknecht's system represents an oversimplification of a complex problem since it is doubtful that behaviors could be so easily classified. But, it served to sensitize researchers to cultural differences.

In recent years, a number of empirical studies about the nature of "normality" and "abnormality" across cultures have been conducted. Martin Katz and his colleagues (e.g., Katz, et al. 1969, 1978) have been leaders in this field. Katz gathered baseline information on areas of problem behavior for both normal (non-clinical) and abnormal (hospitalized) populations from different cultural groups residing in Hawaii.

He then compared the profiles of the normal and abnormal groups across 10 behavior categories including negativism, belligerence, withdrawal, confusion, and so forth. In doing so, he was able to demonstrate what profiles characterized normal samples for a given ethnic group as well as what profiles characterized abnormal samples. His results indicated that cultural variations exist in both normal and abnormal group profiles. Clearly, even for ethnic groups residing in the same geographical area, standards for normality and abnormality differ. The value of this approach is that it provides an empirically-derived standard for defining normality and abnormality in different cultural groups.

Marsella and Tanaka-Matsumi (1976) pursued the problem through the development of baselines for the frequency, intensity, and duration of 60 specific psychiatric symptoms among Caucasian, Japanese-American, and Japanese-National populations. They found group differences across the various parameters for the different symptoms. However, their basic contribution was the fact that with the establishment of symptomatology baselines for different ethnic groups, it would be possible to define "normal" and "abnormal" behaviors within a cultural context.

Yet another approach to the problem of "normality" and "abnormality" has been the efforts by Marsella and his co-workers (e.g., Marsella et al. 1980), to develop problem, cause, treatment interaction matrices for different cultural groups residing in Hawaii. Through the use of cognitive research methods, indigenous conceptions of problems, causes, and treatments are generated for different cultural groups. These conceptions can then be used in clinics by practitioners to evaluate patients from different ethnic backgrounds within the context of their own culture. The research framework for this approach is displayed in Figure 1. Other researchers who have used similar approaches to arrive at indigenous conceptions include Clement (1974) in Samoa, Resner and Hartog (1970) in Malaysia, Edgerton (1966) in Africa, and Boyer (1964) for Apache Indians.

For all of the previous approaches, the conclusion has been that we can no longer impose an arbitrary standard of "normality" and "abnormality" derived

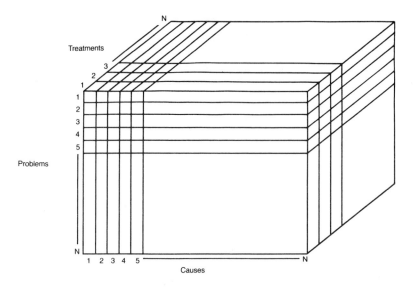

Fig. 1. Research Matrix for Investigating Problem, Cause, Treatment Interactions for Different Cultural Groups (from Marsella 1979).

from one cultural group upon another without risking criticism and perhaps even litigation. Cross-cultural research has clearly demonstrated that the early observations of Edward Sapir, Ruth Benedict, and Irving Hallowell were valid and justified. For one of psychiatry's most basic questions, cross-cultural research has made a basic contribution. Normality and abnormality must be considered within a cultural context!

THE CONCEPT OF MENTAL HEALTH

In addition to influencing our knowledge of the concepts of "normality" and "abnormality", cross-cultural research has also contributed to an expansion of our concept of mental health. In the Western world, mental health has frequently referred to a sense of psychological well-being. In some cases, researchers such as Abraham Maslow (1954) have developed criteria for the concept of "optimum mental health". These criteria concerned numerous psychological and behavioral qualities such as autonomy, democratic values, spontaneity, social interest, and so forth. With the exception of a small number of theorists and practitioners committed to "psychosomatic" orientations, most Western scientists and professionals have tended, in the past, to ignore somatic considerations in their conceptions of mental health. Part of the problem in the West has been the separate institutionalization of roles, facilities, and knowledge for somatic, psychological, and spiritual levels of human functioning. This was due, in part, to our analytical scientific orientation. This tendency is displayed in Figure 2.

Institutional Representations

	Roles	Facilities	Knowledge
Body	Physicians Physical and Biological Scientists Nurses	Hospitals Clinics Laboratories	Medicine Physiology Anatomy Chemistry
Mind	Mental Health Professionals	Hospitals Clinics Rest Homes Laboratories	Psychology Theology Psychiatry
Spirit	Priests Ministers Psychics	Churches Temples Shrines	Philosophy Theology Mysticism

(row label on left side: Levels of Human Functioning)

Fig. 2. The Legacy of Western Science and Technology: Institutionalizing the Separation of Body, Mind and Spirit (from Marsella and Higginbotham 1981).

Today, the Western world is faced with a rather interesting problem. Clearly, the concept of "mental health" has become a valued goal. We frequently find ourselves speaking of "healthy values", "healthy relationships", and "healthy behavior"; we even have mental health associations whose purpose is to promote "mental health". Yet, we seem to be confused about what these things actually mean. We seem to be aware that mental health is not restricted to separate aspects of behavior and experience but rather involves harmonious relationships across all areas of our functioning. But, such holism appears to be alien to our conceptions of human behavior. However, cross-cultural research as well as public exposure to Eastern philosophies and religions, have provided the Western world with the concept of "wholeness" and "harmony among parts". This has given rise to new conceptions of mental health and to new approaches to health problems including "holistic medicine", "behavioral medicine", and "systems theory".

Many traditional Asian healing systems are based on concepts of health which view man as a microcosm, a reflection of the processes at work in the cosmos. For example, Needham (1962), wrote the following regarding the Chinese world view:

Things behaved in particular ways not necessarily because of prior actions or impulsations of other things, but because their position in the ever-moving cyclical universe was such that they were endowed intrinsic natures which made that behavior inevitable for them. If they did not behave in those particular ways they would lose their relational position in the whole (which made them what they were), and in turn into something other than themselves. They were thus parts in existential dependence upon the whole world organism. And they reacted upon one another (Needham 1962:281).

These thoughts are part of ancient Chinese philosophy, but they sound amazingly similar to contemporary Western notions in field theory physics, theoretical biology and organismic psychology.

Within the context of such a philosophy, disorder, whether physical or mental, is viewed as a dysfunction in relationship. Lock (1980) observed,

Sickness ... is not seen so much in terms of an intruding agent, although this aspect of disease causation is acknowledged, but rather due to a pattern of causes leading to disharmony. These causes can be environmental, social, psychological, or physiological .... The function of diagnosis is not to categorize a patient as having a specific disease, but to record the total body state and its relationship to the macrocosm of both society and nature as fully as possible ... the model allows explanations for the benefits of the patient to be in broad psycho/social and environmental terms which are readily understandable and cognitively acceptable. These explanations can be used by the patient to account for the occurrence of suffering in the context of his or her own life history at that moment .... Therapy is designed to act on the whole body — removal of the main symptom is not considered adequate as all parts of the body are thought to be interdependent — in this sense the model is holistic .... It is believed that the functioning of man's mind and body is inseparable .... (Lock 1980:15–17).

Other examples of holistic concepts of mental health are present in Indian, Japanese, and Indonesian philosophy and religion. For example, Setyonegoro (1979) has written about the Javanese concept of *kebathinan. Kebathinan* refers to the search and understanding of the inner self and its harmonious relationship to the world. Setyonegoro stated,

Kebathinan therefore, is a metaphysical search for harmony within one's inner self, harmony between one's fellow men and nature, and harmony with the universe, the almighty God .... One should be aware of the mystical power of communicating with the supernatural (through) which one (will) be able to sense, realize and understand (one's) relation to the environment, the society, and the universe .... To be Javanese means to understand and demonstrate appropriate manners (*pantas dan patut*), to understand and maintain an ordered existence in which persons, matters and things are in their "place", "time", and "space" (*tempat, waktu, dan kedudukannya*), as if everybody and everything and every matter has a predictable "orbit". Disorder and disharmony — ill-health, ill-ness and disease — are hence derangement and confusion of concept and matter (Setyonegoro 1979:1–2).

There are a number of methods for pursuing *Kebathinan* including meditation, fasting, yoga-like exercises, and discussions with a guru.

Clearly, cross-cultural studies have revealed that many non-Western cultures have "enlightened" concepts of mental health which are far more complex, and perhaps, more meaningful, than those in the West. Our recent exposure to non-Western religions and philosophies has greatly increased the popularity of the non-Western concepts and has led to a broader range of therapeutic philosophies and methods. Indeed, it would not be too much of an exaggeration to conclude that many of the "pop psychology" therapies and the various "holistic" philosophies which have swept the Western world in the last decade may be a response to the inadequacies of our Western approaches in the face of the more meaningful concepts of mental health which developed in the East.

THE EPIDEMIOLOGY OF MENTAL DISORDERS

One of the most frequently asked questions in psychiatry concerns cultural variations in the rates and/or patterns of mental disorders. The question is a logical one and certainly deserves study. However, cross-cultural research efforts in this area have taught us that the answer to this question may first require a resolution of the many problems and issues that are inherent in cross-cultural studies of mental disorders including the definition of a "case", the methods used to identify a "case", and the validity of imposing Western classifications of disorder on non-Western people, as discussed in the Introduction to this volume.

According to Opler (1965), the first impetus for psychiatric epidemiological studies was provided by Emerson in 1930, at the First International Congress on Mental Hygiene. Emerson called psychiatric disorders a major public health problem and called for extensive epidemiological efforts similar to those which had been used to help solve other medical problems. Within a brief period of time, studies were initiated in Japan, Germany, and the United States. In subsequent years, the number of epidemiological studies reached enormous proportions. Reviews of the epidemiological literature have been published for mental disorders in general (e.g., Dohrenwend and Dohrenwend 1965, 1969; Schwab and Schwab 1978), for depression (Silverman 1968; Sartorius 1973; Marsella 1978; Bebbington 1978), and for schizophrenia (e.g., Mishler and Scotch 1963; Jablensky and Sartorius 1975).

The epidemiological research indicates that profound cultural variations exist in the rates of mental disorders. However, the comparability of the studies is, as noted previously, questionable. Further, even if comparability were possible, the definitions of mental disorders which have been used, appear to be unwarranted because they ignore indigenous considerations. Marsella (1978) suggested that cross-cultural studies of mental disorders could be improved by implementing new procedures including: (1) An emic determination of mental disorders through the use of cultural methods, (2) the establishment of symptom frequency, duration, and intensity baselines for both normal and abnormal populations, (3) the objective determination of symptom patterns through the use of multivariate statistical cluster methods, and (4) the use of similar case identification methods for different cultural samples. These procedures do not negate the use of Western disorder categories; however, they do emphasize that researchers must be sensitive to "emic" factors.

Thus, what cross-cultural research on the epidemiology of mental disorders has taught us is that comparisons of the rates of mental disorders in different societies requires that prior attention be given to indigenous conceptions of disorder in case identification and comparable research methods. Only then will it be possible to arrive at valid conclusions on cultural variations in rates and/or patterns of mental disorder.

THE MANIFESTATION AND CLASSIFICATION OF MENTAL DISORDERS

Classification is the process by which we arrange, group, or categorize objects or events. It is one of man's basic cognitive operations and it has significant adaptive value. Through classification, man has an opportunity to order his world according to general stimulus configurations. This permits him to observe regularity from which develops understanding and predictability. Science is based on classification. Classification has also been important in the field of mental health.

As early as 400 B.C., Hippocrates suggested a classification system for mental disorders. He categorized them into three main classes: mania, melancholia, and phrenitis (i.e., confusion, delirium). Hippocrates based his system on the symptomatic display of the problem. In the sixteenth century, the German physician Paracelsus, evolved another system of classification based on the causes of mental disorders; he suggested five kinds of insanity: *vesani* (caused by food/beverage impurities), *insani* (caused by genetics), *lunatici* (caused by the moon), *obsessi* (caused by the devil), *melancholi* (caused by constitutional problems). By the eighteenth century, the classification of mental disorder had become a major activity among professionals of the time. Every professional had his own particular system of classification and each system had numerous subtypes and divisions of subtypes. For some, the basis of classification was symptom presentation, while for others it was etiology. From all of this confusion, one system was to emerge as the standard for modern psychiatry. This was the system of classification used by the German psychiatrist, Emil Kraepelin (1855–1926).

Kraepelin was a confirmed organicist. He believed mental disorders were diseases much like tuberculosis or heart trouble, and that with a classification system, the diseases would eventually be easily diagnosed, linked to pathogens, and promptly treated. In spite of the cultural variations in the mental disorders he observed during his around the world trip in 1904, Kraepelin considered mental disorder to be universal.

Kraepelin's legacy, a disease model of mental disorder based on invariant patterns of symptom expression, currently dominates the classification field today. It is the foundation of the American Psychiatric Association's *Diagnostic and Statistical Manual* as well as the *International Classification of Diseases, Number Nine*. But, cross-cultural research has raised a number of questions about the ethnocentricity of these methods of classification.

As was noted in the history section of the current paper, some of the earliest cross-cultural research on mental disorders was concerned with the manifestation of mental disorders in different cultures. As early as the 1890s, researchers pointed out a number of disorders like *latah, mali-mali*, and *myrachit* which had no counterpart in Western systems of diagnosis and classification. As a result these disorders gained the unfortunate rubric of "culture-specific" disorders or "exotic" psychoses. Throughout the years, numerous reports have been published on scores of different "culture-specific" disorders around the world. Yet, Western nosologists have continued to ignore the possibility that their own system was ethnocentric. It was, perhaps, beyond their imagination that their classification system, conceived and developed in Germany, was not universally valid. Yap (1951), even attempted to integrate these disorders into the DSM-I and DSM-II systems as instances of hysterical neuroses. He was unsuccessful.

By the beginning of the twentieth century, Western researchers began to study Western patterns of mental disorder in non-Western countries including New Guinea (e.g., Seligman 1929), India (e.g., Dhunjiboy 1930) and Indonesia (Van Wulfften-Palthe 1936). An interesting finding was the fact that the patterns were hard to apply because of cultural variants in expression. By the mid-twentieth century, casual clinical observations had yielded to more sophisticated quasi-experimental research designs including matched diagnosis, matched samples, international surveys, and factor analytic approaches.

Matched Diagnosis

Matched diagnosis is when individuals from different cultural groups who share a common diagnosis are compared for symptom variations. For example, Opler and Singer (1959) compared Italian and Irish schizophrenic patients and found the Irish tended to have more guilt and sin preoccupations, more systematic delusions, more drinking problems and less affective troubles than the Italians. Enright and Jaeckle (1963) compared Japanese and Filipino paranoid schizophrenics in Hawaii and found that the Filipinos were more active, belligerent, hostile, and agitated while the Japanese were more withdrawn, passive, and cooperative. Sunshine (1971) compared Black and Puerto Rican schizophrenics in New York and found that the latter group were more active, possessed more florid symptomatology, and tended to somatize more often than the former group. A study by DeHoyos and DeHoyos (1965) also found symptom differences between Black and White schizophrenic patients.

Cultural variations in depression have also been reported using the matched diagnosis strategy. For example, Simon et al. (1973) compared Black and White depressive patients and found numerous differences in symptoms leading them to conclude that Blacks "have a quality of their depression different from Whites" (p. 509). Similarly, Kimura (1965) reported variations in the expression of depression between German and Japanese depressives, especially with regard to guilt, suicide, and the quality of depression.

Matched Samples

Matched samples is when individuals from different cultural groups are matched according to such variables as age, education, gender, social class, and rural-urban residence. The different cultural groups are then compared with regard to variations in the frequency or severity of different symptoms. The basic idea is that with these variables held constant, it is possible to attribute any differences in the symptom pictures to cultural factors.

A series of studies comparing matched samples in Argentina and the United States (Fundia et al. 1971) and Japan and the United States (Draguns et al. 1971) found profound differences in the symptom pictures of the contrasting cultures. In general, the differences were in the directions of exaggerations of the normal behavior patterns of the various cultural groups. Stoker et al. (1968) compared symptom profiles of Mexican-American and Anglo-American females and found the Mexican pattern was characterized by greater hostility, hyper-activity, crying, sleeplessness, somatic complaints, and withdrawal. The Anglo pattern was characterized by greater guilt feelings and psycho-motor retardation.

Sechrest (1969) compared patients from Chicago and the National Mental Hospital of the Philippines. A dramatic finding was that only 3% of the Filipino cases were described as depressed. Guilt feelings and suicidal threats and attempts were also quite low in the Philippines. There were also differences in the frequency and content of the hallucinations reported.

International Survey

The international survey approach to studying cultural variations in the manifestation of mental disorders is one of the oldest methods which has been used. In the early 60s, H. B. M. Murphy and Eric Wittkower, two pioneer transcultural psychiatrists, initiated a series of international surveys to compare the symptom pictures associated with schizophrenia and depression in numerous countries around the world. In both instances, cultural differences were found in the expression of the different disorders.

For example, a survey of depression in 30 countries revealed (Murphy et al. 1964), that in nine countries (mainly non-Western), there was a rarity in depressed mood, insomnia, mood variation, and loss of interest in the environment. Yet, these symptoms are considered part of the classic picture of depression in the Western world. A similar survey comparing symptom profiles of schizophrenic patients in different countries also revealed numerous differences in the symptom patterns (Murphy et al. 1963).

A more recent effort by the Division of Mental Health of the World Health Organization examined schizophrenia in nine countries around the world using highly standardized interview forms (World Health Organization, 1973). Although many similarities were found in the symptom profiles of patients from the nine centers, there were also a number of variations. One of the most interesting findings to emerge was that the prognosis or outcome for schizophrenia varied considerably across cultures (Sartorius et al. 1978). Waxler (1979) has also reported cultural variations in prognosis.

It should be noted that the World Health Organization's *International Pilot Study on Schizophrenia* (IPSS) was conducted to determine the feasibility of developing universal criteria for schizophrenic disorders via standardized instruments and interview procedures. The basic instrument was the Present State Examination (see Wing et al. 1973). This interview schedule requires psychiatrists to ask a series of questions related to schizophrenic symptomatology based on various Kraepelinian and Schneiderian concepts of this disorder. The results of the study revealed that investigators could find a core of common symptoms associated with psychotic patients that could be differentiated as schizophrenic. It is, however, important for us to distinguish between reliability and validity in diagnosis.

The IPSS did demonstrate that with careful training and adherence to clear criteria, psychiatrists from different cultures could consistently agree on whether a particular symptom was present or absent. The IPSS, however, did not prove that a symptom has the same meaning across cultures, or the same implications if present. Further, the results of the IPSS revealed that when groups of paranoid schizophrenics from different cultures were compared for the frequency of various "schizophrenic" symptoms, there was considerable cultural variation. For example, autism was very high in Denmark, but virtually absent in India and Nigeria and Taipei. Flat affect was very high in England and Czechoslovakia but was only moderately present in Columbia and Nigeria. Delusions of control were very high in Columbia, Taipei and India, but very low in Denmark, Czechoslovakia and the United States.

Thus, what emerges from the IPSS is the rather interesting finding that symptomatology varies considerably across cultures, even when efforts are made to standardize diagnosis and classification. As the present paper has argued, cultural factors cannot be separated from mental disorders. The latter are not universal phenomena but rather reflect the culture in which they occur with regard to etiology, expression, experience, course, and outcome. Indeed, as the IPSS itself concluded, non-Western countries evidence much better prognoses for "schizophrenic" patients than Western countries. In addition, the course of the disorder is much briefer than in the non-Western countries.

Factor Analysis

The most recent research strategy used to study cultural variations in the manifestation of mental disorders is factor analysis. Throughout psychiatry's history, patterns of disorder have usually been identified through clinical observation. Based on these observations, clinicians suggest clusters of symptoms which appear to fall together. If there is agreement across clinicians, then a syndrome is usually posited. In the case of factor analysis, the clustering of the symptoms is done objectively through a set of mathematical operations rather than subjectively by a clinician. This objective approach often yields different patterns of symptoms from those reported by clinical observation. As a result, factor analysis lends itself to efforts to understand symptom patterns in different cultures, since it reduces the risk of automatically adopting Western notions about the existence of certain patterns of psychiatric disturbance.

For example, using factor analysis, Caudill and Schooler found certain patterns of disorders among Japanese psychiatric patients which were not found among other cultural groups (e.g., *shinkeishitzu*). Similarly, Marsella et al. (1973) found depressive disorders among Chinese-Americans, Japanese-Americans, and Caucasian-Americans differed in terms of symptom profiles. Chinese emphasized somatic complaints while Japanese evidenced more interpersonal dysfunctions (e.g., not wanting to talk to people, not caring for appearance, wanting to have privacy). In contrast, Caucasians presented more existential complaints (e.g., life has no meaning, depressive affect, feelings of worthlessness). Binitie (1978) found cultural variations in depression among Africans and British patients.

CONCEPTUALIZING THE MANIFESTATION OF MENTAL DISORDER ACROSS CULTURES

Regardless of the research strategy used, the results demonstrate that cultures differ in the manifestation of mental disorders. That this is the case should not be surprising! Clearly, there is no reason to believe that cultural variables should have any less influence on deviant behavior patterns than on "normal" behavior patterns. Even if certain biochemical processes may be universally operative in the etiology of mental disorders, it is obvious that the appraisal and behavioral response to these processes must be filtered through culturally conditioned experience. Further, the social response to the behavior pattern must also reflect cultural influences. Certain cultural traditions may, by the response they condition to various behavior patterns, maintain, enhance, and encourage a symptom's development.

For example, with regard to depression, researchers concluded the following. Collomb and Zwingelstein (1961) claimed that Senegalese depressed patients,

... do not appear to be deeply unhappy or miserable; ideas of self accusation and guilt are absent, and suicide is rare; the disorder is characterized rather by ideas of persecution, anxiety, hypochondriasis, and somatic complaints (Quoted by German 1972:461).

Sechrest (1963) in his extensive study of Filipino psychiatric patients, wrote,

... no instances were found of patients complaining of feelings of worthlessness, of hopelessness, of impending doom, and only two instances were found of complaints of being or feeling guilty .... The investigator would conclude, then, that depression is quite infrequent among Filipinos (Sechrest 1963:190).

In a more recent publication, Prince (1980) concluded "In a word, it would appear to me that the typical textbook picture of depression in Western psychiatry is the exception rather than the rule" (Prince 1980:11).

Marsella (1980) in his review of the literature, also concluded that the experience and expression of depressive disorders is not universal. Rather, it varies as a function of Westernization.

The current review of the manifestation of depression across cultures reveals that depression does not assume a universal form. Of special importance is the fact that the psychological representation of depression occurring in the Western world is often absent in non-Western societies. However, somatic aspects do appear quite frequently regardless of culture. Oftentimes, it is only when individuals in non-Western societies become more Westernized that we find similarities in the patterns of depression found in the Western world. This psychological representation involves reports of depressed mood, guilt, and feelings of self-deprecation. The fact that this is absent in many cultures suggests that the epistemic framework of a culture must be considered in evaluating psychiatric disorders. "Depression" apparently assumes completely different meanings and consequences as a function of the culture in which it occurs (Marsella 1980:260–291).

Marsella also observed that without a psychological representation, depressive disorders have different implications. For example, as a somatic problem, it may pass more quickly and be amenable to a wider array of treatments. Further, suicide may not be a consequence. Clearly, our cross-cultural research efforts have forced us to broaden our conception of depressive disorders. Marsella (1980) posited a theoretical model to account for cultural variations in depressive affect and disorder. He suggested that depression cannot be separated from three critical aspects of human experience: *Language* (Abstract, Metaphorical), *Self-Structure* (Diffuse, Individuated), *Representational Mode* (Imagistic, Lexical). Marsella argued that these three components are inter-dependent and serve, in various combinations, to create the basic epistemological orientation toward reality. Since depression, as well as any other form of disorder, cannot occur apart from the experiential processes of an organism, Marsella speculated that the meaning, experience, and manifestation of depression would vary as a function of the culturally-conditioned epistemological orientation of a given group. Those cultural groups which are toward the subjective pole of experience, would have one pattern of depression (e.g., somatic) while those toward the objective pole would have a contrasting pattern (e.g., existential, cognitive).

THE ETIOLOGY OF MENTAL DISORDERS

The effort to reform society as a strategy for dealing with mental disorders lost much of its momentum when an increased reliance on biological and psycho-dynamic models occurred. It is true that voices implicating sociocultural factors in various aspects of mental disorders remained and flourished among some quarters (e.g., Durkheim's theory of anomie based on social disintegration); however, these voices never achieved a major status in the face of the more popular biological, psychodynamic, and later, behavioral models.

But in the author's opinion, the tide of history has changed and a growing pattern of support has emerged for the sociocultural viewpoint among contemporary mental health researchers and professionals. To a large extent, the renewed interest in the sociocultural perspective can be traced to the success of numerous cross-cultural studies which have illuminated the role of sociocultural factors in the etiology, expression, course, and outcome of mental disorders.

Today, there appears to be a growing tolerance for a more eclectic point of view with regard to mental disorders. The commitment to "panaceas" such as medications, electroshock, behavior therapies, and psychoanalysis, has been moderated by a more enlightened viewpoint that mental disorders are a complex phenomena which involve a broad spectrum of interdependent variables. This viewpoint has found some representation in the interactional models of psychopathology (e.g., Marsella et al. 1972; Marsella and Snyder 1981b; Akiskal and McKinney 1976). These models have emphasized the psychobiological representations of externally occurring experiences and events, and thus, they have provided the linkage for relating socioenvironmental phenomena to internal events. This has been an important event for the mental health field since the two dominant professions, psychiatry and clinical psychology, have been almost exclusively associated with biological and psychological variables. Examples of interactional models of psychopathology are presented in Figure 3, which stresses the interdependencies across different categories of variables as well as their simultaneous interactive properties.

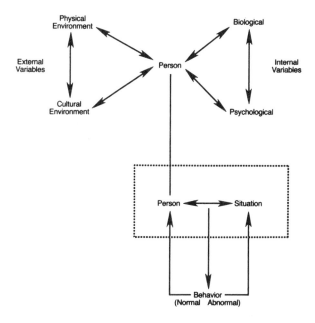

Fig. 3. Interactional model of behavior (from Marsella 1979).

Thus, whereas in the past, many psychiatrists and psychologists tended to reject the notions that variables such as social status, social change, modernization, migration, and so forth could influence mental disorders, there is now more willingness to acknowledge that these variables find their representation in biological and psychological levels of functioning which are structurally associated with behavior. In 1969, the author listed a number of principles related to interactionism. Some examples of these principles include the premises that,

(1) Man and his sociocultural environment are interdependent systems which reflect the attributes of each other. (2) Consideration must be given to the interdependencies of the situation and the individual (as a total organism) if behavior is to be understood. ... No organism exists apart from an environment, and no behavior is independent of the environment in which the organism finds itself (Marsella et al. 1969; Marsella et al. 1972:140).

In brief, cross-cultural research has contributed to the development of new conceptual models of psychopathology which have not only clarified the role of sociocultural factors in mental disorder but have also elaborated the interdependencies among environmental, cultural, psychological, and biological variables.

In addition to this contribution, cross-cultural research has also called our attention to specific socio-cultural variables which should be considered in our efforts to understand, treat, and prevent mental disorder. In one of the first publications, Leighton and Hughes (1959), discussed more than a dozen ways in which cultural factors could be implicated as being causative of mental disorders. These ways ranged from child rearing to dietary and health practices. Many of these variables have subsequently been studied; some of the more popular include: *cultural disintegration* (e.g., Leighton 1959; Leighton et al. 1963a, 1963b); *social status* (e.g., Hollingshead and Redlich 1958; Dohrenwend and Dohrenwend 1969); *social role deprivation* (e.g., Parker and Kleiner 1967; Weissman and Klerman 1978); *modernization* (e.g., Cooper and Sartorius 1977; Marsella 1978); *sociocultural stresses* (e.g., Srole et al. 1962; Marsella et al. 1972; Wittkower and Dubreil 1973; Marsella 1979); *migration* (e.g., Odegaard 1875; Schwab and Schwab 1978; Kavanaugh 1979 for reviews); *social networks* (e.g., Faris and Dunham 1939; Jaco 1954; Cohen and Sokolovsky 1978; Hammer et al. 1978, Hammer 1981; Marsella and Snyder 1981b; Henderson 1977; Henderson et al. 1978); and *social labeling* (e.g., Scheff 1972; Waxler 1974). These and many other sociocultural factors in the etiology of mental disorder have been reviewed extensively by Odegaard (1975), Schwab and Schwab (1978), and Marsella (1979).

In brief, cross-cultural studies have broadened our perspectives on the etiology of mental disorder to include sociocultural variables. Resistance to incorporating these variables into our causal models has been diminished by the adoption of new interactional models of psychopathology which provide for a greater continuity among biological, psychological, and sociocultural variables. No longer do researchers view these variables as being independent of one another. They are now seen as possessing characteristics of continuity through interdependency. Each contains representation properties of the other. Culture is thus inextricably linked with all aspects of mental disorder.

The disease model of mental disorder assumes that the etiology of these disorders, such as schizophrenia and the manic depressive psychosis, resides in a disordered biological substrate. When the disorder develops, it is assumed that it must take a clear course with recognizable and predictable symptoms. But this perspective ignores the obvious fact that any behavior is subsequently modified by the events which follow its occurrence. Figure 4 shows that the final presentation of a problem is a function of formative factors, precipitative factors, exacerbating factors, and maintaining factors. Cultural variables are active at all these levels; thus it is reasonable to expect cultural variations in all aspects of mental disordrs.

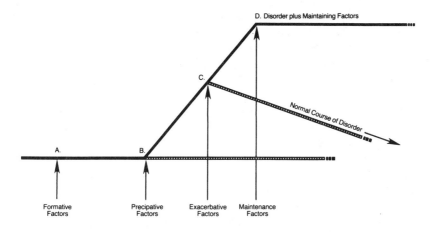

Fig. 4. Comprehensive model of causality for a given problem.

Thus, cross-cultural research has impressed upon contemporary Western psychiatry the likelihood that mental disorders are inextricably linked to socio-cultural factors with regard to their manifestation, clustering, and course and outcome. In doing so, it has undermined the disease model of mental disorder so prevalent during the current century and in the process, has nurtured the alternative that the classification of mental disorders must be sensitive to cultural variations. The new DSM III system, admirable as it may be for its efforts to provide clear standards, is still unresponsive to cultural differences in the expression of mental disorders.

What is needed at this point, in the author's opinion, is a massive international research program, based on ethnographic methods for determining cultural patterns of mental disorder. As individuals become Westernized, their patterns of mental disorders resemble those of Western people (e.g., more cognitive disruption, more existential complaints, etc.). Thus, in non-Western countries, it will be necessary to examine populations at different levels of acculturation to Western life. Researchers such as German (1972) and Marsella 1978, 1980) have pointed out how symptom patterns change along with Westernization.

The scope of such studies, though massive, should not inhibit our efforts to rectify the current situation with regard to classification; the situation is not only invalid but also destructive by virtue of its insensitivity to a patient's cultural experience and a culture's awareness of its own impact upon behavior, be it normal or abnormal.

CULTURE, PSYCHOTHERAPY, AND HEALING

One of the other major areas of interest and concern in the field of culture and mental health is the relationship between culture and psychotherapy. This area first emerged as a popular topic of inquiry with the publication of several books in the early 1960s including Jerome Frank's *Persuasion and Healing* (1961), Ari Kiev's *Magic, Faith and Healing* (1964), and Raymond Prince's *Trance and Possession States* (1968). All three of these books called attention to the role of cultural factors in various psychological interventions around the world. During the same period, a score of articles were published detailing the procedures involved in various healing ceremonies across cultures (e.g., Kondo 1953; Kora 1965; Kennedy 1967; Maupin 1962; Baasher 1967; Wittkower 1970). In the early 1970s, Fuller-Torrey published his controversial book, *The Mind Game: Witchdoctors and Psychiatrists*, in which he traced the many parallels between these two different types of healers. This was followed by a number of other publications which provided both reviews of the issues and concrete examples of psychotherapy and healing across cultures, including William Lebra's *Culture Bound Syndromes, Ethnopsychiatry and Alternative Therapies* (1976), Charles Leslie's Asian Medical Systems (1976), Arthur Kleinman's *Patients and Healers in the Context of Culture* (1980), and Marsella and Pedersen's *Cross-Cultural Counseling and Psychotherapy* (1981). To these books should be added, Prince's excellent review paper which appeared in the *Handbook of Cross-Cultural Psychology: Volume 6, Psychopathology*.

The net result of all this literature has been the recognition that all systems of psychotherapy and healing share some common elements regardless of the cultural context in which they occur. It is clear, however, that certain elements may be more utilized than others, depending upon the specific cultural situation. Basically, the different systems can be grouped around four orientations including those which are (1) *physiologically based* (e.g., rest therapy, massage therapy, exercise therapy, acupuncture); (2) *psychologically based* (e.g., meditation, imagery, problem solving); (3) *socially based* (e.g., family or group involvement, social re-integration), and (4) *supernaturally based* (e.g., exorcism, prayer rituals, divination, possession states). These orientations represent the basic explicit or implicit causal logic that characterizes a given system in a specific culture. What is clear is that these different orientations are found throughout various cultures, although the specific rituals or processes by which they are invoked may differ.

In the final analysis, all forms of behavior change based on psychological principles must be accounted for by some or all of the four principles of learning. These four principles are the only ones which have emerged from decades of study. The four principles include: (1) classical conditioning, (2) operant conditioning, (3) insight, and (4) modeling. Classical conditioning involves the association in time of different stimuli; operant conditioning involves the linkages which are established through behavior and its consequences. Insight learning was first advanced by the Gestalt theorists like Kohler and Wertheimer, who claimed that there can be sudden reorganizations of knowledge with parallel increases in knowledge which exceed the sum of the components involved in the reorganization. Lastly, modeling or imitation learning is based on assumptions that learning can occur through processes of observation with consequent rehearsal of the observed behavior.

Essentially, these four principles of behavior change may operate individually or in various combinations in different types of therapy and healing systems. The social context in which they are utilized can vary considerably and can include any of the following factors: (1) persuasion, (2) hope, (3) catharsis, (4) labeling, (5) expectancy reinforcement, (6) attribution of causality, (7) suggestion, (8) identification with therapist, (9) reduction of uncertainty, (10) information or increased knowledge, (11) unconditional acceptance, (12) guilt reduction, (13) abstraction, (14) perceived support, (15) stimulus overload reduction, (16) fear reduction. All of these factors have been implicated in behavior change via the four principles of learning although the specific relationships have never been articulated. What is clear, however, is that therapists and healers around the world invoke the principles of learning via these different social contexts and interactions to bring about behavior change. Whether we are speaking of a psychoanalyst on Madison Avenue in New York or a witch doctor in the jungles of Africa, learning or behavior change only occurs through a limited number of principles. The cultural context helps determine the particular principles which are used as well as the social contexts (i.e., the above factors) in which they are implemented. Successful behavior change is not limited, however, to one approach and is certainly not limited only to Western methods. Ritchie (1976) stated

Why should we reject exorcism, placebo therapies, or "time out", if these do, in fact, restore a person to functioning. Their use can be no more questionable, no more ethically dubious, no more blindly pragmatic than drug therapy or electroshock therapy (Ritchie 1976:208).

In brief, what I am suggesting is that all forms of psychotherapy and healing acquire their success from the utilization of some of the four basic principles of human learning which are implemented via various interactional contexts or mechanisms. All the systems can be divided into physiological, psychological, sociological, or supernatural orientations with regard to the basic foundations of their logic. In addition, we cannot forget the fact that psychotherapy systems may also acquire their effectiveness by mobilizing various biological mechanisms. For example, Prince (1980) has suggested that therapies may work by increasing levels of endorphins or other endogenous biochemicals.

In the present book, the entire third section is devoted to examples of non-

Western therapy systems including trance, shamanistic, traditional medical, and indigenous psychotherapy forms. These papers provide some concrete examples of successful healing methods, and also articulate the various principles by which these methods may work. In addition, the chapter by Pedersen focuses on the difficulties that emerge when therapy systems from one cultural tradition are used with patients from a different cultural tradition. Through all of this, the reader will do well to recognize that therapy and healing systems reflect the values, assumptions, and themes of the culture. They are cultural products and cultural processes. They serve to reinforce particular cultural tenets, and in this respect they are socializing agents for a culture.

FUTURE DIRECTIONS

Although there have been many important developments in biological psychiatry in the last decade which have served to establish its preeminent position in the field, there also have been a number of critical developments in the sociocultural area which can no longer be ignored by researchers and practitioners. Many of the developments have stemmed from cross-cultural studies of mental health. Some of the more important developments addressed in the papers in this book, which raise issues for further research, include the following:

(1)   The recognition that conceptions of the person and the self vary across cultures. Different cultural traditions hold contrasting views about the nature of personhood and selfhood, and these have implications for mental health and disorder.

(2)   Cultures vary with regard to their epistemological and ontological models of causality about the roots of "madness". Even within the Western cultural tradition, there has been a growing commitment to interactional perspectives which seek to blend biological, psychological, and sociocultural views.

(3)   There is considerable variability with regard to standards of normality and abnormality across cultures which points to the important role cultural experience plays in defining deviancy.

(4)   Extensive research has highlighted cultural variations in the classification and expression of mental disorders. There is an increased awareness that all mental disorders are "culture specific" since none can escape the influence of cultural factors in their emergence, patterns of display, and other clinical parameters.

(5)   Many disorders like "schizophrenia" and "depression" are coming to be viewed within a cultural context which points out their sociocultural roots and definition. Even these disorders are now being considered as disorders of Western culture in terms of their definitions and etiological conceptions.

(6)   The course and outcome of mental disorders has been inextricably

linked to sociocultural factors, both theoretically and empirically. There is an awareness that there is great modifiability in these clinical aspects as a function of the cultural setting in which a disorder occurs.

(7) Measurement of mental disorders is often biased because of reliance on Western instruments which lack conceptual and measurement equivalences across cultures. New instruments are needed which consider cultural factors.

(8) Therapies reflect premises of the culture in which they develop, and are not culture free. Efforts to use therapies derived in one cultural setting on individuals from another cultural setting pose serious ethical and moral problems because of their insidious counter-culture conditioning implications.

(9) New models of mental disorder which focus on cultural variables like the macrosocial, microsocial, and cognitive domains of functioning are gaining increased popularity. They will require integration in the future.

(10) Efforts toward preventing mental disorder must be responsive to sociocultural factors, since the stresses and the resources associated with mental disorder are culturally linked.

(11) The delivery of mental health services to different cultural groups requires sensitivity and accommodation to cultural values and assumptions if the services are to be effective. Indeed, there is a growing interest in integrating indigenous systems with Western systems in many cultures.

(12) The emergence of sub-disciplinary specialties like transcultural psychiatry, medical anthropology, cross-cultural psychology, and public health psychiatry, has resulted in the introduction of cultural variables into professional training programs.

All of these theoretical and practical developments promise to alter the future care and prevention of mental disorder. It is clear that mental health professions can no longer pursue the understanding of mental disorder independent of the sociocultural perspective. To do so runs the risk of ethnocentricity as well as scientific inaccuracy. The current book is part of the growing movement directed toward solving these problems.

(Preparation of this chapter was partially supported by NIMH Research Grant 5R-12-MH 31016-02, *Psychosocial Determinants of Severe Psychatic Disorders*.)

REFERENCES

Ackerknecht, E.
1942 Psychopathology, Primitive Medicine, and Primitive Culture. Bulletin of the History of Medicine 14:30–67.

Akimoto, H., et al.
    1942 Demographische Und Psychiatrische Untersuchung Uber Abgegrenzte Kleinstadt
    Gevolkerung. Psychiatria et Neurologia Japonica: 47:351–374.
Akiskal, H. and W. McKinney
    1975 Overview of Recent Research in Depression. Archives of General Psychiatry 32:
    285–305.
Al-Issa, I.
    1968 Problems in the Cross-Cultural Study of Schizophrenia. Journal of Psychology
    71:143–151.
Baasher, T.
    1967 Traditional Psychotherapeutic Practices in the Sudan. Transcultural Psychiatric
    Research 4:158–160.
Bebbington, P.
    1978 The Epidemiology of Depressive Behavior. Culture, Medicine and Psychiatry
    2:297–343.
Benedict, R.
    1934 Anthropology and the Abnormal. Journal of General Psychology 10:59–80.
Benidict, P. and I. Jacks
    1954 Mental Illness in Primitive Societies. Psychiatry 17:377–389.
Binitie, A.
    1975 A Factor Analytic Study of Depression Across Cultures (African and European).
    British Journal of Psychiatry: 125:559–563.
Boyer, L.
    1964 Folk Psychiatry of the Apaches of the Mescalero Indian Reservation. In Magic,
    Faith and Healing. A. Kiev (ed.). Glencoe, Illinois: Free Press.
Brill, A.
    1913 Pibloktoq or Hysteria Among Perry's Eskimos. Journal of Nervous and Mental
    Disease 40:514–520.
Caudill W. and C. Schooler
    1969 Symptom Patterns and Background Characteristics of Japanese Psychiatric
    Patients. In Mental Health Research in Asia and the Pacific. W. Caudill and T. Y.
    Lin (eds.). Honolulu: East-West Center Press.
Cohen, C. and J. Sokolovsky
    1978 Schizophrenia and Social Newtorks: Ex-patients in the Inner City. Schizophrenia
    Bulletin 4:546–560.
Collomb, H. and J. Zwingelstein
    1961 Depressive States in an African Community (Dakar). In First Pan African Psy-
    chiatric Conference Report. T. Lambo (ed.). Abeokuta, Nigeria.
Cooper, J. and N. Sartorius
    1977 Cultural and Temporal Variations in Schizophrenia: A Speculation on the Impor-
    tance of Industrialization. British Journal of Psychiatry 130:450–455.
Czapligka, M.
    1914 Aboriginal Siberia. Oxford, England: Clarendon Press.
DeHoyos, A. and G. DeHoyos
    1965 Symptomatology Differentials Between Negro and White Schizophrenics. Inter-
    national Journal of Psychiatry 11:245–255.
Devereux, G.
    1940 Primitive Psychiatry. Bulletin of the History of Medicine 8:1194–1213.
    1961 Mohave Ethnopsychiatry and Suicide: The Psychiatric Knowledge and Distur-
    bances of an Indian Tribe. Washington: Smithsonian Institution.
Dhunjiboy, J.
    1930 A Brief Resume of the Types of Insanity Commonly Met With in India. Journal of
    Mental Science 16:254–264.

Dohrenwend, B. and B. Dohrenwend
  1965 The Problem of Validity in Field Studies of Psychological Disorder. Journal of
       Abnormal Psychology 70:52–66.
  1969 Social Status and Psychological Disorder: A Causal Inquiry. New York: John
       Wiley.
Draguns, J.
  1980 Psychological Disorders of Clinical Severity. In Handbook of Cross-Cultural
       Psychology, Volume 5, Psychopathology. H. Triandis and J. Draguns (eds.).
       Boston: Allyn and Bacon.
Draguns, J. and L. Phillips
  1972 Culture and Psychopathology: The Quest for a Relationship. Morristown, N.J.:
       General Learning Press.
Draguns, J., et al.
  1971 Symptomatology of Hospitalized Psychiatric Patients in Japan and in the United
       States: A Study of Cultural Differences. The Journal of Nervous and Mental
       Diseases 152:3–16.
Durant, W. and A. Durant
  1967 The Story of Civilization: Volume X, Rousseau and Revolution. New York:
       Simon and Schuster.
Eaton, J. and R. Weil
  1955 Culture and Mental Disorder. Glencoe, Illinois: Free Press.
Edgerton, R.
  1966 Conceptions of Psychosis in Four East African Societies. American Anthro-
       pologist 68:408–425.
Enright, J. and W. Jaeckle
  1963 Psychiatric Symptoms and Diagnosis in Two Subcultures. International Journal of
       Social Psychiatry 9:12–17.
Fabrega, H.
  1975 Cultural and Social Factors in Depression. In Depression and Human Existence.
       E. Anthony and T. Benedek (eds.). Boston: Little Brown.
Faris, R. and H. Dunham
  1939 Mental Disease in Urban Areas. Chicago: University of Chicago Press.
Frank, J.
  1961 Persuasion and Healing. Baltimore, Maryland: Johns Hopkins Press.
Fundia, T., J. Draguns, and L. Phillips
  1971 Culture and Psychiatric Symptomatology: A Comparison of Argentine and United
       States Patients. Social Psychiatry 6:11–20.
German, A.
  1972 Aspects of Clinical Psychiatry in Sub-Saharan Africa. British Journal of Psychiatry
       121:461–479.
Good, B. J.
  1977 The Heart of What's the Matter: The Semantics of Illness in Iran. Culture, Medi-
       cine and Psychiatry 1:25–58.
Guthrie, G.
  1972 Culture and Mental Disorder. Reading, Mass.: Addison-Wesley.
Hallowell, A.
  1934 Culture and Mental Disease. Journal of Abnormal and Social Psychology 29:
       1–9.
Hammer, M.
  1981 Social Supports, Social Networks, and Schizophrenia. Schizophrenia Bulletin,
       7:45–57.
Hammer, M., L. Makiesky-Barrow, and L. Gutwirth
  1978 Social Networks and Schizophrenia. Schizophrenia Bulletin 4:522–545.

Henderson, S.
  1977 The Social Network, Support, and Neurosis. British Journal of Psychiatry 131: 185–191.
Henderson, S., et al.
  1978 Social Bonds in the Epidemiology of Neurosis. British Journal of Psychiatry 132:463–466.
Higginbotham, H.
  1976 Culture and the Delivery of Mental Health Service: I. Culture and Psychopathology Annotated Bibliography Series. A. J. Marsella (ed.). The Queen's Medical Center, Honolulu, Hawaii.
  1979 The Delivery of Mental Health Services Across Cultures: A Culture Accommodation Model. Unpublished doctoral dissertation. University of Hawaii.
Hollingshead, A. and F. Redlich
  1958 Social Class and Mental Illness. New York: John Wiley.
Jablensky, A. and N. Sartorius
  1975 Culture and Schizophrenia. Psychological Medicine 5:113–124.
Jaco, G.
  1954 The Social Isolation Hypothesis and Schizophrenia. American Sociological Review 19:567–577.
Jarvis, J.
  1969 On the Supposed Increase of Insanity. American Journal of Insanity 8:333–364, 1851. Cited in Rosen, G., Madness in Society. New York: Harper.
Katz, M., H. Gudeman, and K. Sanborn
  1969 Characterizing Differences in Psychopathology Among Ethnic Groups in Hawaii. *In* Social Psychiatry. F. Redlich (ed.). Baltimore: Williams and Wilkins.
Katz, M., et al.
  1978 Ethnic Studies in Hawaii: On Psychopathology and Social Deviance. *In* The Nature of Schizophrenia. L. Wynne, S. Matthyse, and R. Cromwell (eds.). New York: John Wiley and Sons.
Kavanaugh, K.
  1980 Culture, Migration, and Mental Health. Unpublished paper. University of Hawaii, Honolulu.
Kennedy, J.
  1967 Nubian Zar Ceremonies As Psychotherapy. Human Organization 26:185–194.
  1973 Cultural Psychiatry. *In* Handbook of Social and Cultural Anthropology. J. Honigmann (ed.). Chicago: Rand-McNally.
Kiev, A.
  1964 Magic, Faith, and Healing. Glencoe, Illinois: The Free Press.
  1972 Transcultural Psychiatry. New York: Free Press.
Kimura, B.
  1965 Vergleichende Untersuchungen Uber Depressive Erkrankungen in Japan Und In Deutschland. Fortschritte der Neurologie Und Psychiatrie 33:202–215.
King, L.
  1978 Social and Cultural Influences on Psychopathology. Annual Review of Psychology 29:405–433.
Kleinman, A.
  1977 Depression, Somatization, and the "New Transcultural Psychiatry". Social Science and Medicine 11:3–9.
  1980 Patients and Healers in the Context of Culture. Berkeley, California: University of California Press.
Kondo, A.
  1953 Morita Therapy. A Japanese Therapy for Neurosis. American Journal of Psychoanalysis 13:31–37.

Kora, T.
  1965 Morita Therapy. International Journal of Psychiatry 1:611–640.
Kraepelin, E.
  1904 Vergleichende Psychiatric. Zentralblatt Fur Nervenherlkande Und Psychiatrie 15:433–437.
Lebra, W., ed.
  1976 Culture Bound Syndromes, Ethnopsychiatry, and Alternative Therapies. Honolulu: University Press of Hawaii.
Leighton, A.
  1959 My Name is Legion. New York: Basic Books.
Leighton, A. and J. Hughes
  1961 Cultures as Causative of Mental Disorder. In Causes of Mental Disorders: A Review of Epidemiological Knowledge. New York: Milbank Memorial Fund.
Leighton, A., et al.
  1963a Psychiatric Disorder Among the Yoruba. Ithaca: Cornell University Press.
Leighton, D., et al.
  1963b The Character of Danger. New York: Basic Books.
Leslie, C.
  1976 Asian Medical Systems. Berkeley, California: University of California Press.
Lock, M. M.
  1980 East Asian Medicine in Urban Japan. Berkeley: University of California Press.
Marsella, A. J.
  1978a Modernization: Consequences for the Individual. In Overview of Intercultural Education, Training, and Research: Vol. III, Special Research Areas. D. Hoopes, P. Pedersen, and G. Renwick (eds.). La Grange, Ill.: Intercultural.
  1978b Thoughts on Cross-Cultural Studies on the Epidemiology of Depression. Culture, Medicine, and Psychiatry 2:343–357.
  1979 Cross-Cultural Studies of Mental Disorders. In Perspectives in Cross-Cultural Psychology. A. J. Marsella, R. Tharp, T. Ciborowski (eds.). New York; Academic Press.
  1980 Depressive Affect and Disorder Across Cultures. In Handbook of Cross-Cultural Psychology, Volume 5, Psychopathology. H. Triandis and J. Draguns (eds.). Boston: Allyn and Bacon.
  1981 Culture, Self, and Mental Disorder. Paper presented at the "Conference on Culture and Self". University of Hawaii, Honolulu.
Marsella, A. J., M. Escudero, and P. Gordon
  1972 Stresses, Resources, and Symptom Patterns in Urban Filipino Men. In Transcultural Research in Mental Health. W. Lebra (ed.). Honolulu: The University Press of Hawaii.
Marsella, A. J. and H. Higginbotham
  1981 Applications of Traditional Asian Medicine to the Delivery of Mental Health Services in Non-Western Cultures. In Mental Health Services Across Cultures. P. Pedersen, A. Marsella, and N. Sartorius (eds.). Beverly Hills, Calif.: Sage Publications.
Marsella, A. J., F. Hsu, and G. DeVos, eds.
  n.d.   Culture and Self. Forthcoming.
Marsella, A. J., D. Kinzie, and P. Gordon
  1973 Ethnocultural Variations in the Expression of Depression. Journal of Cross-Cultural Psychology 4:435–458.
Marsella, A. J. and P. Pedersen, eds.
  1981 Cross-Cultural Counseling and Psychotherapy. New York: Pergamon Press.
Marsella, A. J. and K. Snyder
  1981 Stressors, Social Supports, and Schizophrenia: Toward an Interactional Model. Schizophrenia Bulletin 7:152–163.

Marsella, A. J. and J. Tanaka-Matsumi
 1976 Frequency, Intensity, and Duration Bases of Psychiatric Symptomatology Among Japanese Nationals, Japanese-Americans and Caucasian-Americans. Unpublished data, University of Hawaii.
Marsella, A. J., et al.
 1980 Psychiatric Problem, Cause, and Treatment Matrices for Ethnic Groups in Hawaii. Unpublished data, University of Hawaii.
Marsella, A. J., et al.
 n.d. Depression Across Cultures. Culture, Medicine, and Psychiatry. in press.
Marsella, A. J., and K. S. Kim
 1973 Social Change and Psychiatric Adjustment in Korea. Unpublished data. University of Hawaii.
Maslow, A.
 1954 Motivation and Personality. New York: Harper and Row.
Maupin, E.
 1962 Zen Buddhism: A Psychological Review. Journal of Consulting Psychology 26: 362–378.
Mishler, E. and N. Scotch
 1963 Sociocultural Factors in the Epidemiology of Schizophrenia. Psychiatry 26:315– 351.
Murphy, H. B. M., et al.
 1963 A Cross-Cultural Survey of Schizophrenic Symptomatology. International Journal of Social Psychiatry 9:237–249.
Murphy, H. B. M., E. Wittkower, and N. Chance
 1964 Cross-Cultural Inquiry Into The Symptomatology of Depression. Transcultural Psychiatric Research Review 1:5–21.
Murphy, J. and A. Leighton, eds.
 1965 Approaches to Cross-Cultural Psychiatry. Ithaca: Cornell University Press.
Needham, J.
 1962 Science and Civilization in China. Cambridge, England: Cambridge University Press.
Obeyesekere, G.
 1977 The Theory and Practice of Psychological Medicine in the Ayurvedic Tradition. Culture, Medicine and Psychiatry 1:155–181.
Odegaard, O.
 1975 Social and Ecological Factors in the Etiology, Outcome, Treatment, and Prevention of Mental Disorders. In Psychiatrie Der Gegenwart. K. P. Kisker, et al. (eds.), pp. 152–198. Heidelberg: Springer-Verlag.
Opler, M.
 1965 Culture, Psychiatry, and Human Values. Springfield, Illinois: Charles V. Thomas.
Opler, M. and J. Singer
 1959 Ethnic Differences in Behavior and Psychopathology: Italian and Irish. International Journal of Social Psychiatry 2:11–23.
Parker, S. and R. Kleiner
 1967 Mental Illness in the Urban Negro Community. New York: Free Press.
Pfeiffer, R.
 1970 Transkulturelle Psychiatrie: Ergebnisse Und Problime. Stuttgart: Thieme.
Prince, R.
 1968a The Changing Picture of Depressive Syndromes in Africa: Is it Fact or Diagnostic Fashion? Canadian Journal of African Studies 1:177–192.
 1980a Some Transcultural Aspects of Adolescent Affective Disorders. Unpublished paper. Montreal, Canada.

1980b Variations in Psychotherapeutic Procedures. *In* Handbook of Cross-Cultural Psychology: Vol. VI, Psychopathology. H. Triandis and J. Draguns (eds.). Boston: Allyn and Bacon.

Prince, R., ed.
   1968b Trance and Possession States. Montreal: R. M. Burke Memorial Society.

Resner, J. and J. Hartog
   1972 Concepts and Terminology of Mental Disorder Among Malays. Journal of Cross-Cultural Psychology 1:369–381.

Reynolds, D.
   1981 The New Psychotherapies. Honolulu, Hawaii: University Press of Hawaii.

Ritchie, J.
   1976 Maori Therapy as Cultural "Time Out." *In* Culture Bound Syndromes, Ethno-psychiatry, and Alternate Therapies. Honolulu, Hawaii: University Press of Hawaii.

Rosen, G.
   1969 Madness in Society. New York: Harper.

Sanua, V.
   1969 Sociocultural Aspects of Schizophrenia. *In* The Schizophrenic Syndrome. L. Bellak and L. Loeb (eds.). New York: Grune and Stratton.
   1980 Schizophrenia Across Cultures. *In* Handbook of Cross-Cultural Psychology: Vol. VI, Psychopathology. H. Triandis and J. Draguns (eds.). Boston: Allyn and Bacon.

Sapir, E.
   1932 Cultural Anthropology and Psychiatry. Journal of Abnormal and Social Psychiatry 27:229–242.

Sartorius, N.
   1973 Culture and the Epidemiology of Depression. Psychiatria, Neurologia, Et Neuro-chirugia 76:479–487.
   1979 Cross-Cultural Psychiatry. *In* Psychiatry Der Gegenwart. K. Kisker et al. (eds.), pp. 711–737. Berlin: Springer-Verlag.

Sartorius, N., A. Jablensky, R. Shapiro
   1978 Cross-Cultural Differences in the Short-term Prognosis of Schizophrenia Psychoses. Schizophrenia Bulletin 4:102–113.

Scheff, T.
   1972 Social Labeling and Deviance. *In* Transcultural Research in Mental Health. W. Lebra (ed.). Honolulu: The University Press of Hawaii.

Schwab, J. and R. Schwab
   1978 Sociocultural Roots of Mental Disorder. New York: Plenum Medical.

Sechrest, L.
   1969 Philippine Culture, Stress, and Psychopathology. *In* Mental Health Research in Asia and the Pacific. W. Caudill and T. Y. Lin (eds.). Honolulu: The University Press of Hawaii.

Seligman, G.
   1929 Temperament, Conflict, and Psychosis in a Stone Age Population. British Journal of Medical Psychology 9:187–202.

Setynegoro, K.
   1979 Some Indonesian Concepts of Mental Health. Paper presented at First International Conference on Traditional Asian Medicine. Canberra, Australia.

Silverman, C.
   1968 The Epidemiology of Depression. Baltimore: The Johns Hopkins Press.

Simon, R. J. Fleiss, B. Gurland, P. Stiller, and L. Sharpe
   1973 Depression and Schizophrenia in Hospitalized Black and White Mental Patients. Archives of General Psychiatry 28:509–512.

Singer, K.
  1975 Depressive Disorders from a Transcultural Perspective. Social Science and Medi-
        cine 9:289–301.
Slotkin, J.
  1955 Culture and Psychopathology. Journal of Abnormal and Social Psychiatry 51:
        269–275.
Srole, L., et al.
  1962 Mental Health in the Metropolis: The Midtown Manhattan Study. New York:
        McGraw Hill.
Stoker, D., L. Zurcher, and W. Fox
  1968 Women in Psychotherapy: A Cross-Cultural Comparison. International Journal of
        Social Psychiatry 14:5–22.
Strauss, J.
  1979 Social and Cultural Influences on Psychopathology. Annual Review of Psychology
        30:397–416.
Sunshine, N.
  1971 Cultural Differences in Schizophrenia. Unpublished doctoral dissertation. City
        University of New York.
Torrey, E.
  1972 The Mind Game: Witchdoctors and Psychiatrists. New York: Emerson Hall.
Uchimura, Y., et al.
  1940 Uber die Vergleichende Psychiatrische Und Erbpathologische Untersuchung Auf
        Einer Japanischen Isel. Psychiatria Et Neurologia Japonica 44:745–782.
Van Brero, P.
  1895 Latah. Journal of Mental Sciences 41:537–538.
Van Loon, F.
  1927 Amok and Latah. Journal of Abnormal and Social Psychology 21:434–444.
Van Wulfften-Palthe, P.
  1936 Psychiatry and Neurology in the Tropics. In A Clinical Textbook of Tropical
        Medicine. Batavia: De Langen.
Waxler, N.
  1974 Culture and Mental Illness: A Social Labeling Perspective. Journal of Nervous and
        Mental Disease 159:379–395.
  1979 Is Outcome For Schizophrenia Better in Non-Industrial Societies. Journal of
        Nervous and Mental Disease:167–144–158.
Weinberg, K., ed.
  1967 The Sociology of Mental Disorders. Chicago: Aldine Press.
Weissman, M. and G. Klerman
  1978 Sex Roles and the Epidemiology of Depression. Archives of General Psychiatry
        34:98–111.
Wing, J., J. Cooper and N. Sartorius
  1974 Description and Classification of Psychiatric Symptoms. London, England:
        Cambridge University Press.
Wittkower, E.
  1970 Trance and Possession States. International Journal of Social Psychiatry 16:153–
        160.
Wittkower, E. and G. Dubreil
  1973 Psychocultural Stress in Relation to Mental Illness. Social Science and Medicine
        7:691–704.
Wittkower, E. and H. Rin
  1965 Transcultural Psychiatry. Archives of General Psychiatry 13:387–394.
Yap, P. M.
  1951 Mental Disease Peculiar to Certain Cultures: A Survey of Comparative Psychiatry.
        Journal of Mental Science 97:313–327.

LIST OF CONTRIBUTORS

Edmund Bourne, Ph.D., Catholic Community Services, San Diego, California.

Dorothy Clement, Ph.D., Department of Anthropology, University of North Carolina, Chapel Hill, North Carolina 27514.

Linda Connor, Ph.D., Department of Anthropology, University of Sydney, Sydney, N.S.W. 2006, Australia.

Horacio Fabrega, M.D., Department of Psychiatry, School of Medicine, University of Pittsburgh, 3811 O'Hara Street, Pittsburgh, Pennsylvania 15261.

Atwood Gaines, Ph.D., M.P.H., Departments of Anthropology and Psychiatry, Duke University, Durham, North Carolina 27706.

Byron Good, Ph.D., Department of Psychiatry, University of California, Davis, Davis, California 94616.

Mary-Jo Del Vecchio Good, Ph.D., Department of Psychiatry, University of California, Davis, California 94616.

Takie S. Lebra, Ph.D., Department of Anthropology, University of Hawaii, Honolulu, Hawaii 96822.

William Lebra, Ph.D., Department of Anthropology, University of Hawaii, Honolulu, Hawaii 96822.

Margaret Lock, Ph.D., Department of the History of Medicine, McGill University, 3665 Drummon Street, Montreal, Quebec, Canada H3G 1Y6.

Anthony Marsella, Ph.D., Department of Psychology, University of Hawaii, Honolulu, Hawaii 96822.

Takao Murase, Ph.D., Department of Psychology, Rikkyo University, Toshima-ku, Tokyo, Japan.

Gananath Obeyesekere, Ph.D., Department of Anthropology, Princeton University, Princeton, New Jersey 08540.

Paul Pederson, Ph.D., Department of Psychology, University of Hawaii, Honolulu, Hawaii 96822.

Richard Shweder Ph.D., Committee on Human Development, Department of Behavioral Sciences, University of Chicago, Chicago, Illinois 60637.

Geoffrey White, Ph.D., Culture Learning Institute, East-West Center, 1777 East-West Road, Honolulu, Hawaii 96848.

David Wu, Ph.D., Culture Learning Institute, East-West Center, 1777 East-West Road, Honolulu, Hawaii 96848.

389

AUTHOR INDEX

Abelson, R., 13, 27, 85
Abram, H., 176
Ackerknecht, E. H., 44, 47, 363–4
Acosta, F., 343
Agar, M., 33
Akimoto, H., 361
Akiskal, H., 375
Albert, M. K., 62
Al-Issa, I., 359
Alland, A., 314
Amarasingham, L., 85, 149
Ambrowitz, D., 344
American Psychological Association, 336
Amir, Y., 334
Andersen, E. S., 65
Anderson, C., 70
Araki, H., 325
Arensberg, C., 179
Areye, S. A., 344
Aronson, H., 343
Arrendondo-Dows, P., 349
Atkinson, D. R., 334, 337, 343–4, 349, 351
Atkinson, P., 149
Aubrey, R. F., 335
Austin, J. L., 103

Baasher, T., 378
Bailey, F., 180
Baldwin, L. M., 108
Balint, M., 324
Bateson, G., 177, 225, 260, 264, 345
Bateson, M. C., 157
Bebbington, P., 368
Beeman, W. O., 157
Behin, M. T., 53
Beiser, M., 10, 72
Belmonte, T., 187
Belo, J., 255, 257, 261
Benedict, P., 359
Benedict, R., 103, 274, 363, 365
Benjamin, L., 7
Berger, P. L., 147
Berlin, B., 74, 99, 101
Berman, J., 343
Berry, J. W., 345–6

Binitie, A., 72, 373
Black, M., 197
Bloombaum, J., 342
Blum, J. D., 27
Blumhagen, D., 149
Boas, F., 195
Boehm, C., 169
Boissevain, J., 179–80
Bolman, W., 344
Bostwick, G. L., 132
Bott, E., 180
Boucher, J., 18, 298
Bourguignon, E., 52, 178, 315
Bourne, E. J., 15–16, 20–2, 24, 86–7, 89, *97–133*, 182, 326
Bourne, P., 181
Boyer, L., 364
Brandt, E., 346
Breedlove, D. E., 74
Bridgman, R., 286
Brill, A., 360
Brislin, R. W., 336
Broverman, I. K., 9
Bruner, J. S., 105, 107, 117
Bryne, R. H., 335
Bryson, L., 343
Bryson, S., 349
Bunkacho, 269
Burton, M., 9, 122

Calhoun, J. F., 336
Calneck, M., 344
Campbell, D., 343
Campbell, J., 180, 187
Caraka, 239–40
Carkhuff, R. R., 343
Carr, J. E., 29, 257
Carroll, J. S., 70
Casas, J. M., 344
Caudill, W., 3, 226, 373
Caughey, J., 29, 86
Chance, N., 386
Chapman, J., 6
Chapman, L., 6
Chen, Pang-Shien, 286
Chen, Ts'un-jen, 290–5

purification in Gedatsu therapy, 278–80

quantitative analysis of cultural knowledge distribution, 78–9

race, confusing use of term, and minority counseling, 334–5
racism in therapists and intercultural context of therapy, 342
rationality, and explanations of insanity, 44, 47–8; vs irrationality in psychiatric research, 167–8
reductionism, in cross-cultural paradigms, 345, 348; in traditional Japanese medicine, 218–21; role of Buddhism, 219–21; the shokanron, 218–19
referential self, Western view of, and psychoanalytic theory, 181–5
reincarnation and self, in Balinese person concept, 261–2
relativism, and mental disorders, 363; of person concept and cross-cultural variation, 98, 102–4, 125–32
religion, church authority in Samoa and context of spirit possession, 199–201, 206–8, 210; impact on Western folk theory, 179–86; Japanese traditions of, and Gedatsu cult therapy, 269–70; and *sunao*, 324–5, 327; related to inflexibility, in case study, 174
religious healing as treatment for supernatural illness, 181
repercussion postulate and interpersonal conflict in Japanese culture, 273
repression of emotion, in Balinese society, 255; and Japanese social order, 227; and stress avoidance, 297–8
responsibility, agency and causality in ethnomedicine, 22–4; cultural definitions of, and mental illness, 70; of doctor to patient in Chinese traditional medicine, 292, 294–6; in illness, 162
ritual, as Balinese therapy, 253, 259–63; as folk representations of folk knowledge, 193–4; medical and illness realities, 162; neglect of, as cause of Balinese madness, 252; in Okinawan culture and shamanism, 304, 308–10; possession, in Gedatsu sect therapy, see Possession ritual; symbolic studies of, 149
role expectations, cultural definitions of, and folk knowledge of mental disorder, 70

role performance, stress of, and susto, 160–1
role substitution and identity interchange in Gedatsu therapy, 276
rootwork, Latin belief in, 180–1

Samkhya philosophy and Ayurvedic medical tradition, 236
Samoa, authority in, 208; causal agents, 79, 84; in mental illness, 23; curing rituals in, and folk theory of illness, 27–8, 30; folk representations, of mental disorder, 193–211, 364; *ma'i aitu* (spirit possession), 200–1; *ma'i valea*, 199–200; mental disorders caused by emotion, 201–3; of social types, 25, 201–3; new mental health program, 206–7; spirit possession, 206–7
Samyogic experimentation and Ayurvedic theory, 246–8
schizophrenia, cross-cultural reviews of, 359; and depression, international surveys of, 371–2; diagnosis and treatment, in case study, 174–5; epidemiological reviews of, 368; International Pilot Study of, and diagnostic style, 9, 371–2; manifestations of, role of culture in, 53–7, 60–1; prognosis for variation across cultures, 371–2; recognition of, 4; across cultures, 72–3, 340; as sensorimotor disorder, 52; treatment outcome and person concept, 88–9; as Western disorder, 56–7, 373–4, 377, 380
schizophrenics, matched diagnosis comparisons, 370
schooling effects on abstract thinking, 107, 111, 117, 119
science, as cultural perspective and manifestations of illness, 55–6; Western, and separation of body, mind and spirit, 365–6
seasons, therapeutic and pathogenic effects of, 238
self, beliefs about and culture-bound disorders, 52; context-dependent, relativist theory of, 125–32; and culture and mental disorder, 362–3, differentiation from others in Naikan therapy, 319–20; and illness, and psychiatric manifestations, 15–16; Iranian view of, 157, and other cultural conceptions of, 177; in ethnomedicine, 21–2; in Gedatsu therapy, 275–9; theory of, and illness, 39;

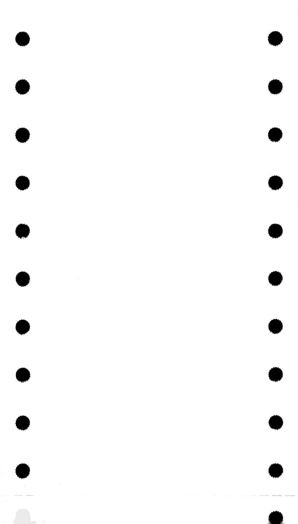

patron's name: SATTLER, DORINDA M

   title:Cultural conceptions of m
   author:Marsella, Anthony J.
   item id:30000000975189
      due:5/29/2004,23:59